PROGRESS IN BRAIN RESEARCH

VOLUME 47

HYPERTENSION AND BRAIN MECHANISMS

EDITED BY

W. DE JONG and A.P. PROVOOST

Rudolf Magnus Institute for Pharmacology, University of Utrecht, Utrecht (The Netherlands)

and

A.P. SHAPIRO

Department of Medicine, University of Pittsburgh School of Medicine, Pittsburgh, Pa. 15261 (U.S.A.)

ELSEVIER SCIENTIFIC PUBLISHING COMPANY

AMSTERDAM/OXFORD/NEW YORK

1977

Published by:

Elsevier/North-Holland Biomedical Press
335 Jan van Galenstraat, P.O. Box 211
Amsterdam, The Netherlands

Sole distributors for the U.S.A. and Canada:

Elsevier/North-Holland, Inc.
52 Vanderbilt Avenue
New York, N.Y. 10017

Library of Congress Cataloging in Publication Data
Main entry under title:

Hypertension and brain mechanisms.

   (Progress in brain research ; vol. 47)
   Bibliography: p.
   Includes index.
   1. Hypertension--Etiology--Congresses. 2. Blood
pressure--Regulation--Congresses. 3. Brain--Congresses.
4. Hypotensive agents--Congresses. I. De Jong, W.
II. Provoost, A. P. III. Shapiro, Alvin P. IV. Series.
[DNLM: 1. Hypertension--Congresses. 2. Brain--Physio-
pathology--Congresses. 3. Brain--Physiology--Congresses.
W1 PR667J v. 47 / WG340 H9945 1976]
QP376.P7 vol. 47 [RC685.H8] 612'.82'08s [616.1'32'071]
ISBN 0-444-41534-3   77-4212

PRINTED IN THE NETHERLANDS

2-9-7

List of Contributors

I. Akiguchi, Department of Internal Medicine, Kyoto University, Kyoto, Japan

Susan M. Barman, Department of Pharmacology, Michigan State University, East Lansing, Mich. 48824, U.S.A.

Claire Baxter, Renal and Hypertension Units, Royal Prince Alfred Hospital, Camperdown, New South Wales 2050, Australia

K.P. Bhargava, Department of Pharmacology, K.G. Medical College, Lucknow 226003, India

W.H. Birkenhäger, Department of Internal Medicine, Zuiderziekenhuis, Rotterdam, The Netherlands

B. Bohus, Rudolf Magnus Institute for Pharmacology, Medical Faculty, University of Utrecht, Utrecht, The Netherlands

P. Bolme, Department of Histology, Karolinska Institute, Stockholm 60, Sweden

D.B. Calne, NINCDS, National Institutes of Health, Bethesda, Md. 20014, U.S.A.

J.P. Chalmers, Department of Medicine, Flinders Medical Center, Bedford Park, Adelaide, South Australia 5042, Australia

C.N. Corder, Departments of Medicine and Pharmacology, University of Pittsburgh, School of Medicine, Pittsburgh, Pa. 15261, U.S.A.

R. Dampney, Istituto di Ricerche Cardiovascolari, Università di Milano, and Centro di Ricerche Cardiovascolari C.N.R., Milan, Italy

W. De Jong, Rudolf Magnus Institute for Pharmacology, Medical Faculty, University of Utrecht, Utrecht, The Netherlands

P.W. De Leeuw, Department of Internal Medicine, Zuiderziekenhuis, Rotterdam, The Netherlands

N. Doba, Laboratory of Neurobiology, Department of Neurology, Cornell University Medical College, 1300 York Avenue, New York, N.Y. 10021, U.S.A.

J-L.A. Elghozi, INSERM U7, Hôpital Necker, 75015 Paris, France

M. Esler, Division of Hypertension, Department of Internal Medicine, University of Michigan Medical School, Ann Arbor, Mich. 48109, U.S.A.

T.D. Fawzi-Meininger, Department of Internal Medicine, Zuiderziekenhuis, Rotterdam, The Netherlands

D.C.E. Ferguson, National Heart and Lung Institute, Bethesda, Md. 20014, U.S.A.

J.T. Fitzsimons, Physiological Laboratory, Cambridge, Great Britain

M. Fukase, Japan Stroke Prevention Center, Izumo, Japan

F. Furby, Renal and Hypertension Units, Royal Prince Alfred Hospital, Camperdown, New South Wales 2050, Australia

K. Fuxe, Department of Histology, Karolinska Institutet, Stockholm 60, Sweden

D. Ganten, Department of Pharmacology, University of Heidelberg, 366 Neuenheimer Feld, 6900 Heidelberg, G.F.R.

Ursula Ganten, Department of Pharmacology, University of Heidelberg, 366 Neuenheimer Feld, 6900 Heidelberg, G.F.R.

G.L. Gebber, Department of Pharmacology, Michigan State University, East Lansing, Mich. 48824, U.S.A.

J.B. Geffen, Departments of Medicine and Physiology, Flinders Medical Centre, Bedford Park, Adelaide, South Australia 5042, Australia

J.J. Groen, Department of Psychobiology, Jelgersma Kliniek, Oegstgeest, The Netherlands

G. Haeusler, Pharmaceutical Research Department, F. Hoffmann-La Roche & Co. Ltd., Basel, Switzerland

B. Hansen, Departments of Psychosomatics, Internal Medicine and Pediatrics University of Ulm, Ulm, G.F.R.

J.P. Henry, University of Southern California, School of Medicine, Department of Physiology, Los Angeles, Calif. 90083, U.S.A.

vi

J.M. Hermann, Departments of Psychosomatics, Internal Medicine and Pediatrics, University of Ulm, Ulm, G.F.R.

S.M. Hilton, Department of Physiology, The Medical School, Vincent Drive, Birmingham B 15 2TI, Great Britain

W.E. Hoffman, Department of Physiology, University of Iowa, Iowa City, Iowa 52242, U.S.A.

T. Hökfelt, Department of Histology, Karolinska Institutet, Stockholm 60, Sweden

R. Horie, Department of Neurosurgery, Kyoto University, Kyoto, and Japan Stroke Prevention Center, Izumo, Japan

J.S. Horvath, Renal and Hypertension Unit, Royal Prince Alfred Hospital, Camperdown, New South Wales 2050, Australia

I.P. Jain, Department of Pharmacology, K.G. Medical College, Lucknow 226003, India

S. Julius, Division of Hypertension, Department of Internal Medicine, University of Michigan Medical School, Ann Arbor, Mich. 48109, U.S.A.

P. Kezdi, Cox Heart Institute, 3525 Southern Boulevard, Dayton, Ohio 45429, U.S.A.

T.L. Kho, Department of Internal Medicine, Zuiderziekenhuis, Rotterdam, The Netherlands

M. Koster, Department of Internal Medicine, Univ. Hospital-Wilhelmina Gasthuis, Amsterdam, The Netherlands

M. Laubie, Département de Pharmacologie, Inst. de Recherches Servier, 14 Rue du Val d'Or, 92 Suresnes, France

F.H.H. Leenen, Department of Medicine, University of Pittsburgh, School of Medicine, 1188 Scaife Hall, Pittsburgh, Pa. 15261, U.S.A.

O. Magnus, Research Unit TNO for Clinical Neurophysiology, Ursula Kliniek, Wassenaar, The Netherlands

R.H. McDonald, Departments of Medicine and Pharmacology, University of Pittsburgh School of Medicine, Pittsburgh, Pa. 15261, U.S.A.

P. Meyer, INSERM-U7, Hôpital Necker, 75015 Paris, France

Y. Nara, Department of Pathology, Kyoto University, Kyoto and Japan Stroke Prevention Center, Izumo, Japan

M.A. Nathan, Laboratory of Neurobiology, Department of Neurology, Cornell University Medical College, 1300 York Avenue, New York, N.Y. 10021, U.S.A.

S. Nicolaïdis, INSERM-U7, Hôpital Necker, 75015 Paris, France

F.P. Nijkamp, Rudolf Magnus Institute for Pharmacology, Medical Faculty, University of Utrecht, Utrecht, The Netherlands

M. Ohtaka, The Center for Adult Diseases, Osaka, and Japan Stroke Prevention Center, Izumo, Japan

M. Palkovits, 1st Department of Anatomy, Semmelweis University Medical School, Tüzoltó utca 58, 1450 Budapest, Hungary

T.G. Pickering, Department of Cardiovascular Medicine, Radcliffe Infirmary, Oxford, Great Britain

C. Piekarski, Department of Internal Medicine, Bonn Medical School, Bonn University, Bonn, G.F.R.

A.J. Porsius, Department of Pharmacy, Division of Pharmacotherapy, University of Amsterdam, Plantage Muidergracht 24, Amsterdam, The Netherlands

A.P. Provoost, Rudolf Magnus Institute for Pharmacology, Medical Faculty, University of Utrecht, Utrecht, The Netherlands

D.P. Redmond, Division of Neuropsychiatry, Walter Reed Army Institute of Research, Washington, D.C., U.S.A.

J.L. Reid, Department of Clinical Pharmacology, Royal Postgraduate Medical School, London W12 OH3, Great Britain

D.J. Reis, Laboratory of Neurobiology, Department of Neurology, Cornell University Medical College, 1300 York Avenue, New York, N.Y. 10021, U.S.A.

N.Th.P. Roozekrans, Department of Pharmacy, Division of Pharmacotherapy, University of Amsterdam, Plantage Muidergracht 24, Amsterdam, The Netherlands

R. Rush, Departments of Medicine and Physiology, Flinders Medical Centre, Bedford Park, Adelaïde, South Australia 5042, Australia

N. Schäfer, Departments of Psychosomatics, Internal Medicine and Pediatrics, University of Ulm, Ulm, G.F.R.

M.A. Schalekamp, Department of Internal Medicine, Academisch Ziekenhuis Dijkzicht, Rotterdam, The Netherlands

P. Schelling, Department of Pharmacology, University of Heidelberg, 366 Neuenheimer Feld, 6900 Heidelberg, G.F.R.

T.H. Schmidt, Departments of Psychosomatics, Internal Medicine and Pediatrics, University of Ulm, Ulm, G.F.R.

H. Schmitt, Département de Pharmacologie, Faculté de Médecine, Broussais Hôtel-Dieu, 15 Rue de l'Ecole de Médecine, 75270 Paris Cedex 06, France

G.E. Schwartz, Department of Psychology, Yale University, New Haven, Conn., U.S.A.

K.H. Selbman, Departments of Psychosomatics, Internal Medicine and Pediatrics, University of Ulm, Ulm, G.F.R.

A.P. Shapiro, Department of Medicine, University of Pittsburgh School of Medicine, Pittsburgh, Pa. 15261, U.S.A.

A. Sjoerdsma, Centre de Recherche Merell International, 16 Rue d'Ankara, F 67000 Strasbourg, France

E. Skinhøj, Department of Neurology, Rigshospitalet, Copenhagen, Denmark

P. Sleight, Department of Cardiovascular Medicine, Radcliffe Infirmary, Oxford, Great Britain

G.W.M. Smeets, Rudolf Magnus Institute for Pharmacology, Medical Faculty, University of Utrecht, Utrecht, The Netherlands

D.W. Snyder, Laboratory of Neurobiology, Department of Neurology, Cornell University Medical College, 1300 York Avenue, New York, N.Y. 10021, U.S.A.

A. Stella, Istituto di Ricerche Cardiovascolari, Università di Milano, and Centro di Ricerche Cardiovascolari, C.N.R., Milan, Italy

Patricia M. Stephens, University of Southern California, School of Medicine, Department of Physiology, Los Angeles, Calif. 90033, U.S.A.

K.K. Tangri, Department of Pharmacology, K.G. Medical College, Lucknow 226003, India India

P.F. Teychenne, N.I.N.C.D.S., National Institutes of Health, Bethesda, Md. 20014, U.S.A.

D.J. Tiller, Renal and Hypertension Units, Royal Prince Alfred Hospital, Camperdown, New South Wales 2050, Australia

P.B.M.W.M. Timmermans, Department of Pharmacy, Division of Pharmacotherapy, University of Amsterdam, Plantage Muidergracht 24, Amsterdam, The Netherlands

J.H.A. Van der Drift, Department of Internal Medicine, University Hospital-Wilhelmina Gasthuis, Amsterdam, The Netherlands

J. Van der Gugten, Rudolf Magnus Institute for Pharmacology, Medical Faculty, University of Utrecht, Utrecht, The Netherlands

R. Vandongen, Department of Internal Medicine, Zuiderziekenhuis, Rotterdam, The Netherlands

A.Th. Van Edixhoven, Department of Internal Medicine, Zuiderziekenhuis, Rotterdam, The Netherlands

P.A. Van Zwieten, Department of Pharmacy, Division of Pharmacotherapy, University of Amsterdam, Plantage Muidergracht 24, Amsterdam, The Netherlands

D.H.G. Versteeg, Rudolf Magnus Institute for Pharmacology, Medical Faculty, University of Utrecht, Utrecht, The Netherlands

A.W. Von Eiff, Department of Internal Medicine, Bonn Medical School, Bonn University, Bonn, G.F.R.

Th. Von Uexküll, Departments of Psychosomatics, Internal Medicine and Pediatrics, University of Ulm, Ulm, G.F.R.

P. Weckmann, Departments of Psychosomatics, Internal Medicine and Pediatrics, University of Ulm, Ulm, G.F.R.

S.M. Weiss, National Heart and Lung Institute, Bethesda, Md. 20014, U.S.A.

A. Wester, Department of Internal Medicine, Zuiderziekenhuis, Rotterdam, The Netherlands

S.W. White, Departments of Medicine and Physiology, Flinders Medical Centre, Bedford Park, Adelaide, South Australia 5042, Australia

L.M.H. Wing, Department of Clinical Pharmacology, Royal Postgraduate Medical School, London W12 OH3, Great Britain

H.J.L.M. Wijnen, Rudolf Magnus Institute for Pharmacology, Medical Faculty, University of Utrecht, Utrecnt, The Netherlands

Y. Yamori, Department of Pathology, Kyoto University, Kyoto and Japan Stroke Prevention Center, Izumo, Japan

G.A. Zaal, Department of Internal Medicine, Zuiderziekenhuis, Rotterdam, The Netherlands

L. Záborsky, 1st Department of Anatomy, Semmelweis University Medical School, Tüzoltó utca 58, 1450 Budapest, Hungary

A. Zanchetti, Istituto di Ricerche Cardiovascolari, Università di Milano and Centro di Ricerche Cardiovascolari, C.N.R., Milan, Italy

P. Zandberg, Rudolf Magnus Institute for Pharmacology, Medical Faculty University of Utrecht, Utrecht, The Netherlands

Preface

In this workshop, held in Utrecht from June 28 to 30, 1976, exciting information has been presented on the control of arterial blood pressure by the brain. The meeting served to enlarge and integrate our understanding of hypertension in relation to brain mechanisms under physiological and pathological conditions. Major aspects ranged from brain neuroanatomy and neurotransmission of cardiovascular control, baroreceptor function, brain damage and hypertension (and the reverse), biofeedback, emotional behavior and psychological as well as drug therapy of hypertension. This reflects the necessary cooperation of workers of different scientific disciplines required to pursue the new developments. The new laboratory and clinical findings already indicate that the study of the central regulation of blood pressure provides important leads for new therapeutic developments. The favorable academic spirit during the conference stimulated a mutual exchange of ideas and future cooperation.

Many people helped to make the workshop a success. I wish to thank all speakers, the chairmen of the different sessions and the different sponsors for making the workshop possible. I am grateful to the Organizing Committee (B. Bohus, A.P. Provoost, A.P. Shapiro, Tj.B. van Wimersma Greidanus, D. De Wied) and other members of the Rudolf Magnus Institute who contributed so much. Special thanks goes to Miss Tine Baas for high level secretarial assistance.

Wybren De Jong
Utrecht (The Netherlands)

Acknowledgements

The Organizing Committee is greatly indebted to the Nederlandse Hartstichting (Dutch Heart Foundation) for acting as the main sponsor of the Workshop "Hypertension and Brain Mechanisms". We also like to express our gratitude for the generous support by the following organizations:

Dr. Saal van Zwanenberg Foundation, Oss

The University of Utrecht and the Medical Faculty, Utrecht

Ministry of Public Health and Environment, The Hague

Merrell International, Strasbourg

Boehringer, Ingelheim

Wellcome Foundation, London

Organon International, Oss

Upjohn, Kalamazoo

Contents

xiv

Session III — Brain Damage and Hypertension: Experimental and Clinical

Session IV — Integrated Brain Function and Hypertension

Session V — Pharmacological Aspects of Central Acting Antihypertensive
  Drugs and Influence on Peripheral Effector Mechanisms

Central Action as a Key to Past and Future Therapy of Hypertension

ALBERT SJOERDSMA

Centre de Recherche Merrell International,
16, rue d'Ankara,
F 67000 Strasbourg (France)

Since the subject of drugs with a central action has been well reviewed recently at a symposium in London (Davies and Reid, 1975), and also expertly by Van Zwieten (1975), it seems appropriate that my remarks be more in the nature of an overview than a review.

LOOKING BACK

With your indulgence, I will first take a brief and rather personal look back to the period of roughly 1949—1962, trusting that others will pick up the subjects of clonidine and the β-blockers which came along later in the 1960's. Prior to and early in this period, a centrally acting drug was actually the mainstay of therapy; this drug, namely phenobarbital, was administered along with reassurance (we had not yet heard of biofeedback). The arterial pressure, however high, was viewed by many with a certain nonchalance, although the unfortunate consequences of uncontrolled hypertension were highly visible on any medical ward. The veratrum alkaloids were available and were the first effective drugs with a central action (via the Bezold—Jarisch reflex) but the therapist needed an emesis basin in one hand and a syringe loaded with atropine in the other to handle untoward effects. I am going to omit the era of ganglion blockade in the current context except to say that both the patient (wearing dark glasses) and the physician had their hands full of antidotes. But at least by working together they put an eventual end to surgical sympathectomy, which had been the only effective treatment.

This was the disillusioning scene I entered in 1953 upon completion of my basic and clinical training. I elected to try some new directions, come what may, and decided to focus my research on the human hypertensive subject and to study the biochemistry of serotonin and other pressor amines in man. Inhibition of the metabolism of these amines by monoamine oxidase (MAO) became a powerful tool in our studies and the paradoxic orthostatic decrease in blood pressure produced by compounds such as iproniazid was intriguing. The next 6 years constituted a very productive period for us and culminated in our introduction into antihypertensive therapy of the MAO inhibitor, pargyline (Horwitz and Sjoerdsma, 1961), and the aromatic amino acid decarboxylase inhibitor, α-methyldopa (Oates et al., 1960). The therapeutic effects of methyldopa were entirely unexpected and were not predictable from enzyme kinetic data and available animal pharmacology. Once we ascertained that the drug had to be decarboxylated to pressor amines to be effective (D-isomer inactive), we felt much better of course since it tended to fit with our general "pressor approach to depressor therapy". I won't give other examples but certainly many of the puzzles were solved with the realization in about 1970 of the central depressor effects of catecholamines (Yamori et al., 1970) and the existence of so-called central α-adrenoreceptors. I am skipping over reserpine, an interesting and exciting drug from the 1950's, although its central and peripheral actions on blood pressure are still worthy of discussion. An interesting additional item from the 1950's concerns the nasal decongestant, tetrahydrazoline (Tyzine®). This pressor amine analogue of clonidine was reported by Finnerty et al. (1957) to produce bradycardia and hypotension in man, later ascribed by Hutcheon et al. (1958) to a central depressant effect on sympathetic nervous tone. I used it frequently at night on my children when they had stuffy noses since it also had sedative effects. I recall contacting the manufacturer (Pfizer and Co.) in the late 1960's on learning of the therapeutic effects of clonidine reasoning that they must have interesting analogues which we could test but nothing came of this.

I would like to add a comment on the question of whether the effects of methyldopa and propranolol as used clinically are produced at least in part by a central action. I am willing to accept this possibility at least in the case of methyldopa but it seems to me that an additional clinical clue, aside from the central depressant effect noted with both drugs, would be whether or not a withdrawal hypertensive rebound is ever observed as commonly noted with clonidine. I think one tends to relate withdrawal responses to centrally acting drugs, obvious examples being the narcotic and hypnotic withdrawal syndromes. It may be relevant therefore that Burden and Alexander (1976) have just reported a fairly convincing case of severe rebound hypertension after acute withdrawal of methyldopa. Similarly, it is now recognized that acute withdrawal of propranolol in patients with angina pectoris is dangerous and may precipitate acute myocardial infarction (cf., Medical Letter, 1976).

LOOKING AHEAD

In assuming the difficult task of making some meaningful suggestions about the future, I would like to quote a maxim of a famous basketball coach in the U.S.; he says that "a pass is not a good pass unless your man catches the ball and scores." If any of my thoughts even come close to enabling one of you to catch the ball and score, so-to-speak, I shall be quite pleased. I believe of course that we will eventually win the game, in other words, that continued progress in our knowledge of central mechanisms of blood pressure control and drug action will lead inevitably to discovery of more effective drugs. However, such a statement, while a nice way to end a scientific paper or a review does not get me off the hook at this point.

Since quite frankly no brilliant predictions have occurred to me, I would like to start out with what might well be labeled daydreaming or wishful thinking. Strictly at a daydreaming level, it seems to me that: (1) if there is one body organ whose functions might be modified by a drug in such a way as to achieve a totally uncomplicated normalization of the blood pressure in hypertensive animals or man, this organ must be the brain, and (2) just as surgical sympathectomy offered an achievable endpoint to be simulated by drugs acting on the peripheral sympathetic nervous system, it would be nice if an invasive procedure of some sort in the brain produced the ideal result which one might hope to simulate with a therapeutic agent. Possibly a detailed investigation of the effects of 6-hydroxydopamine administered centrally is the route to follow, or the effects of noradrenaline applied to the nucleus tractus solitarii, but I would be happier with an even better preparation. Maybe the neuroanatomists and neurophysiologists here can visualize how my daydream could become reality.

In the remainder of the presentation I will offer 3 suggestions of approaches, or if you will, areas of investigation which may lead to new centrally acting antihypertensive drugs. The first and most obvious is the continuation of structure-activity studies by medicinal chemists and pharmacologists. This is of course going on in industrial laboratories worldwide, including our own. I am sure one can count on the synthesis of every conceivable analogue of current antihypertensive drugs as well as of the psychotropic drugs, many of which are known to affect blood pressure control mechanisms in the brain. In this type of work it is important to bear in mind that a drug cannot act on the brain unless it gets into the brain. Thus, it stands to reason that if one synthesizes a new compound with a central site of action in mind, the drug should be administered centrally and not only by injection peripherally or orally. Reliance only on the latter route, while seemingly pragmatic, may result in the loss of a good lead. Van Zwieten (1975) has reviewed the current state of the art, citing various clonidine analogues, as well as the non-neuroleptic pimozide analogue of Janssen, R-28935, which acts centrally but apparently by a mechanism not involving α-adrenoreceptors. Compound BS-100-141, a guanidine analogue of clonidine, is interesting since it appeared to be less sedative in rats than clonidine (Kleinlogel et al., 1975), but has now been reported by Jäättelä (1976) to produce tiredness and dry mouth in patients at a frequency and severity equivalent to that of clonidine. We have been studying a clonidine analogue, lofexidine or 2-[α-(2,6-dichlorophenoxy)-ethyl] Δ-2-imidazoline hydrochloride, because it has a longer duration of action than clonidine and might therefore not be associated with the rebound phenomenon on withdrawal; studies to date are inconclusive. Effective analogues of methyldopa are noteworthy by their absence while quite the reverse is true for propranolol.

My second suggestion is in the direction of a detailed characterization of central adrenoreceptors, regardless of their label as α or β, or whether they exist pre- or postsynaptically. It is becoming clear that central and peripheral α-receptors differ in agonist-antagonist characteristics and that multiple antagonism and/or stimulation is possible. AH-5158 (Labetalol) is a case in point, possessing both α- and β-adrenoreceptor blocking properties peripherally (Farmer et al., 1972); it appears promising in the treatment of hypertension and has recently even been recommended for use in clonidine withdrawal crisis and pheochromocytoma (Brown et al., 1976). In vitro techniques such as those used by Creese et al. (1976) to study antischizophrenic drugs on dopamine receptors in brain membrane preparations should be helpful in studies of α-adrenoreceptors. Williams and Lefkowitz (1976) have recently used [³H]dihydroergocryptine binding as a means of identifying α-adrenergic receptors. Use of this and other radioactive ligands may eventually facilitate our search for centrally acting drugs.

A third approach which I favor is that of enzyme inhibition differing only in detail from that used by us 20 years ago, in that it is now becoming possible to focus more specifically on individual neurotransmitters. Saavedra et al. (1976) may have accomplished this partially using the compound SKF-9698, a tricyclic inhibitor of phenylethanolamine N-methyl transferase, the enzyme required for the methylation of noradrenaline to adrenaline. They found that administration of the compound to rats inhibited the enzyme in certain brain areas and reduced blood pressure in Doca-salt hypertensive animals. Their conclusions had to be qualified by the fact that the compound also has α-adrenergic blocking activity.

We have been interested in employing the approach of catalytic irreversible inhibition promoted by Rando (1974), and applying it to both synthesizing and metabolizing enzymes of individual neurotransmitters. This approach demands that the potential inhibitor be accepted as a substrate by the target enzyme. The enzyme, then, by its normal mode of action converts the inhibitor to a reactive species in its active site, resulting in irreversible inhibition. Such an inhibitor is implicitly enzyme specific as it should only inhibit those enzymes which can accept it as a substrate. The concept is exemplified by the known irreversible inhibitors of MAO, pargyline, clorgyline and deprenil, each containing an acetylenic moiety and exhibiting selectivity against individual monoamine oxidases. In a search for selective, irreversible inhibitors of γ-aminobutyric acid transaminase, Metcalf and Casara (1975) of our center have synthesized the new compounds γ-acetylenic GABA (4-aminohex-5-ynoic acid) and γ-vinyl GABA (4-aminohex-5-enoic acid), which are very potent in vitro and in vivo (Jung et al., 1976), and exhibit antiepileptic properties (Schechter et al., 1976). Their effects on blood pressure are as yet unknown. I feel that this approach will eventually permit selective control of the levels of other neurotransmitters including those involved in blood pressure control and will offer another dimension in our understanding of central control mechanisms.

REFERENCES

Brown, J.J., Rosei, E.A., Lever, A.F., Robertson, A.S., Robertson, J.I.S. and Trust, P.M. (1976) Emergency treatment of hypertensive crisis following clonidine withdrawal. *Brit. med. J.*, 1: 1341.

Burden, A.C. and Alexander, C.P.T. (1976) Rebound hypertension after acute methyldopa withdrawal. *Brit. med. J.*, 1: 1056—1057.

Creese, I., Burt, D.R. and Snyder, S.H. (1976) Dopamine receptor binding predicts clinical and pharmacological potencies of antischizophrenic drugs. *Science*, 192: 481—483.

Davies, D.S. and Reid, J.L. (Eds.) (1975) *Central Action of Drugs in Blood Pressure Regulation*, Pitman Medical Publishing Co., Kent.

Farmer, J.B., Kennedy, I., Levy, G.P. and Marshall, R.J. (1972) Pharmacology of AH 5158; a drug which blocks both α- and β-adrenoreceptors. *Brit. J. Pharmacol.*, 45: 660—675.

Finnerty, F.A., Buchholz, J.H. and Guillaudeu, R.L. (1957) Cardiovascular evaluation of a pressor amine (tetrahydrozyline) showing hypotensive properties in man. *Proc. Soc. exp. Biol. (N.Y.)*, 94: 376—379.

Horwitz, D. and Sjoerdsma, A. (1961) A non-hydrazine monoamine oxidase inhibitor with antihypertensive properties. *Proc. Soc. exp. Biol. (N.Y.)*, 106: 118—120.

Hutcheon, D.E., Scriabine, A. and Niesler, V.N. (1958) The effects of tetrahydrozoline (Tyzine) on cardiac and vasomotor functions. *J. Pharmacol. exp. Ther.*, 122: 101—109.

Jäättelä, A. (1976) Comparison of BS 100-141 and clonidine as antihypertensive agents. *Europ. J. clin. Pharmacol.*, 10: 73—76.

Jung, M., Lippert, B., Metcalf, F., Rieger, B. and Sjoerdsma, A. (1976) A comparison of the biochemical effect of two catalytic inhibitors of mammalian brain GABA transaminase. *Fed. Proc.*, 75: 544.

Kleinlogel, H., Scholtysick, G. and Sayers, A.C. (1975) Effects of clonidine and BS 100-141 on the EEG sleep pattern in rats. *Europ. J. Pharmacol.*, 33: 159—163.

Medical Letter (1976) Should propranolol be stopped before surgery? 18: 41—42.

Metcalf, B.W. and Casara, P. (1975) Regiospecific 1,4 addition of a propargylic anion. A general synthon for 2-substituted propargylamines as potential catalytic irreversible enzyme inhibitors. *Tetrahedron Letters*, 38: 3337—3340.

Oates, J.A., Gillespie, L., Udenfriend, S. and Sjoerdsma, A. (1960) Decarboxylase inhibition and blood pressure reduction by α-methyl-3,4-dihydroxyphenylalanine. *Science*, 131: 1890—1891.

Rando, R.R. (1974) Chemistry and enzymology of Kcat inhibitors. *Science*, 185: 320—324.

Saavedra, J.M., Grobecker, H. and Axelrod, J. (1976) Adrenaline-forming enzyme in brainstem: elevation in genetic and experimental hypertension. *Science*, 191: 483—484.

Schechter, P.J., Jung, M.J., Tranier, Y., Lippert, B. and Sjoerdsma, A. (1976) γ-Acetylenic GABA (amino-4-hex-5-ynoic acid): a GABA transaminase inhibitor with selective antiseizure activity. *Fed. Proc.*, 75: 544.

Van Zwieten, P.A. (1975) Antihypertensive drugs with a central action. *Progr. Pharmacol.*, 1: 1—63.

Williams, L.T. and Lefkowitz, R.J. (1976) Alpha-adrenergic receptor identification by [^{3}H]dihydroergocryptine binding. *Science*, 192: 791—793.

Yamori, Y., Lovenberg, W. and Sjoerdsma, A. (1970) Norepinephrine metabolism in brainstem of spontaneously hypertensive rats. *Science*, 170: 544—547.

NEUROANATOMY AND NEUROPHYSIOLOGICAL MECHANISMS OF CENTRAL CARDIOVASCULAR CONTROL

Chairmen: S.M. Hilton (Birmingham)
P. Kezdi (Dayton, Ohio)

Neuroanatomy of Central Cardiovascular Control. Nucleus Tractus Solitarii: Afferent and Efferent Neuronal Connections in Relation to the Baroreceptor Reflex Arc

MIKLÓS PALKOVITS and LÁSZLÓ ZÁBORSZKY

I. Department of Anatomy, Semmelweis University Medical School, Budapest (Hungary)

INTRODUCTION

There is a large body of neuroanatomical, electrophysiological and neuro-pharmacological evidence that central neurones taking part in the cardio-vascular baroreceptor reflexes are primarily located in the lower part of the brain stem and in the spinal cord. The activity of these cells is to an important degree determined by the nervous impulses carried via primary visceral afferents of the IXth and Xth cranial nerves from several different peripheral baroreceptor sites. A major part of these fibres have their first synapse in the nucleus tractus solitarii (NTS) of the medulla oblongata. The activity of the baroreceptor neurones is influenced by higher control mechanisms originating from cerebral cortex, hypothalamus, limbic system and mesencephalic-pontine structures as well as by the biogenic amine-containing cells in the lower brain stem. Results of studies in this respect can be summarized by using the classical neuroanatomical description of a neuronal reflex arc (Fig. 1).

(I) PRIMARY BARORECEPTOR NEURONES (AFFERENT PATHWAYS)

The cell bodies of the primary baroreceptor neurones which conduct baroreceptor information to the lower brain stem are located in the ganglion nodosum. Specialized axon terminals of these perikarya serve as stretch receptors to detect changes in blood pressure. Such baroreceptive structures are strategically distributed in the carotid sinus, aortic arch (and other great vessels) and cardiac structures. These cells of the ganglion nodosum are of a pseudo-unipolar character, having an axon with peripheral processes connecting the baroreceptive elements to the ganglion, and via the proximal process, to the medulla oblongata (Fig. 1). The proximal fibres of primary baroreceptor neurones travel among the other fibres of the IXth and Xth nerves and reach the medulla oblongata laterally at a level close to the obex. The fibres pass through the nucleus and tractus spinalis nervi trigemini as small branches (Allen, 1923; Foley and DuBois, 1934; Torvik, 1956). Some of the fibres are dorsally located but others in more ventral positions follow the efferent fibres of the vagal nerve (Fig. 1). Both dorsal and ventral afferent fibres reach the tractus solitarius and descend therein to the caudal levels of the medulla oblongata. Some of the fibres in the solitary tract decussate mostly caudal to the obex (Cajal, 1896; Ingram and Dawkins, 1945; Kerr, 1962; Rhoton et al., 1966; Chiba and Doba, 1975; Zaborszky et al., in preparation). The existence of decussating fibres is also shown by electrophysiological studies (Crill and Reis, 1968; Sampson and Biscoe, 1968; Seller and Illert, 1969).

The distribution and topography of the IXth and Xth cranial nerves including the primary baroreceptor afferents can be demonstrated by means of light microscopic nerve degenerating techniques and by electron microscopy a few days after removal of the nodose ganglion or after transection of the IXth and Xth nerves proximal to this ganglion. Fine silver dots representing degenerated axon fragments can be followed from the roots of the vagal nerve throughout the dorsal part of the tractus spinalis of the Vth nerve. The fibres which pass through the ventral part of the nucleus and tractus spinalis of the Vth nerve may contain most of the primary baroreceptor afferents (Fig. 1). Both the dorsal and the ventral fibres have their first synapse in the NTS. Hypertension develops immediately after bilateral transections, lateral to the NTS, are made sufficiently deep to cut the ventrally located afferent (as well as efferent) fibres. No changes in blood pressure were observed when only the dorsal fibres were interrupted (De Jong and Palkovits, 1976). Similarly, transection of the tractus solitarius at the level of the obex failed to cause a change in blood pressure in rabbits (Fallert and Bucher, 1966) or in rats (De Jong et al., 1975b; De Jong and Palkovits, 1976).

The termination of the fibres of the Vth, VIIth, IXth and Xth cranial nerves within the NTS has been described in various species (Torvik, 1956; Kerr, 1962; Cottle, 1964; Rhoton et al., 1966). These neuroanatomical studies are paralleled by a large body of electrophysiological data, which provide further support for the anatomical observations (Oberholzer, 1955; Smith and Pearce, 1961; Hellner and von Baumgarten, 1961; Humphrey, 1967; Crill and Reis, 1968; Miura and Reis, 1969; Seller and Illert, 1969; Biscoe and Sampson, 1970a, 1970b; Lipski et al., 1972; Miura and Reis, 1972; Kumada and Nakajima, 1972; Mezenich and Brugg, 1973; Sessle, 1973). The afferent fibres reach the tractus solitarius and descend through the medulla oblongata just rostral to the level of C_1 and C_2 of the spinal cord (Cajal, 1896; Torvik, 1956; Kerr,

Fig. 1. Schematic drawing of the baroreceptor reflex arc. Frontal sections at the level of the pons (A), medulla oblongata (B and C) and spinal cord (D). Indications of colours: green = primary baroreceptor afferent neurones; blue = secondary baroreceptor neurones from the nucleus tractus solitarii; orange = fibre connections with modulatory centres; red = efferent baroreceptor neurones; yellow = biogenic amine fibres (solid line = noradrenergic; dotted line = serotonergic fibres). Abbreviations: NTS = nucleus tractus solitarii; C = pars commissuralis of the NTS; A = nucleus ambiguus; A1 = nucleus reticularis lateralis; TV = tractus spinalis of Vth; Vth = nucleus tractus spinalis of Vth; LC = locus coeruleus; m = nucleus raphe magnus; rg = nucleus reticularis gigantocellularis; rpv = nucleus reticularis parvocellularis; rpo = nucleus reticularis pontis caudalis; rd = nucleus reticularis medullae oblongatae, pars dorsalis; rv = nucleus reticularis medullae oblongatae, pars ventralis; P = pyramidal tract; DF = dorsal funiculus; LF = lateral funiculus; VF = ventral funiculus; i = nucleus intermedio-lateralis; S = sympathetic ganglion; IX. = ganglion petrosum; X. = ganglion nodosum.

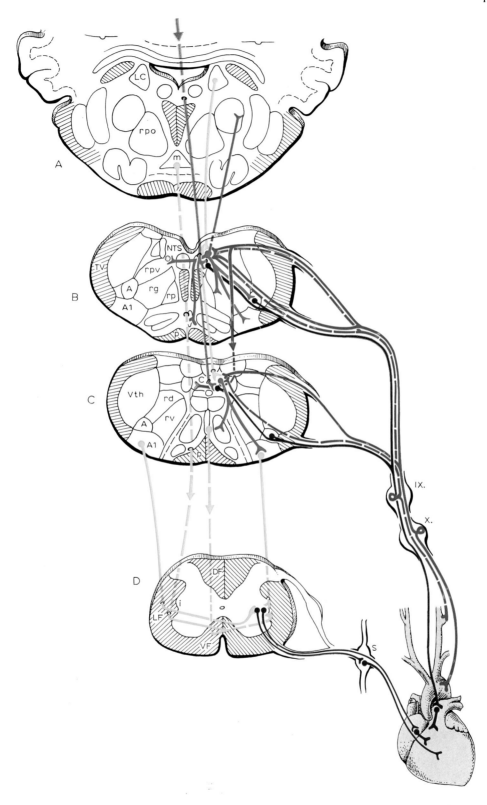

12

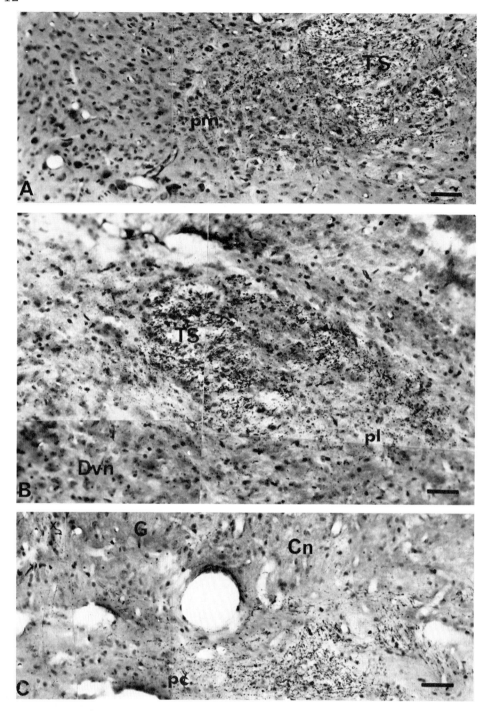

Fig. 2. Degenerating axons and nerve terminals in the tractus solitarius (TS) and in the nucleus tractus solitarii 4 days after removal of the nodose ganglion (Fink—Heimer silver impregnation technique). A = 6.3 mm, B = 7.0 and C = 8 mm behind the interauricular line. TS = tractus solitarius; pm = pars medialis of the NTS; pl = pars lateralis of the NTS; pc = pars commissuralis of the NTS; Dvn = dorsal vagal nucleus; G = funiculus gracilis; Cn = nucleus cuneatus. In part C of the figure the midline is indicated by x. Bar scale = 50 μm.

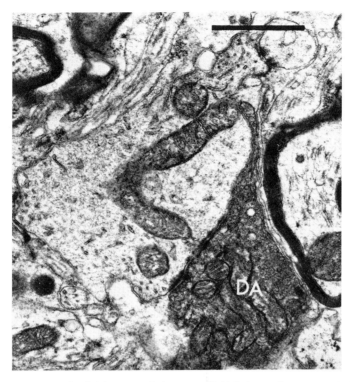

Fig. 3. Degenerating axo-dendritic synaptic bouton (DA) 2 days after removal of the nodose ganglion, in the pars commissuralis of the nucleus tractus solitarii. Bar scale = 1 μm.

1962). Four days after removal of the ganglion nodosum or transection of the IXth and Xth cranial nerves, massive degeneration is seen over the whole length of the tractus solitarius and the NTS between the level of the obex and the caudal end of the tract. Fig. 2 shows an example obtained by means of the Fink—Heimer silver degeneration technique*. Degenerating axo-dendritic synaptic boutons can be identified in the caudal part of the NTS and in the nucleus commissuralis by electron microscopy (Fig. 3). Two to three days after transection of the IXth and Xth nerves, degenerated axon terminals amounted to about 15—20% of the total population (Chiba and Doba, 1975).

Nerve degeneration was not observed in any other cell group of the brain stem after either extirpation of the ganglion nodosum or transection of the IXth and Xth nerves. This finding agrees with earlier studies performed in different species (Foley and DuBois, 1934; Ingram and Dawkins, 1945; Torvik, 1956; Kerr, 1962; Cottle, 1964; Rhoton et al., 1966). Neuroanatomical studies with nerve degeneration techniques did not support the electrophysiological observations, suggesting that primary baroreceptor fibres would also terminate just ventral to the NTS in the nucleus reticularis paramedianus (Miura and Reis, 1968, 1969, 1972; Homma et al., 1970; Calaresu and Thomas, 1971; Miura,

*Figures and experimental data presented in this paper are from studies performed in Wistar rats.

1975). Few degenerating axons, however, were found ventral to the NTS; they belong to the A2-catecholaminergic cell group rather than to the paramedian reticular nucleus. Other electrophysiological observations (Spyer and Wolstencroft, 1971) as well suggest that there is no direct input from the sinus nerve to the paramedian reticular nucleus. In the rat no depressor response was obtained from sites ventral to the NTS (De Jong et al., 1975a, b).

The present findings and the data from the literature clearly demonstrate that the NTS serves as the primary relay station of the cardiovascular reflex arc.

(II) NUCLEUS TRACTUS SOLITARII (NTS) (PRIMARY SYNAPTIC SITES OF AFFERENT FIBRES OF THE BARORECEPTOR REFLEX ARC)

Viscerosensory nerve cells receiving projections of the Vth, VIIth, IXth and Xth cranial nerves constitute the elongated nucleus of the NTS which extends over the whole length of the medulla oblongata (Fig. 4). Cell bodies are located both medially and laterally to the solitary tract. Cranial nerve fibres terminating in the NTS occupy relatively distinct parts of the nucleus (Torvik, 1956). The rostral part of the NTS (rostral to the level of the obex) contains cells which are mostly connected with the Vth and VIIth nerves; primary fibres of the IXth and Xth cranial nerves terminate in the caudal part of the nucleus.

The perikarya of the medial and lateral parts of the NTS have different cellular characteristics and different functions. The lateral part of the NTS (which is also referred to as the nucleus parasolitarius) has been implicated as a primary cell station of afferent respiratory fibres (von Euler et al., 1973a, 1973b). The cells in this part of the nucleus are less densely packed than the cells in the medial part (Fig. 5). Perikarya in this subdivision are relatively large. The lateral part of the NTS ends caudally, at the level of the area postrema (Fig. 4). In human and higher mammal neuroanatomy only this part of the NTS is described as the nucleus tractus solitarii. The medial part of the NTS is larger. In the rostrocaudal direction, the NTS shifts more and more medially (Fig. 4) and at a short distance rostral to the obex it touches the basal surface of the fourth ventricle (Fig. 4_6). At the closing of the IVth ventricle (obex) the left and the right part of the NTS come closer and closer to each other and finally, 800—900 μm behind the obex, the NTS cells constitute the nucleus commissuralis in the midline (Figs. 4 and 5). On the basis of the character of the cells, the nucleus commissuralis can be considered as a mere topographical caudal continuation of the NTS.

Fig. 4. Frontal serial sections of the dorsal part of the medulla oblongata of the rat. Luxol fast blue—cresyl violet staining. Distances between two neighbouring sections are 200 μm (calculated for the living state in a 200 g rat). Distance between picture 9 and 10 is only 100 μm). 1 = 12.9 mm behind the bregma (5.5 mm behind the interauricular line or 1.5 mm rostral to the obex). Obex level is between pictures 8 and 9. T = tractus solitarius; m = pars medialis of the nucleus tractus solitarii (NTS); l = pars lateralis of the NTS; c = pars commissuralis of the NTS; d = dorsal vagal nucleus; i = intercalate nucleus; XII = motor nucleus of the XIIth cranial nerve; AP = area postrema; FLM = fasciculus longitudinalis medialis; G = nucleus gracilis; Cu = nucleus cuneatus; F = fibrae arcuatae internae; ph = nucleus prepositus hypoglossi. Magnification = x 40.

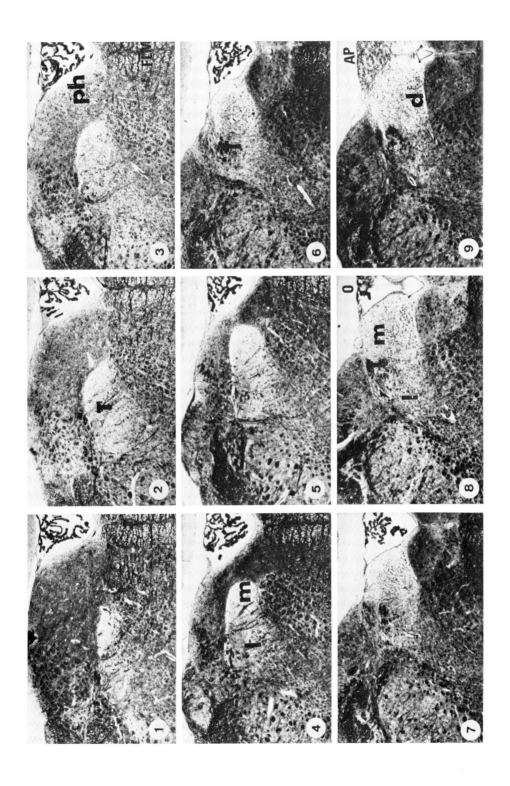

16

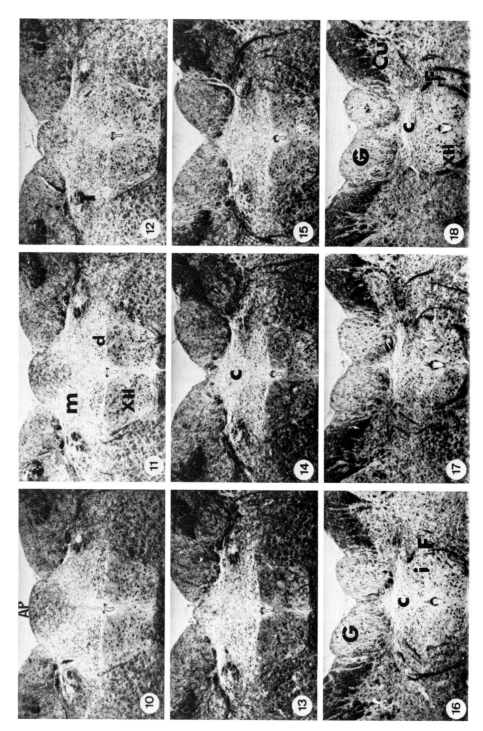

Fig. 4. For legend see p. 14.

17

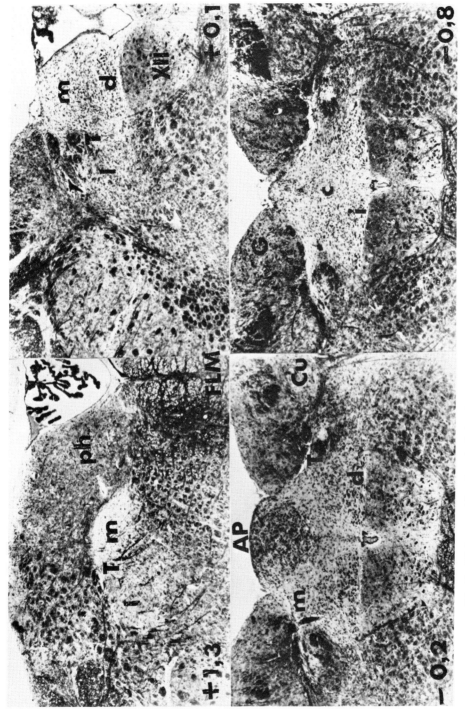

Fig. 5. High magnification (× 60) of Fig. 4_2, 4_8, 4_{10} and 4_{13}. Numbers indicate distances rostral (+) and caudal (−) to the obex in mm. For abbreviations see legend of Fig. 4.

In human anatomy the medial part of the NTS is designated as the nucleus alae cinereae lateralis. This name would be logical on the basis of the anatomical localization of these cells but they are connected with the tractus solitarius as well. We suggest, that in view of the neuroanatomical and neurophysiological studies in which this region is commonly called nucleus tractus solitarii (NTS), it would be correct and helpful to use the term independently of the cell type for all cells and cell groups connected with the tractus solitarius. The NTS should be subdivided into 3 parts (Fig. 5) : (1) pars medialis, (2) pars lateralis, and (3) pars commissuralis (generally called nucleus commissuralis without any reason other than a topographical one). The pars medialis can be further divided into a rostral part which is rostral to the level of the obex and contains mainly projections from the Vth and VIIth cranial nerves (Fig. 4_{1-7}) and a caudal part (Fig. 4_{8-12}). The caudal part and probably also the pars commissuralis form the primary medullary centre for the cardiovascular reflex arc. Lesions of this particularly small area of the NTS proper caused acute hypertension in both cats and rats (Doba and Reis, 1973; De Jong et al., 1975b; De Jong and Palkovits, 1976), while electrical stimulation of this region resulted in hypotension and bradycardia (Oberholzer, 1955; Hellner and von Baumgarten, 1961; De Jong et al., 1975a, b).

The fibres of the IXth and Xth nerves terminate in both the medial and lateral parts of the NTS. Degenerating nerve terminals were also found in the pars commissuralis after removal of the nodose ganglion or transections of the IXth and Xth fibres extra- or intramedullary (Foley and DuBois, 1934; Ingram and Dawkins, 1945; Torvik, 1956; Kerr, 1962; Cottle, 1964; Chiba and Doba, 1975, 1976; Záborszky et al., in preparation; Palkovits et al., in preparation).

Only a few reports have appeared about the ultrastructure of the neurones of the NTS (Fuxe et al., 1965; Chiba and Doba, 1975, 1976). Three major neuronal cell populations can be distinguished in the medial and commissural parts of the NTS by means of light and electron microscopy (Mészáros et al., in preparation). The majority of the cells are multiangular with 2—3 long dendrites having a number of spines which invade the medial part of the NTS deeply (Fig. 6). Axons originate mostly from the perikarya and can be followed into different parts of the reticular formation, for example to the nucleus ambiguus (Fig. 8C). Axo-somatic, axo-dendritic (Chiba and Doba, 1975) and also axo-axonic synaptic terminals can be observed by electron microscopy (Fig. 7). Transections of the IXth and Xth nerves resulted in degeneration in the axo-dendritic and axo-somatic but not of the axo-axonic nerve terminals (Chiba and Doba, 1975; Mészáros et al., in preparation). The other relay neurones are the fusiform cells. These cells have two main dendrites with less spines than the former cells. The axons originate from one of the dendrites and are relatively short. They ramify somewhere in the vicinity of the solitary tract. Primary axons of the IXth and Xth nerve terminate with axo-dendritic synaptic boutons on these cells. Intramedullary transection of these nerve fibres caused degeneration of synaptic terminals in the caudal and commissural parts of the NTS (Palkovits et al., in preparation). There is a third type of cells in the NTS which can be recognized as Golgi 2nd cells (Fig. 6C). Axons of these cells make axo-axonic contacts with the multiangular cells (Fig. 6B).

The fact that only 15—20% of the total amount of synaptic terminals degenerated following complete transection of the IXth and Xth cranial nerves may point to a high degree of intrinsic nerve connections in the NTS. Electrophysiological studies also indicate the presence of a high number of interneurones in the NTS. This may mean that the structure consists of a highly organized neuronal network.

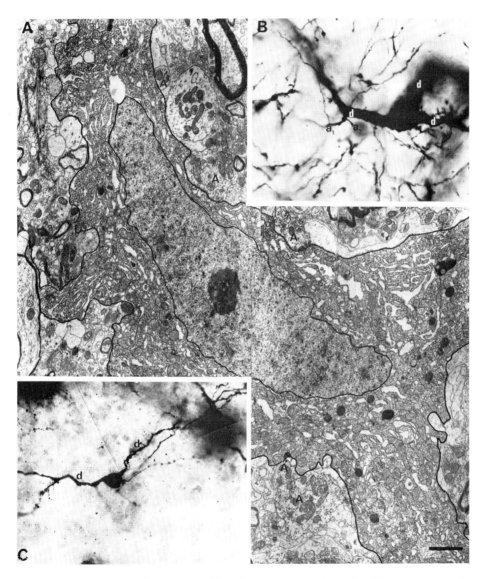

Fig. 6. Electron microscopic montage (A) of the main cell type (multiangular cell) of the nucleus tractus solitarii (pars commissuralis). B, multiangular; C, Golgi 2nd cells impregnated with rapid Golgi technique. A = axo-somatic synapses; a_1 = parent axon; a_2 = axo-axonic synapse; d = dendrite. Bar scale = 1 μm.

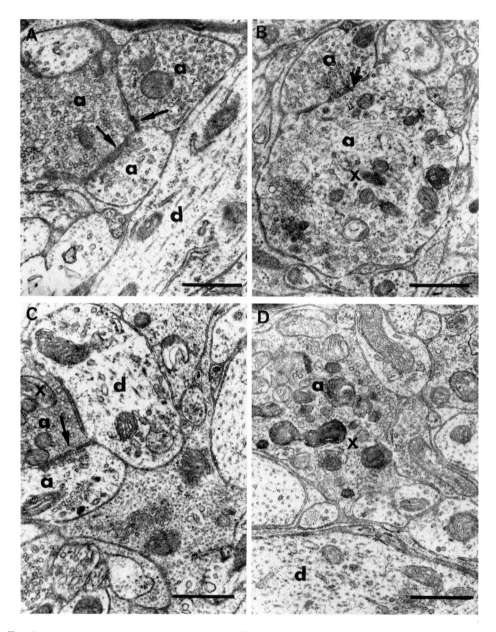

Fig. 7. Axo-axonic nerve terminals in the medial-caudal part of the nucleus tractus solitarii in intact (A) and in 6-OHDA treated rats (B, C, D). Arrows point to the synaptic thickenings from the postsynaptic side. d = dendrite; a = axons; x indicates degenerating axons. Bar scale = 1 μm.

(III) EFFERENT NEURONAL CONNECTIONS OF THE NUCLEUS TRACTUS SOLITARII (SECONDARY NEURONES OF THE BARORECEPTOR REFLEX ARC)

Both the neuroanatomical and the electrophysiological aspects of secondary neurones of the baroreceptor reflex arc are difficult to study. Electrophysiological observations provide indirect evidence for neuronal connections. Experimental neuroanatomical studies in general have not been suitable enough to allow interventions to be made limited to NTS structures. Earlier data thus require critical evaluation in this respect.

Following a very small lesion in the medial part of the NTS we observed axon and preterminal degeneration in the dorsal vagal nucleus, in the intercalate nucleus and also in the different subdivisions of the NTS. A diffuse pattern of degenerating fibres could be followed in a ventral direction and terminal degenerations were also observed in the nucleus reticularis lateralis (Fig. 8A). This region contains the A1 catecholaminergic cells. Nerve terminal degeneration was also observed in the nucleus reticularis medullae oblongatae, in the nucleus reticularis gigantocellularis (Fig. 8B) and there was fairly dense degeneration around the motor neurones of the nucleus ambiguus (Fig. 8C).

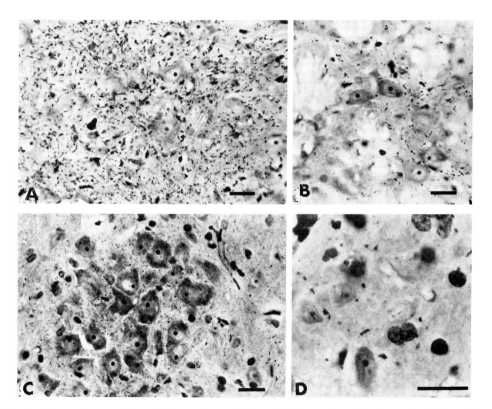

Fig. 8. Nerve degeneration 4 days after a lesion of the nucleus tractus solitarii in: (A) nucleus reticularis gigantocellularis, (B) nucleus reticularis lateralis (A1 catecholaminergic cell group), (C) nucleus ambiguus, and (D) substantia grisea centralis mesencephali. Fink—Heimer silver impregnation technique. Bar scale = 25 μm.

Similar findings using the Nauta silver degenerating technique in cats were published by Morest (1967) and also by Cottle and Calaresu (1975) after a lesion involving the dorsal part of the NTS and the tractus solitarius. The degeneration observed in the intact part of the NTS after a small lesion in another part of the nucleus might reflect the intensive intrinsic connections of the NTS cells. It would also provide anatomical evidence for a multisynaptic organization within the NTS as suggested by electrophysiological studies (Humphrey, 1967; Miura and Reis, 1969).

Spinal projections from the NTS have been reported to originate mainly from the lateral part of the nucleus (Torvik, 1957; von Euler et al., 1973a, 1973b). After a lesion restricted to the medial part of the NTS, degenerating fibres could be followed only to the medullary—spinal cord junction. Descending fibres are mostly located medially among the fibres of the medial longitudinal fasciculus (Morest, 1967).

With nerve degenerating techniques, ascending fibres from the NTS cannot be followed further rostrally than the genu of the facial nerve in the pons. These fibres and also probably nerve terminals were observed within the nucleus prepositus hypoglossi (Morest, 1967). However, the lesion used extended rostrally and damaged the rostral part of the NTS. Other lesions, which caused destruction more laterally in the gracilis and cuneatus nuclei, resulted in degenerating axons and nerve terminals in the central gray of the mesencephalon (Fig. 8D) and in thalamic nuclei. These systems do not seem to be directly related to the central vasomotor control mechanisms.

Lesions in the NTS caudal to the obex destroy noradrenergic (Dahlström and Fuxe, 1964) and adrenergic cells (Hökfelt et al., 1973) located in the caudal part of the NTS, in the pars commissuralis and in the dorsal vagal nucleus. Catecholaminergic cells have a great number of axon collaterals and synaptic terminals which can innervate various regions of the CNS. Degenerating nerve terminals were observed in the hypothalamus and in the median eminence after an electrolytic lesion in the A2 catecholaminergic region (Palkovits et al., in press). Therefore, for the interpretation of studies using lesions in the NTS region the probable consequences of damage to catecholaminergic cells have to be taken into account.

(IV) EFFERENT BARORECEPTOR NEURONES (SITE OF ORIGIN OF EFFERENT BARORECEPTOR FIBRES IN THE IXTH AND XTH CRANIAL AND IN THE SPINAL NERVES)

Preganglionic cells of the efferent cardiovascular baroreceptor fibres are located in the medulla oblongata (vagal cardio-inhibitory) and in the spinal cord (preganglionic sympathetic). Axons of these cells have synaptic contacts with sympathetic ganglion cells or intramural ganglionic cells which constitute the final neuronal stage in the baroreceptor reflex arc to the heart and the vascular bed (Fig. 1).

(a) Efferent neurones in the medulla oblongata

Cell bodies of the baroreceptor efferent axons have not been convincingly localized in the medulla oblongata. Perikarya might be located in the visceromotor vagal nucleus which is called the nucleus originis dorsalis vagi (dorsal vagal nucleus). After a lesion of the dorsal vagal nuclei, fine foci of degeneration have been observed in the vagal nerve in the cat (Calaresu and Cottle, 1965; Morest, 1967). Electrical stimulation of this region, however, failed to induce bradycardia (Calaresu and Pearce, 1965)

The dorsal vagal nucleus begins only a few μm rostral to the obex level (Fig. 4_7) and can be followed (intercalate nucleus) to near the caudal end of the medulla oblongata (Fig. 4_{1-6}). The cells are bordered by the NTS dorsally and by the motor nucleus of the XIIth cranial nerve ventrally. The nucleus is much smaller than the NTS (Fig. 4). Perikarya of this nucleus, like the other visceromotor cells, are of a medium size which distinguishes them from the small cells of the NTS and also from the large somatomotor cells of the XIIth nerve (Fig. 5). The nucleus is penetrated by the cells of the A2 catechol-aminergic cell group (Dahlström and Fuxe, 1964; Palkovits and Jacobowitz, 1974) and is extremely rich in catecholaminergic and serotonergic terminals (Fuxe, 1965).

It has also been suggested that efferent baroreceptor neurones may be located in the nucleus ambiguus (Gunn et al., 1968; McAllen and Spyer, 1976). This nucleus is in fact a rostrocaudal column of somatomotor cells belonging to the IXth, Xth and XIth cranial nerves. The nucleus ambiguus receives fibres from the NTS (Fig. 8C). More direct data are required to establish the direct involvement of these neurones in the baroreceptor reflex arc.

The nucleus intercalatus can be considered as the caudal continuation of the dorsal vagal nucleus and is also located in the vicinity of the NTS (Fig. 4). The nucleus intercalatus as well has been suggested as being a part of the central cardiovascular reflex mechanisms. Smith (1965) proposed that descending hypothalamic pathways inhibit the putative cardio-inhibitory neurones of this nucleus. Calaresu and Henry (1970) showed cardio-acceleratory responses following stimulation of the intercalate nucleus and the surrounding region. The nucleus has been reported to receive primary vagal and glossopharyngeal fibres. The major function of this nucleus, however, has been linked with taste.

(b) Preganglionic efferent neurones in the spinal cord

The intermedio-lateral cell column between the Th_1 and L_2 segments are the site of perikarya of the cardiovascular preganglionic sympathetic neurones (Henry and Calaresu, 1972a, b). Axons of these cells leave the spinal cord via the ventral spinal roots and terminate either in the sympathetic or peripheral ganglia on the postganglionic neurones which constitute the final stage in the baroreceptor reflex arc (Fig. 1).

Henry and Calaresu (1974a) demonstrated that nuclei such as the nucleus reticularis pontis caudalis, the nucleus reticularis gigantocellularis, the nucleus reticularis parvocellularis, the nucleus reticularis paramedianus, the nucleus reticularis medullae oblongatae pars ventralis and dorsalis project directly to the intermedio-lateral nucleus of the spinal cord. Descending fibres from the nucleus reticularis lateralis (Torvik and Brodal, 1957; Henry and Calaresu, 1974a) have been shown to be noradrenergic (Dahlström and Fuxe, 1965) and those fibres from the (magnus, obscurus and pallidus) raphe nuclei (Brodal et al., 1960) to be serotonergic (Dahlström and Fuxe, 1965). No direct neuronal connection from the medial part of the NTS to the spinal cord could be seen when nerve degenerating techniques were used. The terminations of the secondary neurone fibres from the NTS on various nuclei of the reticular formation in the medulla oblongata may suggest that baroreceptor reflexes could reach the spinal cord by a multisynaptic pathway: via the NTS — reticular formation — intermedio-lateral nucleus of the spinal cord (Fig. 1).

Inhibitory fibres from medullary nuclei to the intermedio-lateral nucleus descend mostly in the lateral (both in dorsal and in ventral positions) and partly in the ventral funiculus of the spinal cord (Kerr and Alexander, 1964; Illert and Seller, 1969; Illert and Gabriel, 1970, 1972; Henry and Calaresu, 1974b; Coote and Macleod, 1974, 1975). Excitatory fibres to the preganglionic sympathetic cells probably descend in the dorsolateral funiculus (Kell and Hoff, 1952; Henry and Calaresu, 1974b). The preganglionic sympathetic neurones also receive inputs from the contralateral medulla: fibres from the nucleus reticularis gigantocellularis and nucleus reticularis paramedianus cross the midline in the caudal medulla and descend in the contralateral ventral funiculus (Henry and Calaresu, 1974c). Serotonergic fibres from the lower raphe nuclei descend in the medial part of the ventral funiculus and after decussation terminate in the intermedio-lateral nucleus (Dahlström and Fuxe, 1965). Fibres from the nucleus reticularis lateralis descend in the dorsolateral and ventral funiculi (Fig. 1) and cross the midline in the spinal cord before termination (Henry and Calaresu, 1974c). These fibres are inhibitory and probably catecholaminergic. (Aminergic fibre connections will be discussed on the forthcoming pages.)

(V) MODULATORY NEURONAL MECHANISMS OF THE CARDIOVASCULAR REFLEX ARC

The cardiovascular reflex arc is influenced by neuronal inputs of higher brain regions at the level of the medulla and at the spinal cord, as demonstrated by transection of the lower brain stem (Wang and Chai, 1962; Chai et al., 1963; Leibowitz et al., 1963; Doba and Reis, 1973). Higher modulatory centres receive information carried via primary afferents of the IXth and Xth cranial nerves using an ascending multisynaptic neuronal pathway originating from the secondary baroreceptor neurones in the NTS (Fig. 1). In the same manner, neuronal outputs from the higher brain regions do not directly effect the peripheral sympathetic neurones but modulate the activities of baroreceptor efferent neurones both in the medulla oblongata and in the spinal cord (Fig. 1). The existence of the higher modulatory mechanisms on the cardiovascular reflexes has been demonstrated in a number of electrophysiological studies, but there are only a few direct neuroanatomical observations of the topographical localization of the cells or of the ascending and descending neuronal pathways.

The hypothalamus has been implicated as a possible site of the higher cardiovascular control mechanisms (Wang and Ranson, 1939, 1941; Hilton, 1963; Smith, 1965; Peiss, 1965; Chai and Wang, 1968; Hilton and Spyer, 1971; Thomas and Calaresu, 1972; Hilton, 1975; McAllen, 1976). Electrical stimulation in the anterior hypothalamus and in the preoptic area elicits bradycardia and hypotension (Wang and Ranson, 1939, 1941; Hilton and Spyer, 1971) and inhibits the baroreceptor reflexes (Hilton, 1963; McAllen, 1976). Bilateral lesions of these areas reduce the response to baroreceptor afferent stimulation (Hilton and Spyer, 1971). However, the cells involved are situated, according to the maps of Hilton and Spyer (1971), in the nucleus interstitialis striae terminalis rather than in the hypothalamus. This nucleus is supposed to be a relay station between the amygdala and the hypothalamus and contains catecholamines in extremely high concentrations (Brownstein et al., 1974). Catecholaminergic fibres run from the nucleus interstitialis striae terminalis to the amygdala which is also proposed to be a neuronal region influencing cardiovascular responses (Hilton and Zbrożyna, 1963). The importance of the nucleus interstitialis striae terminalis in the baroreceptor control mechanisms is supported by the observation that injection of noradrenaline into the area of this nucleus induces a fall in blood pressure and heart rate. These effects are probably due to stimulation of alpha adrenergic receptors by noradrenaline as both bradycardia and hypotension could be induced by phenylephrine and could be antagonized by phentolamine (Struyker Boudier et al., 1974).

Direct fibres from the hypothalamus cannot be followed by neuroanatomical techniques further caudally than the ponto-mesencephalic border (Magoun, 1940; Crosby and Woodburne, 1951). Hypothalamic vasodepressor and pressor pathways may be multisynaptic: fibres from the posterior hypothalamus terminate in the locus coeruleus (Enoch and Kerr, 1967a, b; Mizuno and Nakamura, 1970) from which fibres (probably noradrenergic fibres) descend through the ventrolateral medulla to the A1 neurones (Ward and Gunn, 1976). Smith (1965) suggested, however, that a direct pathway from the hypothalamus descends to the medulla and to the spinal cord. Preterminal degenerating fibres were traced to the intercalate nucleus, to the nucleus reticularis lateralis and to the intermedio-lateral nucleus after lesions of sites in the posterior hypothalamus. This observation, however, could not be corroborated by others, and the possibility of damage of the corticofugal fibres which descend through the diencephalon and terminate in the NTS (Brodal et al., 1957) or in the spinal cord cannot be excluded.

It is possible that the locus coeruleus and its neighbouring area may influence cardiovascular mechanisms. Electrical stimulation of this region elicits changes in arterial pressure (Chai and Wang, 1962; Fallert and Polc, 1970; Ward and Gunn, 1976a) and modulates cardiovascular activity (Ward and Gunn, 1976b). The locus coeruleus sends descending projections to the medulla oblongata (Dahlström and Fuxe, 1964; Loizou, 1969; Chu and Bloom, 1974). These fibres as well as neurones in the locus coeruleus were shown to be noradrenergic. The major descending pathway from the locus coeruleus is the lateral tegmento-reticular tract to the nucleus reticularis lateralis (Russell, 1955). An additional descending pathway from the locus coeruleus follows the midline both dorsally and ventrally to the nucleus reticularis paramedianus (Russell, 1955). Ward et al. (1975) showed a descending projection from the locus coeruleus to the immediate vicinity of the NTS. The identification of the exact terminations of those fibres requires further electron microscopic studies. It is postulated that the fibres which originate in the locus coeruleus terminate in areas identical to or located just in the vicinity of the medullary catecholaminergic cell groups (A1 and A2 regions). On the other hand, these areas also have close topographical connections with the possible efferent medullary baroreceptor arc neurones (dorsal vagal and ambiguus nuclei).

(VI) BRAIN STEM BIOGENIC AMINE NEURONES AND THE BARORECEPTOR REFLEX ARC

There is considerable evidence that brain biogenic amines participate in baroreceptor control of the blood pressure and in the development of neurogenic hypertension (Chalmers and Wurtman, 1971; Chalmers and Reid, 1972; De Jong, 1974; Doba and Reis, 1974; Chalmers, 1975; De Jong et al., 1975a, 1975b; Saavedra et al., 1976). Elevations in the catecholamine levels in various regions of the central nervous system were also observed in spontaneously hypertensive rats (Versteeg et al., 1976b). Chalmers (1975) defined the role of central catecholaminergic neurones with regard to cardiovascular activity as inhibitory on the medullary and as excitatory on the spinal level.

Regions connected with cardiovascular regulation in the medulla oblongata are especially rich in catecholamines. The alteration of catecholamine levels or their synthesis with changes in blood pressure was demonstrated recently (Saavedra et al., 1976; Versteeg et al., 1976; Palkovits et al., in preparation). Local injection of noradrenaline or alteration of catecholamine levels or their synthesis in the NTS by injection of 6-hydroxydopamine (6-OHDA) caused changes of blood pressure and heart rate (De Jong, 1974; Doba and Reis, 1974; Chiba and Doba, 1975; De Jong et al., 1975a, 1975b).

(a) Biogenic amines in the medullary baroreceptor sites

Both the NTS and the dorsal vagal nucleus are highly innervated by catecholamine- and serotonin-containing nerve terminals (Dahlström and Fuxe, 1964; Fuxe, 1965). Fluorescence intensity (Fuxe, 1965), catecholamine levels (Van der Gugten et al., 1976; Versteeg et al., 1976a, b) as well as the phenylethanolamine N-methyl transferase activity (Saavedra et al., 1974) of these regions are much higher than those in the other nuclei of the medulla oblongata. Within the NTS high catecholamine levels were found only in regions which are primarily involved in the baroreceptor reflex arc (Van der Gugten et al., 1976; Versteeg et al., 1976b).

Serotonin concentration of the NTS only slightly exceeded the average level measured in the medulla oblongata (Palkovits et al., 1974).

Two noradrenergic (and perhaps also adrenergic) cell groups in the medulla oblongata may play an important role in modulating the baroreceptor reflex arc. Noradrenergic neurones of the A1 cell group (Dahlström and Fuxe, 1964) and adrenergic neurones of the C1 cell group (Hökfelt et al., 1973) are located within the nucleus reticularis lateralis and send fibres to the spinal cord. A high number of catecholaminergic terminals in the NTS and dorsal vagal nucleus originate from the A2 cell group. These cells are located mostly within the NTS but mainly behind the area postrema level (Palkovits and Jacobowitz, 1974).

Cells are also scattered in neighbouring regions such as the dorsal vagal nucleus and the reticular formation. Adrenergic cells (C2 cell groups) have also been demonstrated in the NTS (Hökfelt et al., 1973).

NTS cells are innervated by axo-axonic synapses of A2 neurones (Chiba and Doba, 1976). After local injection of 6-OHDA into the A2 region, degenerating axo-axonic synapses are observable in the pars medialis of the NTS both ipsi- and contralaterally (Figs. 7B, C, D and 9).

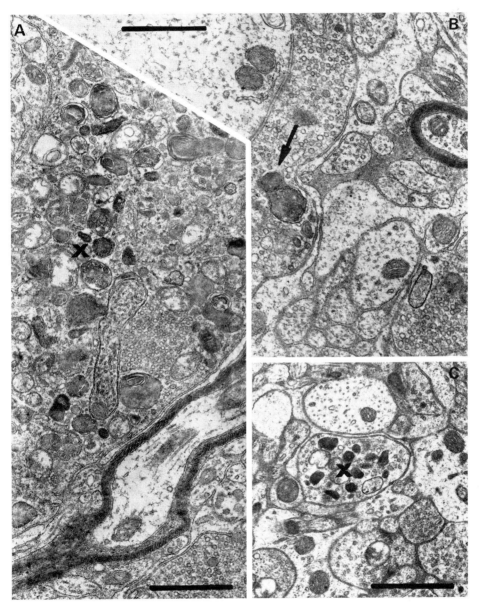

Fig. 9. Degenerating axon profiles filled with lysosomes (arrow) and dense bodies (X) in the contralateral medial part of the nucleus tractus solitarii 24 h after locally injected 6-hydroxydopamine in the A2 catecholaminergic cell group. Bar scale = 1 μm.

Studies of nerve degeneration after intramedullary transection of IXth and Xth fibres show that the A2 cells have a direct connection with fibres of these cranial nerves (Palkovits et al., in preparation). However, no terminal degeneration was found in the A1 cell group after removal of the nodose ganglion, but extensive degeneration occurred in the A1 region following a lesion of the NTS (Fig. 8A). This observation may suggest that baroreceptor nerve information to the A1 catecholaminergic cells is not carried by the primary but by the secondary neurones of the baroreceptor reflex arc (Fig. 1). Neither histofluorescence nor electron microscopic studies distinguish adrenergic nerve elements from the noradrenergic ones. The similarity in localization of these two kinds of cells suggests a similarity in their innervation patterns as well. So far, no data are available about the cellular origin and functional importance of the relatively high concentration of dopamine in the NTS (Versteeg et al., 1976a). Serotonin terminals in the NTS and dorsal vagal nucleus (Fuxe, 1965) arise from cells of the medullary raphe nuclei (Dahlström and Fuxe, 1964).

(b) Biogenic amines in the spinal cord

The most dense termination of both catecholamine- and serotonin-containing neurones in the spinal cord were found in the intermedio-lateral nucleus where they appear to make intimate synaptic contact with sympathetic preganglionic neurones (Carlsson et al., 1964; Dahlström and Fuxe, 1965). The highest concentrations of catecholamines and serotonin in thoracic segments of the spinal cord were also found in the lateral horn (Andén, 1965; Zivin et al., 1975).

Recent results of Neumayr et al. (1974) provide evidence that sympathetic preganglionic neurones are reciprocally controlled by bulbospinal noradrenaline (excitatory) and serotonin (inhibitory) pathways. However, other electrophysiological studies suggested that both noradrenergic and serotonergic pathways which descend to the spinal cord from the medulla were inhibitory to sympathetic outflow (Coote and Macleod, 1974, 1975; Henry and Calaresu, 1974c). Sympatho-inhibitory tracts have been located within the dorsolateral, ventral and ventrolateral funiculi (Illert and Seller, 1969; Illert and Gabriel, 1970, 1972; Henry and Calaresu, 1974b, 1974c; Coote and Macleod, 1974, 1975).

According to histofluorescence and electrophysiological studies, the A1 cell group is the site of origin of descending noradrenergic fibres to the intermedio-lateral nucleus (Carlsson et al., 1964; Dahlström and Fuxe, 1965; Henry and Calaresu, 1974c; Coote and Macleod, 1975). Fibres run in the lateral and ventral ipsilateral funiculi and cross the midline in the spinal cord close to their level of termination.

Serotonergic cells innervating the intermedio-lateral nucleus of the spinal cord are located in the medullary raphe nuclei (magnus, obscurus and pallidus raphe nuclei). Fibres descend in the medial part of the ventral funiculus and in the lateral funiculus to terminate on the cells of the intermedio-lateral nucleus after decussation (Dahlström and Fuxe, 1965; Coote and Macleod, 1974, 1975).

The origin of adrenaline and dopamine of the intermedio-lateral nucleus (Zivin et al., 1975) is still unknown.

FINAL REMARKS

Neuroanatomical data about the central organization of the control and modulation of cardiovascular baroreceptor reflexes are mostly descriptive. However, they provide a topographical basis for experimental studies. Better knowledge of cardiovascular control mechanisms requires further neuro-anatomical studies to analyze possible neuronal connections. More adequate methods, e.g., immunohistochemistry, autoradiography and electron microscopy and also investigations with antero- and retrograde nerve degeneration, are needed for these studies. Such fine qualitative neuroanatomical studies should be followed by a synthesis of the data obtained from quantitative analysis. Elucidation of the synaptic organization of the baroreceptor reflex arc and a neuronal network model based on solid anatomical data would be fruitful for further functional studies.

SUMMARY

The neuroanatomy of the baroreceptor reflex arc is reviewed and relevant new data are presented. The baroreceptor reflex arc consists of a multisynaptic neuronal chain. Primary neurones have perikarya in the nodose ganglion and they connect the peripheral baroreceptor sites with the nucleus tractus solitarii (NTS) via fibres in the IXth and Xth cranial nerves. The first synapse in the baroreceptor reflex arc and also the origin of the secondary neurones are located in the caudal and partly in the commissural parts of the NTS. Neuroanatomical topography of the NTS and neighbouring medullary nuclei in the rat is presented and detailed. The fibres of the secondary neurones terminate in various medullary nuclei (dorsal vagal, ambiguus, lateralis reticularis, gigantocellularis reticularis nuclei) and probably reach, directly or by multisynaptic pathways, higher regions which may modulate the baroreceptor reflex arc. A discussion is presented of the possible site of these modulatory centres in the hypothalamus and in the brain stem and of the "loop" of the descending fibres from these regions to the medullary and spinal baroreceptor neurones. The efferent preganglionic neurones of the baroreceptor reflex arc are located in the medulla oblongata and in the intermedio-lateral nucleus of the spinal cord. An outline is given of the possible interrelationship between the modulatory biogenic amine-containing neurones and the baroreceptor reflex arc.

REFERENCES

Allen, W.F. (1923) Origin and distribution of the tractus solitarius in the guinea pig. *J. comp. Neurol.*, 35: 171–204.

30

Andén, N.-E. (1965) Distribution of monoamines and dihydroxy-phenylalanine decarboxylase activity in the spinal cord. *Acta physiol. scand.*, 64: 197—203.

Biscoe, T.J. and Sampson, S.R. (1970a) Field potentials evoked in the brain stem of the cat by stimulation of the carotid sinus, glossopharyngeal, aortic and superior laryngeal nerves. *J. Physiol. (Lond.)*, 209: 341—358.

Biscoe, T.J. and Sampson, S.R. (1970b) Responses of cells in the brain stem of the cat to stimulation of the sinus, glossopharyngeal, aortic and superior laryngeal nerves. *J. Physiol. (Lond.)*, 209: 359—373.

Brodal, A., Szabó, T. and Torvik, A. (1956) Corticofugal fibers to sensory trigeminal nuclei and nucleus of solitary tract. An experimental study in the cat. *J. comp. Neurol.*, 106: 527—556.

Brodal, A., Taber, E. and Walberg, F. (1960) The raphe nuclei of the brain stem in the cat. II. Efferent connections. *J. comp. Neurol.*, 114: 239—259.

Brownstein, M., Saavedra, J.M. and Palkovits, M. (1974) Norepinephrine and dopamine in the limbic system of the rat. *Brain Res.*, 79: 431—436.

Cajal, S. Ramón y (1896) *Beitrag zum Studium der Medulla oblongata, des Kleinhirns und des Ursprungs der Gehirnnerven*, Barth, Leipzig, pp. 1—139.

Calaresu, F.R. and Cottle, M.K. (1965) Origin of cardiomotor fibres in the dorsal nucleus of the vagus in the cat. A histological study. *J. Physiol. (Lond.)*, 176: 252—260.

Calaresu, F.R. and Henry, J.R. (1970) The mechanism of the cardioacceleration elicited by electrical stimulation of the parahypoglossal area in the cat. *J. Physiol. (Lond.)*, 210: 107—120.

Calaresu, F.R. and Pearce, J.W. (1965) Electrical activity of efferent vagal fibres and dorsal nucleus of the vagus during reflex bradycardia in the cat. *J. Physiol. (Lond.)*, 176: 228—240.

Calaresu, F.R. and Thomas, M.R. (1971) The function of the paramedian reticular nucleus in the control of heart rate in the cat. *J. Physiol. (Lond.)*, 216: 143—158.

Carlsson, A., Falck, B., Fuxe, K. and Hillarp, N.-Å. (1964) Cellular localization of monoamines in the spinal cord. *Acta physiol. scand.*, 60: 112—119.

Chai, C.Y. and Wang, S.C. (1962) Localization of central cardiovascular control mechanisms in lower brain stem of the cat. *Amer. J. Physiol.*, 202: 25—30.

Chai, C.Y. and Wang, S.C. (1968) Integration of sympathetic cardiovascular mechanisms in medulla oblongata of the cat. *Amer. J. Physiol.*, 215: 1310—1315.

Chai, C.Y., Share, N.N. and Wang, S.C. (1963) Central control of sympathetic cardiac augmentation in lower brain stem of the cat. *Amer. J. Physiol.*, 205: 749—753.

Chalmers, J.P. (1975) Brain amines and models of experimental hypertension. *Circulat. Res.*, 36: 469—480.

Chalmers, J.P. and Reid, J.L. (1972) Participation of central noradrenergic neurones in arterial baroreceptor reflexes in the rabbit: a study with intracisternally administered 6-hydroxy-dopamine. *Circulat. Res.*, 31: 789—804.

Chalmers, J.P. and Wurtman, R.J. (1971) Participation of central noradrenergic neurones in arterial baroreceptor reflexes in the rabbit. *Circulat. Res.*, 28: 480—491.

Chiba, T. and Doba, N. (1975) Catecholaminergic axon varicosities and their synaptic structure in the nucleus tractus solitarii: possible roles in the regulation of the cardiovascular reflexes. *Brain Res.*, 84: 31—46.

Chiba, T. and Doba, N. (1976) Catecholaminergic axo-axonic synapses in the nucleus of the tractus solitarius (pars commissuralis) of the cat: possible relation to presynaptic regulation of baroreceptor reflexes. *Brain Res.*, 102: 255—265.

Chu, N.-S. and Bloom, F.E. (1974) The catecholamine-containing neurons in the cat dorsolateral pontine tegmentum: distribution of the cell bodies and some axonal projections. *Brain Res.*, 66: 1—22.

Coote, J.H. and Macleod, V.H. (1974) The influence of bulbospinal monoaminergic pathways on sympathetic nerve activity. *J. Physiol. (Lond.)*, 241: 453—475.

Coote, J.H. and Macleod, V.H. (1975) The spinal route of sympathoinhibitory pathways descending from the medulla oblongata *Pflügers Arch. ges. Physiol.*, 359: 335—347.

Cottle, M.K.W. (1964) Degeneration studies of primary afferents of IXth and Xth cranial nerves in the cat. *J. comp. Neurol.*, 122: 329—345.

Cottle, M.K.W. and Calaresu, F.R. (1975) Projections from the nucleus and tractus solitarius in the cat. *J. comp. Neurol.*, 161: 143—158.

Crill, W.E. and Reis, D.J. (1968) Distribution of carotid sinus and depressor nerves in cat brain stem. *Amer. J. Physiol.*, 214: 269—276.

Crosby, E.C. and Woodburne, R.T. (1951) The mammalian midbrain and isthmus regions. II. The fiber connections. c. The hypothalamotegmental pathways. *J. comp. Neurol.*, 94: 1—32.

Dahlström, A. and Fuxe, K. (1964) Evidence for the existence of monoamine neurones in the central nervous system. I. Demonstration of monoamines in the cell bodies of brain stem neurons. *Acta physiol. scand.*, 62, Suppl. 232: 1—55.

Dahlström A. and Fuxe, K. (1965) Evidence for the existence of monoamine neurones in the central nervous system. II. Experimentally induced changes in the intraneuronal amine levels of bulbospinal neuron systems. *Acta physiol. scand.*, 64, Suppl. 247: 1—36.

De Jong, W. (1974) Noradrenaline: central inhibitory control of blood pressure and heart rate. *Europ. J. Pharmacol.*, 29: 179—181.

De Jong, W. and Palkovits, M. (1976) Hypertension after localized transection of brain stem fibres. *Life Sci.*, 18: 61—64.

De Jong, W., Nijkamp, F.P. and Bohus, B. (1975a) Role of noradrenaline and serotonin in the central control of blood pressure in normotensive and spontaneously hypertensive rats. *Arch. int. Pharmacodyn.*, 213: 272—284.

De Jong, W., Zandberg, P. and Bohus, B. (1975b) Central inhibitory noradrenergic cardiovascular control. In *Hormones, Homeostasis and the Brain, Progr. Brain Res.,* Vol. 42, W.H. Gispen, Tj.B. van Wimersma Greidanus, B. Bohus and D. De Wied (Eds.), Elsevier, Amsterdam, pp. 285—298.

Doba, N. and Reis, D.J. (1973) Acute fulminating neurogenic hypertension produced by brainstem lesions in the cat. *Circulat. Res.*, 32: 584—593.

Doba, N. and Reis, D.J. (1974) Role of central and peripheral adrenergic mechanisms in neurogenic hypertension produced by brainstem lesions in rat. *Circulat. Res.*, 34: 293—301.

Enoch, D.M. and Kerr, F.W.L. (1967a) Hypothalamic vasopressor and vesicopressor pathways. I. Functional studies. *Arch. Neurol. (Chic.)*, 16: 290—306.

Enoch, D.M. and Kerr, F.W.L. (1967b) Hypothalamic vasopressor and vesicopressor pathways. II. Anatomic studies of their course and connections. *Arch. Neurol. (Chic.)*, 16: 307—320.

Euler, C. von, Hayward, J.N., Marttila, I. and Wyman, R.J. (1973a) Respiratory neurones of the ventrolateral nucleus of the solitary tract of cat: vagal input, special connections and morphological identification. *Brain Res.*, 61: 1—22.

Euler, C. von, Hayward, J.N., Marttila, I. and Wyman, R.J. (1973b) The spinal connections of the inspiratory neurones of the ventrolateral nucleus of the cat's tractus solitarius. *Brain Res.*, 61: 23—33.

Fallert, M. und Bucher, M.V. (1966) Lokalisation eines blutdruckaktiven Substrats in der Medulla oblongata des Kaninchens. *Helv. physiol. pharmacol. Acta*, 24: 139—163.

Fallert, V.U. und Polc, P. (1970) Blutdruckreizeffekte aus dem Locus coeruleus, dem pontobulbaren Raphe-System und der medullaren Formation reticularis beim Kaninchen. *Arch. Kreisl.-Forsch.*, 62: 153—166.

Foley, J.O. and DuBois, F.S. (1934) An experimental study of the rootlets of the vagus nerve in the cat. *J. comp. Neurol.*, 60: 137—156.

Fuxe, K. (1965) Evidence for the existence of monoamine neurones in the central nervous system. IV. The distribution of monoamine terminals in the central nervous system. *Acta physiol. scand.*, 64, Suppl. 247: 38—85.

Fuxe, K., Hökfelt, T. and Nilsson, O. (1965) A fluorescence microscopical and electron microscopic study on certain brain areas rich in monoamine terminals. *Amer. J. Anat.*, 117: 33—46.

Gunn, C.G., Sevelius, G., Puiggari, M.J. and Myers, F.K. (1968) Vagal cardiomotor mechanisms in the midbrain of the dog and cat. *Amer. J. Physiol.*, 214: 258—262.

Gutman, J., Leibowitz, U. and Bergmann, F. (1962) Effect of brain stem transections on blood pressure responses to medullary stimulation. *Arch. int. Physiol.*, 70: 671—681.

32

Hellner, K. und Baumgarten, R. von (1961) Über ein Endigungsgebiet afferenter, kardiovasculärer Fasern des Nervus vagus im Rautenhirn der Katze. *Pflügers Arch. ges. Physiol.*, 273: 223—243.

Henry, J.L. and Calaresu, F.R. (1972a) Distribution of cardioacceleratory sites in intermediolateral nucleus of the cat. *Amer. J. Physiol.*, 222: 700—704.

Henry, J.L. and Calaresu, F.R. (1972b) Topography and numerical distribution of neurones of the thoraco-lumbar intermedio-lateral nucleus in the cat. *J. comp. Neurol.*, 144: 205—214.

Henry, J.L. and Calaresu, F.R. (1974a) Excitatory and inhibitory inputs from medullary nuclei projecting to spinal cardioacceleratory neurons in the cat. *Exp. Brain Res.*, 20: 485—504.

Henry, J.L. and Calaresu, F.R. (1974b) Pathways from medullary nuclei to spinal cardioacceleratory neurons in the cat. *Exp. Brain Res.*, 20: 505—514.

Henry, J.L. and Calaresu, F.R. (1974c) Origin and course of crossed medullary pathways to spinal sympathetic neurons in the cat. *Exp. Brain Res.*, 20: 515—526.

Hilton, S.M. (1963) Inhibition of baroreceptor reflexes on hypothalamic stimulation. *J. Physiol. (Lond.)*, 165: 56—57P.

Hilton, S.M. (1975) Ways of viewing the central nervous control of the circulation — old and new. *Brain Res.*, 87: 213—219.

Hilton, S.M. and Spyer, K.M. (1971) Participation of the anterior hypothalamus in the baroreceptor reflex. *J. Physiol. (Lond.)*, 218: 271—293.

Hilton, S.M. and Zbrożyna, A.W. (1963) Amygdaloid region for defence reactions and its efferent pathway to the brain stem. *J. Physiol. (Lond.)*, 165: 160—173.

Hökfelt, T., Fuxe, K., Goldstein, M. and Johansson, O. (1973) Evidence for adrenergic neurons in the rat brain. *Acta physiol. scand.*, 89: 286—288.

Homma, S., Miura, M. and Reis, D.J. (1970) Intracellular recording from paramedian reticular neurons monosynaptically excited by stimulation of the carotid sinus nerve. *Brain Res.*, 18: 185—188.

Humphrey, D.R. (1967) Neuronal activity in the medulla oblongata of cat evoked by stimulation of the carotid sinus nerve. In *Baroreceptors and Hypertension*, P. Kezdi (Ed.), Pergamon, Oxford, pp. 131—168.

Illert, M. and Gabriel, M. (1970) Mapping the cord of the spinal cat for sympathetic and blood pressure responses. *Brain Res.*, 23: 274—276.

Illert, M. and Gabriel, M. (1972) Descending pathways in the cervical cord of cats affecting blood pressure and sympathetic activity. *Pflügers Arch. ges. Physiol.*, 335: 109—124.

Illert, M. and Seller, H. (1969) A descending sympathoinhibitory tract in the ventrolateral column of the cat. *Pflügers Arch. ges. Physiol.*, 313: 343—360.

Ingram, W.R. and Dawkins, E.A. (1945) The intramedullary course of afferent fibers of the vagus nerve in the cat. *J. comp. Neurol.*, 32: 157—168.

Kell, J.F. and Hoff, E.C. (1952) Descending spinal pathways mediating pressor responses of cerebral origin. *J. Neurophysiol.*, 15: 299—311.

Kerr, F.W.L. (1962) Facial, vagal and glossopharyngeal nerves in the cat. Afferent connections. *Arch. Neurol. (Chic.)*, 6: 264—281.

Kerr, F.W.L. and Alexander, R.S. (1964) Descending autonomic pathways in the spinal cord. *Arch. Neurol. (Chic.)*, 10: 249—261.

Kumada, N. and Nakajima, H. (1972) Field potentials evoked in rabbit brainstem by stimulation of the aortic nerve. *Amer. J. Physiol.*, 233: 575—582.

Leibowitz, U., Bergmann, F. and Korczyn, D. (1963) Effect of brain stem transections on vasomotor responses to nerve stimulation. *Arch. int. Physiol.*, 71: 662—673.

Lipski, J., McAllen, R.M. and Spyer, K.M. (1972) Localization of sinus nerve afferent endings in the brain stem. *J. Physiol. (Lond.)*, 225: 30—31.

Loizou, L.A. (1969) Projections of the nucleus locus coeruleus in the albino rat. *Brain Res.*, 15: 563—566.

Magoun, H.W. (1940) Descending connections from the hypothalamus. *Ass. Res. nerv. Dis. Proc.*, 20: 20—36.

McAllen, R.M. (1976) Inhibition of the baroreceptor input to the medulla by stimulation of the hypothalamic defence area. *J. Physiol. (Lond.)*, 257: 45P.

McAllen, R.M. and Spyer, K.M. (1976) The location of cardial preganglionic motoneurones in the medulla of the cat. *J. Physiol. (Lond.)*, 258: 187—204.

Mezenich, M.M. and Brugg, J.F. (1973) Neuronal activity with cardiac periodicity in the medulla oblongata of cat. *Brain Res.*, 50: 275—296.

Miura, M. (1975) Postsynaptic potentials recorded from nucleus of the solitary tract and its subjacent reticular formation elicited by stimulation of the carotid sinus nerve. *Brain Res.*, 100: 437—440.

Miura, M. and Reis, D.J. (1968) Electrophysiological evidence the carotid sinus nerve fibres terminate in the bulbar reticular formation. *Brain Res.*, 9: 394—397.

Miura, M. and Reis, D.J. (1969) Termination and secondary projections of carotid sinus nerve in the cat brainstem. *Amer. J. Physiol.*, 217: 142—153.

Miura, M., and Reis, D.J. (1972) Role of the solitary and paramedian reticular nuclei in mediating cardiovascular reflex responses from carotid baro- and chemoreceptors. *J. Physiol. (Lond.)*, 223: 525—548.

Mizuno, N. and Nakamura, Y. (1970) Direct hypothalamic projections to the locus coeruleus. *Brain Res.*, 19: 160—162.

Morest, D.K. (1967) Experimental study of the projections of the nucleus of the tractus solitarius and the area postrema in the cat. *J. comp. Neurol.*, 130: 277—293.

Neumayr, R.J., Hare, B.D. and Franz, D.N. (1974) Evidence for bulbospinal control of sympathetic preganglionic neurons by monoaminergic pathways. *Life Sci.*, 14: 793—806.

Oberholzer, R.J.H. (1955) Lokalisation einer Schaltstelle für den Depressorreflex in der Medulla Oblongata des Kaninchens. *Helv. physiol. pharmacol. Acta*, 13: 331—353.

Palkovits, M. and Jacobowitz, D.M. (1974) Topographic atlas of catecholamine and acetylcholinesterase-containing neurons in the rat brain. II. Hindbrain (mesencephalon, rhombencephalon). *J. comp. Neurol.*, 157: 29—42.

Palkovits, M., Brownstein, M. and Saavedra, J.M. (1974) Serotonin content of the brain stem nuclei in the rat. *Brain Res.*, 80: 237—249.

Palkovits, M., Léránth, Cs., Záborszky, L. and Brownstein, M.J. (in press) Nerve terminal degenerations in the median eminence following various brain stem lesions.

Palkovits, M., De Jong, W., Zandberg, P., Versteeg, D.H.G., Van der Gugten, J. and Léránth, Cs. (in press) Central hypertension and catecholamine content of the nucleus tractus solitarii after surgical cuts in the medulla oblongata of the rat. *Brain Res.*, 127 (1977). 307—312.

Peiss, C.N. (1965) Concepts of cardiovascular regulation: past, present and future. In *Nervous Control of the Heart*, W.C. Randall (Ed.), Williams and Wilkins, Baltimore, Md., pp. 154—197.

Rhoton, A.L., O'Leary, J.L. and Ferguson, J.P. (1966) The trigeminal, facial, vagal and glossopharyngeal nerves in the monkey. *Arch. Neurol. (Chic.)*, 14: 530—540.

Russell, G.V. (1955) The nucleus locus coeruleus (dorsolateralis tegmenti). *Tex. Rep. Biol. Med.*, 13: 939—988.

Saavedra, J.M., Palkovits, M., Brownstein, M.J. and Axelrod, J. (1974) Localization of phenylethanolamine N-methyl transferase in the rat brain nuclei. *Nature (Lond.)*, 248: 695—696.

Saavedra, J.M., Grobecker, H. and Axelrod, J. (1976) Adrenaline-forming enzyme in brainstem: elevation in genetic and experimental hypertension. *Science*, 191: 483—484.

Sampson, S.R. and Biscoe, T.J. (1968) Electrical potentials evoked in the brain stem by stimulation of the sinus nerve. *Brain Res.*, 9: 398—402.

Seller, H. and Illert, M. (1969) The localization of the first synapse in the carotid sinus baroreceptor reflex pathway and its alteration of the afferent input. *Pflügers Arch. ges. Physiol.*, 306: 1—19.

Sessle, B.J. (1973) Excitatory and inhibitory inputs to single neurons in the solitary tract nucleus and adjacent reticular formation. *Brain Res.*, 53: 319—331.

Smith, O.A., Jr. (1965) Anatomy of central neural pathways mediating cardiovascular functions. In *Nervous Control of the Heart*, W.C. Randall (Ed.), Williams and Wilkins, Baltimore, Md., pp. 34—52.

Smith, R.E. and Pearce, J.W. (1961) Microelectrode recordings from the region of the nucleus solitarius in the cat. *Canad. J. Biochem.*, 39: 933—939.

Spyer, K.M. and Wolstencroft, J.H. (1971) Problems of the afferent input to the paramedian reticular nucleus, and the central connections of the sinus nerve. *Brain Res.*, 26: 411—414.

Struyker Boudier, H.A.J., Smeets, G.W.M., Brouwer, G.M. and Van Rossum, J.M. (1974) Hypothalamic alpha adrenergic receptors in cardiovascular regulation. *Neuropharmacology*, 13: 837—846.

Thomas, M.R. and Calaresu, F.R. (1972) Responses of single units in the medial hypothalamus to electrical stimulation of the carotid sinus nerve in the cat. *Brain Res.*, 44: 49—62.

Torvik, A. (1956) Afferent connections to the sensory trigeminal nuclei, the nucleus of the solitary tract and adjacent structures. An experimental study in the cat. *J. comp. Neurol.*, 106: 51—141.

Torvik, A. (1957) The spinal projection from the nucleus of the solitary tract. An experimental study in the cat. *J. Anat. (Lond.)*, 91: 314—322.

Torvik, A. and Brodal, A. (1957) The origin of reticulospinal fibres in the cat. An experimental study. *Anat. Rec.*, 128: 113—137.

Van der Gugten, J., Palkovits, M., Wijnen, H.L.J.M and Versteeg, D.H.G. (1976) Regional distribution of adrenaline in rat brain. *Brain Res.*, 107: 171—175.

Versteeg, D.H.G., Palkovits, M., Van der Gugten, J., Wijnen, H.L.J.M., Smeets, G.W.M. and De Jong, W. (1976a) Catecholamine content of individual brain regions of spontaneously hypertensive rats (SH-rats). *Brain Res.*, 112: 429—434.

Versteeg, D.H.G., Van der Gugten, J., De Jong, W. and Palkovits, M. (1976b) Regional concentrations of noradrenaline and dopamine in rat brain. *Brain Res.*, 113: 563—574.

Wang, S.C. and Chai, C.Y. (1962) Central control of sympathetic cardio-acceleration in the medulla oblongata of the cat. *Amer. J. Physiol.*, 202: 31—34.

Wang, S.C. and Ranson, S.W. (1939) Descending pathways from the hypothalamus to the medulla and spinal cord. Observations on blood pressure and bladder responses. *J. comp. Neurol.*, 71: 457—472.

Wang, S.C. and Ranson, S.N. (1941) The role of the hypothalamus and preoptic region in the regulation of heart rate. *Amer. J. Physiol.*, 132: 5—8.

Ward, D.G. and Gunn, C.G. (1976a) Locus coeruleus complex: elicitation of a pressor response and a brain stem region necessary for its occurrence. *Brain Res.*, 107: 401—406.

Ward, D.G. and Gunn, C.G. (1976b) Locus coeruleus complex: differential modulation of depressor mechanisms. *Brain Res.*, 107: 407—411.

Ward, D.G., Baertschi, A.J. and Gunn, D.S. (1975) Activation of solitary nucleus neurons from the locus coeruleus and vicinity. *Neurosci. Abstr.*, 1: 424.

Záborszky, L., Mészáros, T. and Léránth, Cs. (in preparation) Afferent fiber connections and intranuclear structure of the nucleus alae cinereae lateralis of the cat.

Zivin, J.A., Reid, J.L., Saavedra, J.M. and Kopin, I.J. (1975) Quantitative localization of biogenic amines in the spinal cord. *Brain Res.*, 99: 293—301.

Baroreceptors in Normotension

PAUL KEZDI

Cox Heart Institute, Dayton, Ohio 45429 (U.S.A.)

INTRODUCTION

Reflex regulation of cardiovascular functions is extremely complicated as we have learned by the enormous quantity of research generated since the discovery of the depressor nerves (Cyon and Ludwig, 1866), the carotid sinus nerves (Hering, 1927), the cardiac receptors (Jarisch and Richter, 1939), and the vasomotor center (Owsjannikow, 1871; Dittmar, 1873). The reflex arc is composed of (1) the receptors located in strategic areas of the cardiovascular system responding to strain as the result of deformation; (2) the afferent nerves: carotid sinus (IX), aortic depressor (X) and cardiac vagal afferents; (3) central synapses passing mainly through the tractus and nucleus solitarius; (4) medullary vasomotor neurons; (5) efferent nerves to effector organs such as the heart, blood vessels, and viscera; and (6) the adrenergic and cholinergic end-plates producing the appropriate neurotransmitter to complete the reflex effect on the end-organs.

When considering baroreceptor reflex mechanisms, the condition and function of the following segments of the reflex arc are usually analyzed: (1) the vascular wall or cardiac structures respectively where the receptors are located; (2) the receptors themselves; (3) the afferent pathways; (4) the central synapses and interactions with higher centers; (5) the distribution of baroreceptor afferents to the medullary vasomotor neurons; (6) the distribution of efferent pathways and reflex effects from vasomotor neurons to end-organs; (7) the neurotransmitter system; (8) the state of the smooth muscles in the vascular walls or viscera and the heart muscle or pacemaker (sinus node), respectively.

Recent years of research have shown that baroreceptor reflexes mediated through the autonomic nervous system do not operate uniformly and indiscriminately. Their action on effector pathways is qualitatively similar but varies quantitatively, resulting in differing reflex responses in the cardiovascular target organs.

It would be impossible to list in this brief review all the research findings to date on the baroreceptor control of normal circulation, let alone research in abnormal cardiovascular states. Much is being presented on this subject in subsequent papers. I would like to restrict my remarks to certain aspects of the baroreceptor reflex control which we have investigated.

VASCULAR WALL AND RECEPTORS

In the vascular walls, receptors of the baroreceptor system are located in the adventitia and between the adventitia and the media between elastic fibers and connective tissue paralleling smooth muscles. The strategically located baroreceptor areas are somewhat modified arterial structures with a high elastic fiber content. The receptors are similar to the Pacinian corpuscles of other types of mechanoreceptors. Two factors may influence their response to deformation of the arterial wall, namely (1) the condition of the arterial wall, its stiffness and the radius of its lumen; and (2) the ionic balance of the receptors. Many investigators have studied these factors (Peterson et al., 1960; Peterson, 1961, 1964; Jones et al., 1964; Aars, 1968a,b, 1969, 1971; Bagshaw and Peterson, 1972; Koushanpour and Kelso, 1972; Kezdi et al., 1973) and I would like to present some of our findings.

We have studied the stress-strain characteristics of excised 1 mm wide rings of the carotid sinus from dogs (Fig. 1). The rings were stretched by increasing loads in steps of 2 g and the resulting increase in diameter was measured. Photomicrographs with 10 times magnification of the freely floating rings were used to measure the unstretched vessel thickness and the exact diameter of the ring. Assuming an isotropic strain with Poisson's ratio of 0.5, the applied force in grams was converted to equivalent mm Hg using Laplace's formula.

$$P = \frac{T \cdot \delta}{r} = \frac{\left(\dfrac{\frac{1}{2}F_a}{w \cdot \delta}\right)\delta}{L_a/\pi} = \frac{\pi}{2} \cdot \frac{F_a}{w \cdot L_a}$$

In the equation, F_a is the force applied and L_a is the resulting length of the vessel ring; δ is the radial thickness of the ring and w the width of the ring in the longitudinal direction.

Prior to excision of the ring some nerve fiber activity of the carotid sinus was recorded in the same isolated sinus with increasing pressures. The actual nerve activity in microvolts was plotted as a function of the intracarotid pressure. To obtain the pressure-circumference data for the same set of pressures, a linear interpolation of the calculated pressure and circumference changes to a given load was computed (Fig. 2).

As in hypertensive states, stretching of the elastic, connective and smooth muscle tissue results in hypertrophy of the arterial wall. Concomitant changes

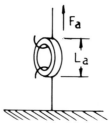

Fig. 1. Schematic drawing of a force (F_a) in grams applied to a carotid sinus vascular ring.

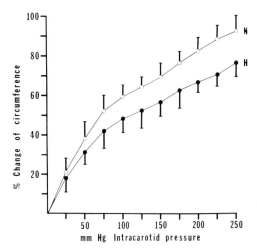

Fig. 2. Circumference changes of carotid sinus vascular rings plotted as funtion of equivalent pressure from 9 normotensive and 6 hypertensive dogs. (From P. Kezdi et al., 1973.)

in ionic and water composition further alter the stress-strain characteristics of the wall. This leads to a shift of the nerve activity curve to the right. Jones et al. (1964) and Tobian and Redleaf (1958) found increased sodium and water in the walls of hypertensive common carotid arteries. We have shown a similar increase in the sodium content in carotid sinus arterial walls without, however, the simultaneous increase in water content (Table I). This may be due to a difference in the compositions of the common carotid artery and the carotid sinus, the latter being much less muscular. This suggests that the sodium increase was partially at least intracellular both in the carotid sinus and probably the receptors. Sodium increase could modify (decrease) receptor sensitivity and contribute to resetting.

In addition, the calculated elasticity modulus (E') is increased in hypertension indicating increased stiffness (Table II). Receptor response is decreased to a given intrasinus pressure as demonstrated by McCubbin and co-workers (1956), Kezdi (1967), Aars (1968b), Angell-James (1973) and others. The modified stress-strain characteristics are probably due to initial changes in the

TABLE I

WATER, SODIUM AND POTASSIUM CONTENT OF EXCISED CAROTID SINUS ARTERIAL WALLS FROM NORMOTENSIVE AND RENAL HYPERTENSIVE DOGS

Type of carotid sinus	No. of car. sin. analyzed	Water (%)	Sodium in mEquiv./g tissue	Potassium mEquiv./ 100 g
Normotensive	13	67.6 ± 5.7**	39.7 ± 2.2	9.3 ± 1.6
Hypertensive	18	62.0 ± 7.5	43.5 ± 2.7*	6.6 ± 3.3*

*Difference significant at $P < 0.05$ level.
**Mean ± S.D.

TABLE II

DYNAMIC ELASTIC MODULUS (Ep) OF CAROTID SINUS RINGS CALCULATED FROM
IN VITRO MEASUREMENTS OF PRESSURE/CIRCUMFERENCE IN NORMOTENSIVE
AND HYPERTENSIVE DOGS

$$Ep = \Delta P/\Delta \epsilon, \Delta P = \text{pulse pressure}$$
$$\Delta \epsilon = \Delta D/\overline{D} = \Delta C/\overline{C}, \Delta \epsilon = \text{incremental change in strain}$$
$$\Delta D = \text{incremental change in diameter}$$
$$\overline{D} = \text{mean diameter}$$
$$\Delta C = \text{incremental change in circumference}$$
$$\overline{C} = \text{mean circumference}$$

	Normotensive	Hypertensive
Ep (g/sq. cm) for 125 mm Hg mean pressure	899	902
Ep (g/sq. cm) for 175 mm Hg mean pressure	1,421	1,559

ionic composition of the receptors (increased Na^+) upon which the effect of increased stiffness is later superimposed.

A decreased response in the baroreceptors was also found in congestive heart failure. Increased stiffness of the vascular wall has not been found in non-hypertensive congestive heart failure. Some ionic changes in the receptors with the intracellular shift of sodium could in part be responsible for both decreased baroreceptor sensitivity and catecholamine depletion of the heart as shown by Higgins et al. (1972).

RESPONSE OF BARORECEPTORS IN DIFFERENT LOCATIONS OF THE CARDIOVASCULAR SYSTEM

The principal stimulus of baroreceptors located in different areas of the vascular system is always the degree of strain resulting from deformation due to intravascular pressure changes. However, there are differences in the level of intravascular pressure at which threshold activity and saturation of baro-receptor nerve activity occur (Table III). Differences in the threshold of carotid

TABLE III

THRESHOLD PRESSURE IN ISOLATED CAROTID SINUS AND AORTIC ARCH
AT WHICH CAROTID SINUS AND AORTIC NERVE ACTIVITY CAN FIRST BE
DETECTED IN NORMOTENSIVE AND RENAL HYPERTENSIVE DOGS

Ramp pressure increase; multifiber nerve preparation.

Location of pressure increase and nerve recording	No. of recordings	Normotensive mm Hg mean threshold pr.	No. of recordings	Hypertensive mm Hg mean threshold pr.
Carotid sinus	8	73 ± 15*	6	125 ± 12*
Aortic arch	21	91 ± 13*	12	147 ± 22*

*Difference significant at $P < 0.05$ level.
**Mean ± S.D. (Kordenat, 1967).

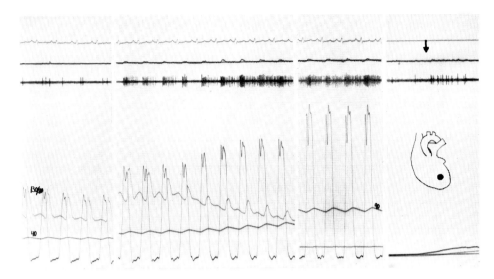

Fig. 3. Vagal afferent nerve activity before (left panel) and after (two center panels) balloon occlusion of the ascending aorta with simultaneous left ventricular and femoral artery pressure recordings. Note sparse activity on the right, increased systolic synchronous activity in left center and continuous activity right of center. Receptor location identified by pressing (arrow) with hemostat the area shown on the right.

sinus and aortic depressor nerve activity have also been observed by others (Pelletier et al., 1972). Separation of the nerve activity curves by increasing and decreasing pressures has also been shown, thus indicating hysteresis of the arterial wall. Different thresholds for carotid sinus and aortic receptors, resulting in varying degrees of strain for a given pressure, are probably due to differences in the structure of arterial walls.

In the case of ventricular mechanoreceptors the stimulus is exerted by distension of the ventricle. While these receptors are often quiescent during normal resting pressure they become activated with increasing ventricular pressure (Fig. 3). First there is synchronous activity with systole and then later, as diastolic pressure increases, a continuous activity is present. A saturation of activity is related to the increased level of diastolic pressure as well as a rise in left ventricular mean pressure. The ventricular mechanoreceptors thus have an even higher threshold than both the carotid sinus and aortic baroreceptors and probably function normally as safeguard reflexes to prevent overloading or excessive distension of the ventricles.

EFFECTOR ORGAN RESPONSE

It has been shown that the effector responses to loading or unloading different baroreceptors vary considerably. For instance, the skeletal muscular vascular system, the renal vascular system, the splanchnic and the skin vascular system as well as heart rate show quantitatively different responses to stimulation or withdrawal of various baroreceptors. The differences appear to be due to the number of different contacts of various baroreceptors with vasomotor neuron pools rather than to qualitative differences in receptor response (Little et al., 1975; Pelletier and Shepherd, 1975a).

In the studies of Little et al. (1975), reflex responses to stimulation of ventricular receptors conducted in cardiac nerve afferents were compared to stimulation of carotid sinus baroreceptors in different vascular beds. The low frequency stimulation of the cardiac afferents produced pronounced responses in the renal vascular system and only submaximal responses in the skeletal muscular system. In contrast, high pressure stimulation of the isolated carotid sinus induced maximum reflex responses in both the renal system and the skeletal muscular system. High frequency stimulation of the cardiac afferents elicited maximal reflex renal vessel responses but had only a submaximal effect on muscle vessels and heart rate. Cardiac nerve afferents have therefore a less dense contact with vasomotor neuron pools innervating the skeletal muscular system, and a more dense contact with neuron pools innervating the renal vascular system.

It was also shown that there is an interaction between the chemoreceptor and baroreceptor reflexes. Pelletier and Shepherd (1975b) have studied muscle, skin and renal vascular responses to bilateral carotid occlusion during control conditions and during stimulation of the chemoreceptors by reducing oxygen tension in the blood. They found that hypoxia caused a marked potentiation of renal sympathetic nerve activity and renal vasoconstrictor responses to carotid occlusion. Constriction of the skeletal muscle blood vessels increased only slightly in response to carotid occlusion during hypoxia. They conclude that the level of intrinsic activity in the vasomotor neurons innervating the renal circulation is normally low. Stimulation of chemoreceptors, however, causes intrinsic activity to increase following the release of neurons from the carotid sinus baroreceptor restrain. Therefore the increase in sympathetic outflow to the kidney is much larger during hypoxia than in the absence of chemoreceptor stimulation. On the other hand, Pelletier and Shepherd (1975b) also state that the neurons controlling resistance vessels in the skeletal muscular system appear to discharge at the maximal physiological rate when they are released from the inhibitory effect of carotid sinus baroreceptors, however, little further increase in activity occurs with hypoxia.

In contrast, tonic activity of the medullary vasomotor neurons is inherently low for those neurons controlling a vascular system of glands such as the kidney. The high activity vasomotor neurons on the other hand control vascular beds involving cardiovascular homeostasis. Reflex mechanisms maintaining blood pressure control therefore do not markedly interfere with renal circulation or arteriovenous anastomosis of the skin. These vascular beds are involved in other homeostatic mechanisms such as regulation of salt and water balance and body temperature rather than in control of blood pressure. Only in emergency situations when other superimposed stimulations of the vasomotor neurons occur, such as from the chemoreceptors, will the renal vascular system contribute to the maintenance of the circulation of other vital organs by increasing its resistance. These interactions between baroreceptors and chemoreceptors play an important role in the overall regulation of the cardiovascular system (Wennergren et al., 1976).

SUMMARY

Reflex regulation of the cardiovascular system by baroreceptors involves multiple components of the reflex arc. The state of the vascular wall and/or the heart muscle where the receptors are located is an important determining factor of receptor response. The ionic balance (Na^+ content) of the receptors themselves is also a possible factor.

The differences in effector organ response to loading or unloading of different baroreceptors indicate that the distribution and contact of systemic and cardiac baroreceptors between different vasomotor neuron pools are not uniform. Interaction between baro- and chemoreceptors in potentiating the effect of baroreceptor withdrawal is more pronounced in the case of certain effector organs (for instance the kidney) than in others. Regulation of the cardiovascular system by baroreceptors is highly differentiated by their contact and interaction with vasomotor neuron pools.

ACKNOWLEDGEMENT

The work reported here has been supported by Grant Nr. HL 15004 of the National Institute of Health, U.S. Public Health Service.

REFERENCES

Aars, H. (1968a) Aortic baroreceptor activity in normal and hypertensive rabbits. *Acta physiol. scand.*, 72: 298—309.

Aars, H. (1968b) Aortic baroreceptor activity during permanent distension of the receptor area. *Acta physiol. scand.*, 74: 183—194.

Aars, H. (1969) Relationship between aortic diameter and aortic baroreceptor activity in normal and hypertensive rabbits. *Acta physiol. scand.*, 75: 406—414.

Aars, H. (1971) Effects of altered smooth muscle tone on aortic diameter and aortic baroreceptor activity in anesthetized rabbits. *Circulat. Res.*, 28: 254—262.

Angell-James, J.E. (1973) Characteristics of single aortic and right subclavian baroreceptor fiber activity in rabbits with chronic renal hypertension. *Circulat. Res.*, 32: 149—161.

Bagshaw, R.J. and Peterson, L.H. (1972) Sympathetic control of the mechanical properties of the canine carotid sinus. *Amer. J. Physiol.*, 222: 1462—1468.

Cyon, E. und Ludwig, C. (1866) Die Reflexe eines der sensiblen Nerven des Herzens auf die motorischen der Blutgefasse. *Verh. Kgl. ges. Wiss. (Lpz.)*, 18: 307—328.

Dittmar, C. (1873) Ueber die Lage des sogenannten Gefasscentrums in der Medulla oblongata. *Verh. Kgl. ges. Wiss. (Lpz.)*, 25: 449—469.

Hering, H.E. (1927) *Die Karotissinusreflexe auf Herz and Gefasse*, Theodor Steinkopff, Dresden und Leipzig.

Higgins, C.B., Vatner, S.F., Eckberg, D.L. and Braunwald, E. (1972) *J. clin. Invest.*, 51: 715—724.

Jarisch, A. und Richter, H. (1939) Die afferenten Bahnen des Veratrin-effektes in den Herznerven. *Naunyn-Schmiedeberg's Arch. exp. Path. Pharmak.*, 193: 355—371.

Jones, A.W., Feigl, E.O. and Peterson, L.H. (1964) Water and electrolyte content of normal and hypertensive arteries in dogs. *Circulat. Res.*, 15: 386—392.

Kezdi, P. (1967) Resetting of the carotid sinus in experimental renal hypertension. In *Baroreceptors and Hypertension*, P. Kezdi (Ed.), Pergamon Press, Oxford, pp. 301—308.

Kezdi, P., Spickler, J.W. and Kordenat, R.K. (1973) Neurogenic factors in renal hypertension. In *Hypertension: Mechanisms and Management*, G. Onesti, K.E. Kim and J.H. Moyer (Eds.), Grune and Stratton, New York, pp. 681—692.

Kordenat, R.K. (1967) Aortic nerve activity in normal and renal hypertensive dogs. In fulfillment of requirements of Master of Science, University of Cincinnati.

Koushanpour, E. and Kelso, D.M. (1972) Partition of the carotid sinus baroreceptor response in dogs between the mechanical properties of the wall and the receptor elements. *Circulat. Res.*, 31: 831—845.

Little, R., Wennergren, G. and Oberg, B. (1975) Aspects of the central integration of arterial baroreceptor and cardiac ventricular receptor reflexes in the cat. *Acta physiol. scand.*, 93: 85—96.

McCubbin, J.W. (1967) Interrelationship between the sympathetic nervous system and the renin-angiotensin system. In *Baroreceptors and Hypertension*, P. Kezdi (Ed.), Pergamon Press, Oxford, pp. 323—327.

Owsjannikow, Ph. (1871) Die tonischen und reflectorischen Centren der Gefassnerven. *Verh. Kgl. ges. Wiss. (Lpz.)*, 23: 135—147.

Pelletier, C.L. and Shepherd, J.T. (1975a) Relative influence of carotid baroreceptors and muscle receptors in the control of renal and hind limb circulations. *Canad. J. Physiol. Pharmacol.*, 53: 1042—1049.

Pelletier, C.L. and Shepherd, J.T. (1975b) Effect of hypoxia on vascular responses to the carotid baroreflex. *Amer. J. Physiol.*, 22: 331—336.

Pelletier, C.L., Clement, D.L. and Shepherd, J.T. (1972) Comparison of afferent activity of canine aortic and sinus nerves. *Circulat. Res.*, 31: 557—568.

Peterson, L.H. (1961) The mechanical properties of the blood vessels and hypertension. In *Proc. World Health Organization: Symp. on Pathogenesis of Essential Hypertension*, State Med. Publ. House, Prague, pp. 295—313.

Peterson, L.H. (1964) Vessel wall stress-strain relationship. In *Pulsatile Blood Flow*, E.O. Attinger (Ed.), McGraw-Hill, New York, pp. 263—274.

Peterson, L.H., Jensen, R.E. and Parnell, J. (1960) Mechanical properties of arteries in vivo. *Circulat. Res.*, 8: 622—639.

Tobian, L. and Redleaf, P.D. (1958) Ionic composition of the aorta in renal and adrenal hypertension. *Amer. J. Physiol.*, 192: 325—330.

Wennergren, G., Little, R. and Oberg, B. (1976) Studies on the central integration of excitatory chemoreceptor influences and inhibitory baroreceptor and cardiac receptor influences. *Acta physiol. scand.*, 96: 1—18.

Baroreceptors and Hypertension

T.G. PICKERING and P. SLEIGHT

Department of Cardiovascular Medicine,
Radcliffe Infirmary, Oxford (Great Britain)

INTRODUCTION

Ever since the discovery of the aortic depressor nerves by Cyon and Ludwig in 1866, there has been speculation as to the role of the baroreceptors in hypertension. Since the pressure is elevated both in the systemic arteries and in the left ventricle during systole, there must be some alteration of the functioning of the baroreceptors in these regions to permit the development of hypertension; pressures in the venous system, pulmonary circulation and atria are usually normal in hypertension, and there is as yet no particular reason to suppose that cardiovascular reflexes from these lower pressure areas are functioning any differently from normal.

In principle, hypertension could produce secondary changes in the baroreceptors or some other part of the baroreflex arc, or the hypertension might itself be caused by abnormalities in baroreflex control. Since essential hypertension in man is probably caused by more than one factor, it is necessary to consider all these possibilities and how the baroreflexes could interact with other factors likely to be important in the genesis of hypertension.

CHANGES IN THE BAROREFLEX IN EXPERIMENTAL HYPERTENSION

The normal stimulus to the baroreceptors is distortion: the pulsatility of the pressure wave distending the sinus is reflected both in the changes of diameter of the carotid sinus and in the electroneurogram in the sinus nerve (Fig. 1). The curve relating impulse frequency to distending pressure is virtually linear, but flattens out as impulse frequency reaches a maximum; this limitation in impulse frequency could be either due to failure of the arterial wall to distend further at high pressures, or to saturation of the receptor endings. Koushnapour and Kelso (1972) found that the pressure—strain (distortion) relation was linear up to a pressure of 250 mm Hg in the carotid sinus of dogs, whereas the maximum impulse frequency was reached at less than 200 mm Hg; they concluded that saturation of the receptor endings was responsible for the limitation of impulse frequency. In these experiments dimension changes were measured by photography of markings on the sinus wall; the recording of nerve

44

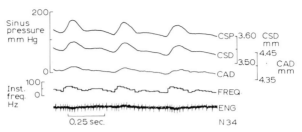

Fig. 1. Simultaneous recordings of carotid sinus pressure (CSP), carotid sinus diameter (CSD), carotid artery diameter (CAD), and impulse frequency (FREQ.) in carotid sinus nerve. ENG = electroneurogram. Note that profile of impulse frequency parallels changes of pressure and diameter, and greater pulsatility of CS compared with CA (Bergel et al., 1976; unpublished figure).

activity and dimension was not simultaneous. We have recently recorded carotid sinus dimensions using an ultrasound micrometer (Bertram, 1974) simultaneously with nerve activity, and our results (Fig. 2) show that the firing is limited by the distensibility of the sinus rather than by the receptors themselves (Bergel et al., 1975, 1976). The mechanical properties of the sinus region are such that sudden changes of pressure produce a more rapid change of diameter in the sinus region than in the less distensible carotid artery (Fig. 3).

These findings are likely to be of relevance in hypertension. It has been known since the work of McCubbin et al. in 1956 that the impulse frequency in the sinus nerve of dogs with renal hypertension is relatively normal, despite the higher distending pressures. Subsequent workers confirmed this also for the rat (Krieger and Marseillan, 1966), the rabbit (Aars, 1968a) and the dog (Sleight et al., 1975). This is not surprising, as it is well known that the

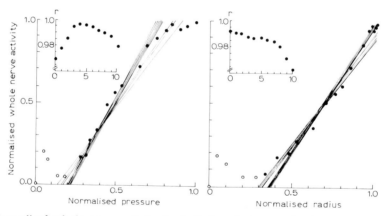

Fig. 2. Normalised whole nerve activity is plotted against normalised carotid sinus pressure (A) and normalised sinus dimension change (B). Low pressure points are ignored (open circles). The lines represent successive linear regressions, initially on all remaining points (closed circles); subsequent regressions were done by progressively removing one point at a time from the top of the curve. Inset figures show for either case the correlation coefficients (ordinate) against the number of points removed (abscissa). Note that in A the highest correlation occurs when 4 points are removed, whereas in B the relation is linear over the whole range. (Reproduced with permission from Bergel et al., 1976.)

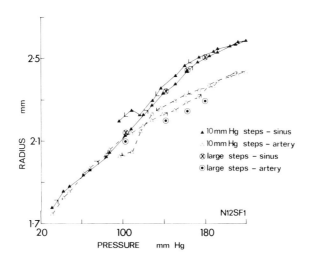

Fig. 3. Pressure—radius relation for dog's carotid sinus (solid symbols) and carotid artery (open symbols). Sinus shows greater distensibility. For large increments of pressure sinus immediately reaches steady-state radius, whereas artery does not. Radius measured 60 sec after pressure increment (Bergel et al., 1976; unpublished figure).

baroreceptors show adaptation, in common with other mechanoreceptors (Landgren, 1952). What is not yet clear is whether this is due to changes in the mechanical properties of the arterial wall, or to changes in the receptors themselves. The curve relating impulse frequency and pressure is not only reset to the higher level of pressure, so that the threshold pressure is increased, but the sensitivity of the baroreceptors to changes of pressure is also less (Aars, 1968a; Angell James, 1973; Sleight et al., 1975), and the maximum firing frequency is also lower (Sleight et al., 1975). These changes are illustrated in Fig. 4. Such changes appear to be a direct effect of the higher distending pressure rather than to any effect of circulating hormones or sympathetic innervation of the receptors, because if one sinus is protected from the raised pressure by being anastomosed to the jugular vein, it does not show any resetting (Kezdi et al., 1972). Such resetting takes place within hours (Krieger, 1970) or days (Aars, 1968a; Liard et al., 1974) of the increase of pressure, and for relatively short elevations is reversible if the arterial pressure is restored to normal (Salgado and Krieger, 1973; Sleight et al., 1975). It took longer than 4 days to occur in the dog's carotid sinus and appeared to be related both to the level of pressure and the duration of hypertension (Sleight, Robinson and Brooks, unpublished).

There is no doubt that the dynamic properties of the arterial wall are altered in hypertension. These changes may be due to changes in water and electrolyte distribution (Tobian et al., 1969), and to deposition of increased amounts of elastin and collagen in the media (Wolinsky, 1970). Kezdi et al. (1972) found that there was an increased sodium concentration in the sinus exposed to a raised arterial pressure, but not in the protected sinus. The hypertensive sinus was in fact more distensible than normal in his experiments. Conversely, Aars (1968b) and Angell James (1973) both found that the aorta from hypertensive

46

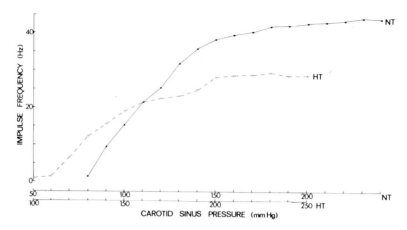

Fig. 4. Curves relating impulse frequency to carotid sinus pressure in a normotensive (NT) and hypertensive (HT) dog. Axes of pressure have been shifted so that unanaesthetized resting mean arterial pressures were the same (100 mm Hg for NT, 150 for HT). Note (a) higher threshold for HT, (b) reduced receptor sensitivity, (c) same impulse frequency at animal's normal pressure, (d) reduced maximal impulse frequency for HT.

rabbits was stiffer than normal, and that this could account for the resetting of the baroreceptors (Aars, 1969).

The fact that resetting of the receptors occurs, and is reversible, has two important implications. First, it implies that the arterial baroreceptors will only effectively oppose a sustained change of pressure in either direction for a matter of hours or days. Secondly, it implies that the resetting is initially unlikely to be primarily due to damage of the receptor endings, which has been reported to occur in hypertension by some workers (Hilgenberg, 1958; Abraham, 1969), but not others (Rees et al., 1976). These conflicting results may be due to differences in the duration of hypertension.

Most of these experiments have been done on animals with renal hypertension; spontaneous hypertension in rats is also associated with a resetting of the baroreceptors (Nosaka and Wang, 1972). Angell James (1974a, b) has also examined rabbits' aortic baroreceptor activity in situations where there are more pronounced structural changes in the aortic wall. Thus experimentally induced vitamin D sclerosis in rabbits impaired both baroreceptor sensitivity and aortic arch distensibility (Angell James, 1974a). A high cholesterol diet resulted in mild hypertension, an impairment of baroreceptor sensitivity, and a reduction of aortic distensibility; there was also evidence of degeneration of receptor endings (Angell James, 1974b).

There is also some evidence to suggest that there are changes in the central connections of the baroreflex in experimental hypertension. Thus Griffith and Schwartz (1964) found that prolonged stimulation of the carotid sinus nerve produced only a transient reduction of pressure in normal dogs, but a prolonged fall in dogs with renal hypertension. Finally, it must not be forgotten that the effector response to a given change in sympathetic nerve stimulation is likely to be quantitatively different in hypertension (Folkow, 1971).

CHANGES IN THE BAROREFLEX IN HUMAN HYPERTENSION

Evidence from human studies generally supports the findings in experimental animals. Kezdi (1953) showed that local anaesthesia of the carotid sinus region in hypertensive patients produced a further elevation of pressure, indicating that the reflex was still tonically active. Efferent sympathetic activity is qualitatively normal in hypertension, but is inhibited at higher pressures than normal (Wallin et al., 1973; Fig. 5). Since baroreceptor stimulation is a potent inhibitor of efferent sympathetic activity, this finding is compatible with the resetting of the receptors found in animals.

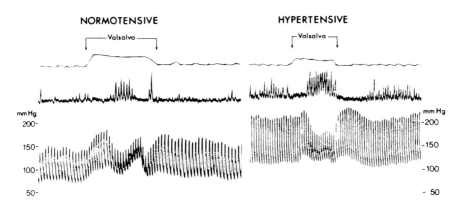

Fig. 5. Effects of Valsalva's manoeuvre on muscle nerve sympathetic activity in a normotensive and a hypertensive subject. Top trace: respiratory movements. Middle: integrated muscle nerve sympathetic activity recorded from peroneal nerve. Bottom: blood pressure. (Reproduced with permission from Wallin et al., 1973.)

A quantitative estimation of the sensitivity of the cardiac limb of the baroreflex arc can be obtained by relating the reflex bradycardia to the rise of arterial pressure produced by an intravenous bolus of phenylephrine (Smyth et al., 1969). Patients with hypertension show both a resetting and a diminished reflex sensitivity (Bristow et al., 1969). Increasing age results in a loss of reflex sensitivity independently of the effect of pressure (Gribbin et al., 1971; Fig. 6). Borderline hypertension is also associated with a loss of reflex sensitivity (Takeshita et al., 1975; Fig. 7). Patients with renal hypertension on haemodialysis show an even greater impairment of reflex sensitivity than those with essential hypertension with similar pressures and ages (Pickering et al., 1972). This would favour the view that this loss of reflex sensitivity is a consequence rather than a cause of the hypertension; patients with end-stage renal disease are particularly prone to vascular disease which, as we have seen above, may impair baroreceptor function. The loss of reflex sensitivity in human hypertension is not necessarily reversible, for when the pressures of patients on haemodialysis are restored to normal (e.g. by nephrectomy), there is no improvement in reflex sensitivity, at any rate over a one year period (Pickering et al. 1972; Fig. 8). The studies of Heath et al. (1973) suggest that

48

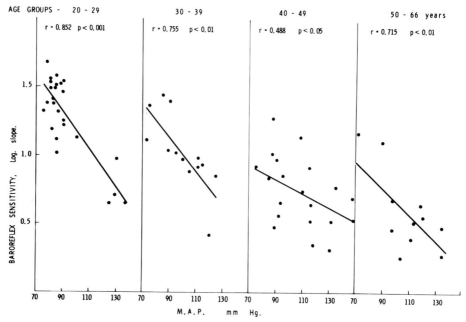

Fig. 6. Correlation of baroreflex sensitivity and resting mean arterial pressure (MAP) in a group of 81 untreated subjects with different ages and pressures. Subjects are grouped according to age, and the solid lines are the regression lines of MAP on log of reflex sensitivity. (Reproduced with permission from Gribbin et al., 1971.)

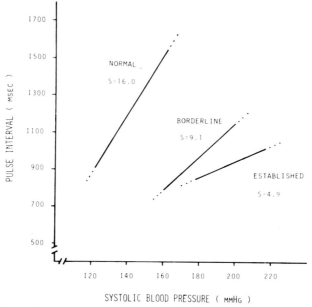

Fig. 7. Comparison of the mean slopes of linear regression relating baroreceptor sensitivity developed by an elevation of arterial pressure with phenylephrine in normal subjects, patients with borderline hypertension, and those with established hypertension. S indicates the mean slope of linear regression. The baroreceptor slope in patients with borderline hypertension is reduced as compared to that in normal subjects ($P < 0.01$), but greater than that in patients with established hypertension ($P < 0.01$). (Reproduced with permission from Takeshita et al., 1975.)

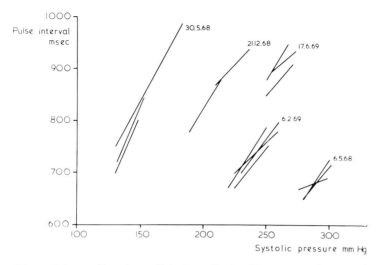

Fig. 8. Resetting of baroreflex in a dialysis patient without any change of sensitivity. Results are from one subject tested on 5 different occasions (dates given by lines). Each line represents one injection of phenylephrine. Reflex sensitivity is represented by slope of lines. Between 6.5.68 and 30.5.68 this patient had a bilateral nephrectomy. (Reproduced with permission from Pickering et al., 1972.)

this could be due to fixed changes of intimal fibrosis and atheroma of the sinus wall.

NEUROGENIC HYPERTENSION

Many early studies claimed to have demonstrated sustained hypertension in animals subjected to sinoaortic denervation (Heymans and Neil, 1958). The hallmark of such hypertension is its variability. External stimuli produce a large rise of pressure, but when the animal is at rest or asleep the pressure may be normal or low. The hypertension is largely due to an increased sympathetic tone, for there is an increased turnover of catecholamines (De Quattro et al., 1969) and sympathectomy can abolish it (Grimson, 1941). The existence of neurogenic hypertension as a significant entity has recently been discounted by Cowley et al. (1973), who measured blood pressure continuously in dogs with sinoaortic denervation. The chief effect of the denervation was a greatly increased variability of pressure, with a relatively small (11 mm Hg) rise in the average level. They suggested that the earlier results showing bigger changes were largely spurious, on the grounds that the psychic stimuli associated with the measurement procedures had themselves produced a temporary elevation of pressure. This dismissal of neurogenic hypertension can be criticised on several grounds: first, in other species (e.g. cats), pressures after deafferentation are higher both during wakefulness and sleep, although significantly lower during REM sleep (Zanchetti et al., 1967). Doba and Reis (1973) produced fatal pulmonary oedema and hypertension in rats following electrolytic lesions of the tractus solitarius. Ferrario et al. (1969) also recorded arterial pressure directly from dogs with sinoaortic deafferentation while the animals were "fully relaxed and resting", and found an average rise of pressure of 31 mm Hg following denervation. Surprisingly, the pressure rose during slow-wave sleep in these animals. Sleight et al. (1976) have shown that the sinus nerve activity of dogs with renal hypertension at the dogs' own arterial pressure is the same as in normal animals at their own pressures. This could suggest equally well that the baroreceptors had completely reset passively, or that the level of pressure in experimental renal hypertension is determined by the neural activity in these reset baroreceptors.

The influence of psychic stimuli should probably not be discounted, for there is suggestive evidence that they may be important in the genesis of hypertension (reviewed by Gutmann and Benson, 1971; Henry and Cassel, 1969). The very high pressures that may occur transiently in these animals might be sufficient to produce arterial damage, e.g. in the kidney and baroreceptor areas, which could further exacerbate hypertension.

Denervation of the baroreceptors has been found by some workers to augment renal hypertension (Kezdi, 1960; Lawrence and Dickinson, 1964), although others (Cowley and Guyton, 1975) have found that the eventual level of pressure in renal hypertension is unaffected by sinoaortic denervation, the principle effect of which was to accelerate the rise of pressure. These discrepancies could be due to the differences in the methods of inducing the renal hypertension.

RELEVANCE OF NEUROGENIC HYPERTENSION TO HUMAN HYPERTENSION

Hering (1927) was one of the first to suggest that impairment of the baroreflex could lead to hypertension in man. The carotid sinus region is a favoured site for atheromatous deposits, which could interfere with the distensibility of the arterial wall and hence of baroreceptor function, as found experimentally by Angell James (1974b). Denervation of the carotid sinus has occasionally been tried in man as a treatment for epilepsy or asthma. Capps and De Takats (1938) reported moderate hypertension for a week following this procedure in two patients, and Sleight et al. (unpublished) noted a progressive rise of pressure in a patient who had had bilateral carotid body removal, and who showed no reflex cardiac slowing in response to a rise of arterial pressure (Fig. 9). The absence of any permanent rise of pressure following this operation does not disprove the possibility that hypertension can be induced in this way, since the aortic baroreceptors will still be functioning. The same may apply to the observation of Lowe (1961), who found that patients with bilateral common carotid occlusion do not have particularly high blood pressures.

The converse situation to neurogenic hypertension is the treatment of hypertension by prolonged electrical stimulation of the carotid sinus nerve by "baropacing" (Fig. 10), which may produce a sustained reduction of blood pressure in some patients (Dunning, 1971). A possible pharmacological analogy to this is the finding that clonidine may exert some of its antihypertensive

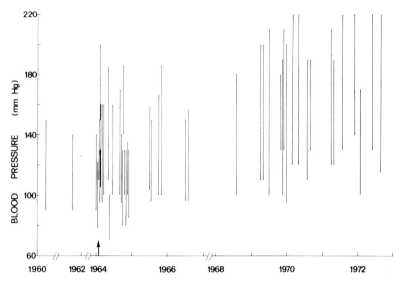

Fig. 9. Hypertension following bilateral carotid denervation (marked by arrow) in one patient. Pressure appears more labile following denervation, with a progressive rise subsequently.

action by a central sensitisation of the baroreflex. This has been demonstrated in animals by Korner et al. (1975) (Fig. 11), and also in man using the phenylephrine method (Sleight and West, 1975).

If baroreceptor dysfunction were a cause of essential hypertension in man, we might expect that the early stages of essential hypertension, or "borderline" hypertension, would resemble neurogenic hypertension in animals. In particular, we would make the following predictions. First, blood pressure should be more variable than in other types such as renal hypertension. Most of the reports of so-called "labile" hypertension are based on a few isolated measurements of pressure and are of negligible value in establishing the

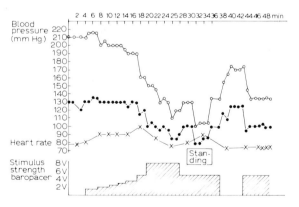

Fig. 10. Effect of carotid sinus nerve stimulation in a patient with refractory essential hypertension shortly after the implantation of a stimulator ("baropacer"). (Reproduced with permission from Dunning, 1971.)

52

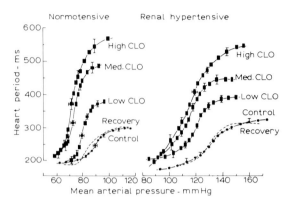

Fig. 11. Baroreflex lines relating pressure and heart period in normotensive and hypertensive rabbits. Pressure was changed by aortic balloon inflation. With progressively larger doses of clonidine (LOW CLO., MED. CLO. and HIGH CLO.) sensitivity of reflex (slope of line) is increased in both groups of rabbits. (Reproduced with permission from Korner et al., 1975.)

variability of arterial pressure. Bevan et al. (1969) using 24 hr continuous measurement of blood pressure found that percentage variations were smaller in those with higher pressures, but absolute variations were greater. A more recent analysis by Littler et al. (1976) has shown no correlation between the 24 hr level of diastolic pressure and its variability. There is no convincing evidence that hypertension goes through a "labile" phase. The second prediction would be that sympathetic tone should be increased in this type of hypertension. This again is difficult to answer confidently. Older methods of measuring sympathetic tone, such as estimations of urinary catecholamines and catecholamine turnover, have given conflicting results (reviewed by De Quattro and Miura, 1973). Newer methods, such as estimations of plasma catecholamine levels, have found that levels are frequently elevated in patients with established essential hypertension, but not so much in those with borderline hypertension (De Quattro and Chan, 1972; Louis et al., 1973). Dopamine-β-hydroxylase (DBH) levels are more difficult to interpret, and may be raised (Stone et al., 1974; Alexandre et al., 1975) or normal (Geffen et al., 1973).

Renin levels are probably normal in neurogenic hypertension (Bliddal et al., 1965) and normal or high in borderline hypertension (Esler et al., 1975).

Finally, we should expect that baroreflex sensitivity should be reduced in borderline hypertension. Takeshita et al. (1975) did find this to be the case, but not as much as in established essential hypertension.

Many of the circulatory changes in borderline hypertension could thus be due to some abnormality of autonomic regulation. Baroreflex dysfunction is one of a number of possible causes of this, but the findings could be equally well explained by some primary central nervous system abnormality.

INTERACTIONS BETWEEN THE BAROREFLEX AND THE BRAIN

It is becoming increasingly clear that the baroreflex arc is not a fixed entity, but is subject to modulation by the CNS (Moruzzi, 1940; Reis and Cuénod,

1965). Thus stimulation of the hypothalamic "defence area" may reset the reflex to a higher pressure level (Humphreys and Joels, 1972) and inhibit the reflex vagal bradycardia from carotid sinus stimulation (Gebber and Snyder, 1970). The cardiac component of the baroreflex is also inhibited during exercise in man (Bristow et al., 1971), which may represent a similar phenomenon. It is clearly teleologically absurd for the reflex to oppose a rise of arterial pressure where this is physiologically appropriate, such as occurs during isometric exercise (where baroreflex sensitivity is inhibited to a greater extent than during dynamic exercise (Cunningham et al., 1972). An example of this central modulation of the reflex can be seen in patients with high cervical cord transections, in whom the only direct efferent communication between the brain and the cardiovascular system is via the vagus, sympathetic outflow being interrupted by the transection (Fig. 12). In such patients a learned voluntary rise of pressure can be produced by a withdrawal of vagal tone, whereas an involuntarily produced one (e.g. following noxious stimulation below the level of the cord transection) is brought about by activation of

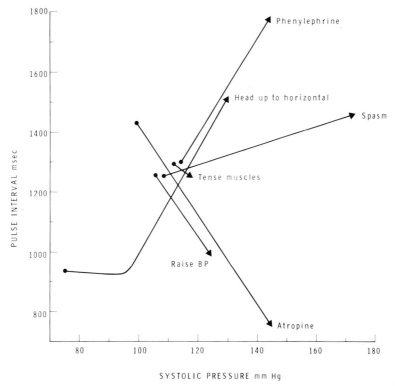

Fig. 12. Relation between systolic pressure (SP) and pulse interval (PI) during different situations in a tetraplegic subject. Solid circles show conditions at rest, and arrows direction of change. Phenylephrine line shows normal baroreflex response, which is also seen when he was tilted from the head up to horizontal position. During spontaneous muscle spasms slope of line is flatter because of activation of sympathetic centres in the spinal cord, which counteract the reflex bradycardia. During voluntary blood pressure raising, and attempted muscle tensing, line follows the line obtained during atropinisation, indicating that the changes here are due to vagal withdrawal (Pickering et al., 1976).

sympathetic centres in the isolated cord, so that the rise of pressure causes a reflex vagal bradycardia (Pickering et al., 1976). Thus in the former case the reflex must be inhibited (both rate and pressure increasing), while in the latter it opposes the pressure rise. One reason why such patients may show very large and sudden increases of arterial pressure could be due to disinhibition of spinal sympathetic reflexes. In cats with high cervical cord transection, Malliani et al. (1975) found that distension of the thoracic aorta produced a rise of arterial pressure. They suggested that a positive feedback loop of this sort could play a role in the maintenance of hypertension.

The relevance of this central modulation of the reflex to hypertension remains uncertain. Stimuli that evoke the defence reflex produce cardiovascular effects similar to those of hypothalamic stimulation, and as mentioned above, have been implicated in the genesis of hypertension. Intermittent stimulation of the defence area may produce a sustained elevation of pressure in rats (Folkow and Rubinstein, 1966), and Brod (1963) has compared the circulation in essential hypertension to a state of preparedness for flight. In these circumstances the cardiac limb of the baroreflex is likely to be inhibited. This hypothalamic inhibition has been considered to be an advantageous interaction, because the suppression of vagal cardiac inhibition ensures a maximal cardiac output and perfusion of skeletal muscles without much increase in arterial pressure (Kylstra and Lisander, 1970). The reflex bradycardia from ventricular receptor stimulation is inhibited in the same way (Wennergren et al., 1976).

Interaction between the brain and the baroreflex also takes place in the opposite direction. Stimulation of the baroreceptors may cause synchronisation of the EEG (Bonvallet et al., 1954), and in decorticate cats carotid occlusion can provoke outbursts of sham rage (Bartorelli et al., 1960). "Experimental neurosis", i.e. an impaired behavioural responsiveness in a conflict situation, is more easily induced in rats with carotid sinus denervation than in control rats (Szekely et al., 1963). A possible interpretation of these findings is that under normal circumstances the rise of pressure accompanying a conflict situation may induce a reduction of the level of arousal via the baroreceptors. When baroreceptor function is impaired this buffering action would be less, leading to heightened levels of arousal and further elevations of arterial pressure.

THE BAROREFLEX AND THE KIDNEY

Guyton et al. (1970) have proposed that the baroreflex is only of importance in the short term buffering of changes of arterial pressure, and that it is the relation between fluid balance and the kidney which determines arterial pressure over the long term. Pressor agents will only produce sustained elevations of pressure if they alter this relationship, e.g. by inducing renal vasoconstriction, because a rise of pressure will induce a diuresis which will return the pressure to normal. This relationship will, however, be altered by changes of sympathetic tone, which normally exerts a tonic influence on the kidney — hence the phenomenon of denervation diuresis (Kaplan et al., 1953). There has been some confusion as to the effects of the baroreceptors on the renal circulation, partly because autoregulation plays a major role in maintaining renal blood flow. Renal sympathetic nerve activity is reduced at high levels of arterial pressure (Ninomiya et al., 1971), and carotid sinus nerve stimulation also reduces it (Wilson et al., 1971). Nevertheless Kirchheim (1976) concluded that in the conscious animal, alterations in renal vascular resistance are largely due to autoregulation. Stimulation of ventricular and cardiopulmonary baroreceptors has a much more potent effect on the renal circulation than stimulation of the arterial baroreceptors (Little et al., 1975; Mancia et al., 1975b), but little is known about the functioning of these receptors in hypertension.

There is less information about the effects of the baroreflex on urine flow. Carotid sinus denervation impairs the diuresis that normally follows expansion of the plasma volume, and it has been suggested that this is because of increased ADH secretion (Gilmore and Weisfeldt, 1965). Cowley et al. (1974) have recently emphasised the importance of ADH in blood pressure regulation: denervation of the baroreceptors in dogs produced an enormous increase in the pressor response to infusions of ADH. Keeler (1974) found that traction of the carotid sinus area could increase sodium and water excretion with little effect on arterial pressure. This appeared to be mediated humorally.

Although renin secretion is partly under sympathetic control, the arterial baroreceptors do not appear to have any important effects on plasma renin activity, other than via their effects on arterial pressure (Brennan et al., 1974). Receptors from the cardiopulmonary region, however, do exert an important tonic effect on renin release (Mancia et al., 1975a).

CONCLUSIONS

Any consideration of the circulation in hypertension must include the baroreceptors. Much attention has been paid to the receptors themselves, but it must be remembered that it is the baroreflex, not the baroreceptors, which is of physiological importance. Most of the acute experimental evidence favours the view that the chief role of the reflex is to buffer short term changes of pressure, and that over the long term they exert a permissive role by virtue of their resetting. Hypertension from any cause will produce secondary changes in the baroreflex, since the observed changes appear to be a direct consequence of the raised pressure. A primary disturbance of baroreflex function leading to hypertension has been mooted for many years, but the chief feature of this type of hypertension, namely a greatly increased lability, has so far not been observed in human hypertension. Thus animals with experimental neurogenic hypertension show an abnormally low pressure at times, which is not a feature of borderline hypertension in man.

At the present time the roles of the kidney and the brain in hypertension are receiving considerable attention. The chief role of the kidney is the maintenance of body fluid balance, with changes of arterial pressure probably occurring secondarily to this. The renal circulation is under nervous control, and the baroreceptors, particularly from the cardiopulmonary region, exert an important influence on renal sympathetic nerve activity, and may have humoral effects on the kidney as well.

The baroreflex is not a fixed entity, but can be modulated by the brain to suit the prevailing physiological needs. To what extent this modulation is involved in the development of hypertension is uncertain, but there is no doubt that the central connections of the reflex are intimately related to areas of the brain subserving the defence reflex and level of arousal. If the baroreflex has any important role in the development of human essential hypertension it is likely to be through a combination of receptor dysfunction due to degenerative changes in the sinus wall, a very common occurrence in middle aged Western man, coupled with central inhibition of the reflex arc by environmental conditions which activate the defence reflex.

SUMMARY

Baroreceptors are deformation receptors whose output is limited by wall strain.

Experimental hypertension in animals is associated with a resetting of the baroreceptors such that the threshold pressure and set point are raised, and gain decreased. These changes begin within a few days, are reversible, and are probably due to a splinting of the receptors by a stiffer arterial wall. The pulsatile pattern of impulse activity in the sinus nerve is maintained. Studies of the baroreflex arc in hypertensive man using the phenylephrine method have shown both resetting and a diminished sensitivity; the same changes occur with ageing.

Neurogenic hypertension produced by baroreceptor denervation remains controversial, possibly due to species differences. Deafferentation may augment renal hypertension. Interaction between the baroreflex and the brain works both ways: situations where there is a heightened level of arousal may be associated with an inhibition of the cardiac limb of the reflex, while baroreceptor stimulation tends to lower the level of arousal.

Malfunction of the baroreceptors might exacerbate hypertension by (a) impairing the buffering of pressor stimuli, and (b) by altering renal arterial resistance, resetting the relation between pressure and urine flow.

Essential hypertension in man does not show the same degree of lability seen in experimental neurogenic hypertension in animals, but impairment of the reflex could be related to changes in distensibility of the sinus wall.

REFERENCES

Aars, H. (1968a) Aortic baroreceptor activity in normal and hypertensive rabbits. *Acta physiol. scand.*, 72: 298—309.

Aars, H. (1968b) Static load-length characteristics of aortic strips from hypertensive rabbits. *Acta physiol. scand.*, 73: 101—110.

Aars, H. (1969) Relationship between blood pressure and diameter of ascending aorta in normal and hypertensive rabbits. *Acta physiol. scand.*, 75: 397—405.

Abraham, A. (1969) *Microscopic Innervation of the Heart and Blood Vessels in Vertebrates including Man*, Pergamon, Oxford.

Alexandre, J.M., London, G.M., Chevillard, C., LeMaire, P., Safar, M.E. and Weiss, Y. (1975) The meaning of dopamine-β-hydroxylase in essential hypertension. *Clin. Sci. molec. Med.*, 49: 573—579.

Angell James, J.E. (1973) Characteristics of single aortic and right subclavian baroreceptor fiber activity in rabbits with chronic renal hypertension. *Circulat. Res.*, 32: 149—161.

Angell James, J.E. (1974a) Pathophysiology of aortic baroreceptors in rabbits with vitamin D sclerosis and hypertension. *Circulat. Res.*, 34: 327—338.

Angell James, J.E. (1974b) Arterial baroreceptor activity in rabbits with experimental atherosclerosis. *Circulat. Res.*, 34: 27—39.

Bartorelli, C., Bizzi, E., Libretti, A. and Zanchetti, A. (1960) Inhibitory control of sinocarotid pressoceptive afferents on hypothalamic autonomic activity and sham rage behavior. *Arch. ital. Biol.*, 98: 308—326.

Bergel, D.H., Bertram, C.D., Brooks, D.E., MacDermott, A.J., Robinson, J.L. and Sleight, P. (1975) Simultaneous recording of the carotid sinus dimensions and the baroreceptor nerve in the anaesthetized dog. *J. Physiol. (Lond.)*, 252: 15—16P.

Bergel, D.H., Brooks, D.E., MacDermott, A.J., Robinson, J.L. and Sleight, P. (1976) The relation between carotid sinus dimension, nerve activity and pressure in the anaesthetised greyhound. *J. Physiol. (Lond.)*, In press.

Bertram, C.D. (1974) Ultrasound arterial diameter measurement. *J. Physiol. (Lond.)*, 241: 85—87P.

Bevan, A.T., Honour, A.J. and Stott, F.H. (1969) Direct arterial pressure recording in unrestricted man. *Clin. Sci.*, 36: 329—344.

Bliddal, J., Masson, G.M.C. and McCubbin, J.W. (1965) Renin-like activity in kidneys of dogs with neurogenic and nephrogenic hypertension. *Amer. J. Physiol.*, 208: 1078—1082.

Bonvallet, M., Dell, P. et Hiebel, G. (1954) Tonus sympathique et activité électrique corticale. *Electroenceph. clin. Neurophysiol.*, 6: 119—144.

Brennan, L.A., Henninger, A.L., Jochim, K.E. and Malvin, R.L. (1974) Relationship between carotid sinus pressure and plasma renin level. *Amer. J. Physiol.*, 227: 295—299.

Bristow, J.D., Honour, A.J., Pickering, G.W., Sleight, P. and Smyth, H.S. (1969) Diminished baroreflex sensitivity in high blood pressure. *Circulation*, 39: 48—54.

Bristow, J.D., Brown, E.B., Cunningham, D.J.C., Howson, M.G., Strange Petersen, E., Pickering, T.G. and Sleight, P. (1971) Effect of bicycling on the baroreflex regulation of pulse interval. *Circulat. Res.*, 28: 582—592.

Brod, J. (1963) Haemodynamic basis of acute pressor reactions and hypertension. *Brit. Heart J.*, 25: 227—245.

Capps, R.B. and De Takats, G. (1938) The late effects of bilateral carotid sinus denervation in man. *J. clin. Invest.*, 17: 385—389.

Cowley, A.W. and Guyton, A.C. (1975) Baroreceptor reflex effects on transient and steady-state hemodynamics of salt-loading hypertension in dogs. *Circulat. Res.*, 36: 536—546.

Cowley, A.W., Liard, J.-F. and Guyton, A.C. (1973) Role of the baroreceptor reflex in daily control of arterial pressure and other variables in dogs. *Circulat. Res.*, 32: 564—576.

Cowley, A.W., Monos, E. and Guyton, A.C. (1974) Interaction of vasopressin and the baroreceptor reflex system in the regulation of arterial blood pressure in the dog. *Circulat. Res.*, 34: 505—514.

Cunningham, D.J.C., Strange Petersen, E., Peto, R., Pickering, T.G. and Sleight, P. (1972) Comparison of the effect of different types of exercise on the baroreflex regulation of heart rate. *Acta physiol. scand.*, 86: 444—455.

Cyon, E. and Ludwig, C. (1866) Die Reflexe eines der sensiblen Nerven des Herzens auf die motorischen der Blutgefässe. *Verh. Kgl. ges. Wiss. (Lpz.)*, 18: 307—328.

De Quattro, V. and Chan, S. (1972) Raised plasma catecholamines in some patients with primary hypertension. *Lancet*, 1: 806—809.

De Quattro, V. and Miura, Y. (1973) Neurogenic factors in human hypertension: mechanism or myth? *Amer. J. Med.*, 55: 362—378.

De Quattro, V., Nagatsu, T., Maronde, R. and Alexander, N. (1969) Catecholamine synthesis in rabbits with neurogenic hypertension. *Circulat. Res.*, 24: 545—555.

Doba, N. and Reis, D.J. (1973) Acute fulminating neurogenic hypertension produced by brainstem lesions in the rat. *Circulat. Res.*, 32: 584—593.

Dunning, A.J. (1971) *Electrostimulation of the Carotid Sinus Nerve in Angina Pectoris*, Excerpta Medica, Amsterdam.

58

Esler, M.D., Julius, S., Randall, O.S., Ellis, C.N. and Kashima, T. (1975) Relation of renin status to neurogenic vascular resistance in borderline hypertension. *Amer. J. Cardiol.*, 36: 706—715.

Ferrario, C.M., McCubbin, J.W. and Page, I.H. (1969) Hemodynamic changes of chronic experimental neurogenic hypertension in unanesthetized dogs. *Circulat. Res.*, 24: 911—922.

Folkow, B. (1971) The haemodynamic consequences of adaptive structural changes of the resistance vessels in hypertension. *Clin. Sci.*, 41: 1—12.

Folkow, B. and Rubinstein, E.H. (1966) Cardiovascular effects of acute and chronic stimulations of the hypothalamic defence area in the rat. *Acta physiol. scand.*, 68: 48—57.

Gebber, G.L. and Snyder, D.W. (1970) Hypothalamic control of baroreceptor reflexes. *Amer. J. Physiol.*, 218: 124—131.

Geffen, L.B., Rush, R.A., Louis, W.J. and Doyle, A.E. (1973) Plasma dopamine-beta-hydroxylase and noradrenaline amounts in essential hypertension. *Clin. Sci.*, 44: 617—620.

Gilmore, J.P. and Weisfeldt, M.L. (1965) Contribution of intravascular receptors to the renal responses following intravascular volume expansion. *Circulat. Res.*, 17: 144—154.

Gribbin, B., Pickering, T.G., Sleight, P. and Peto, R. (1971) Effect of age and high blood pressure on baroreflex sensitivity in man. *Circulat. Res.*, 29: 424—431.

Griffith, L.S.C. and Schwartz, S.I. (1964) Reversal of renal hypertension by electrical stimulation of the carotid sinus nerve. *Surgery*, 56: 232—239.

Grimson, K.S. (1941) The sympathetic nervous system in neurogenic and renal hypertension. *Arch. Surg.*, 43: 284—305.

Gutmann, M.C. and Benson, H. (1971) Interaction of environmental factors and systemic arterial blood pressure: a review. *Medicine (Baltimore)*, 50: 543—553.

Guyton, A.C., Coleman, T.G., Bower, J.D. and Granger, H.J. (1970) Circulatory control in hypertension. *Circulat. Res.*, 26—27, Suppl. II: 135—147.

Heath, D., Smith, P., Harris, P. and Winson, M. (1973) The atherosclerotic human carotid sinus. *J. Path. Bact.*, 110: 49—58.

Henry, J.P. and Cassel J.C. (1969) Psychosocial factors in essential hypertension. Recent epidemiologic and animal experimental evidence. *Amer. J. Epidemiol.*, 90: 171—200.

Hering, H.E. (1927) *Die Karotissinusreflexe auf Herz und Gefässe vom normalphysiologischen, pathologisch-physiologischen und klinischen Standpunkt*, Steinkopff, Dresden.

Heymans, C. and Neil, E. (1958) *Reflexogenic Areas of the Cardiovascular System*, Churchill, London.

Hilgenberg, F. (1958) Neurohistologische Studien über die Pressorezeptoren des Carotissinus bei Hypertonikern. *Acta neuroveg. (Wien)*, 19: 1—14.

Humphreys, P.W. and Joels, N. (1972) The vasomotor component of the carotid sinus baroreceptor reflex in the cat during stimulation of the hypothalamic defence area. *J. Physiol. (Lond.)*, 226: 57—78.

Kaplan, S.A., West, C.O. and Forman, S.J. (1953) Effects of unilateral division of the splanchnic nerve on the renal excretion of electrolytes in unanaesthetised and anaesthetised dogs, the mechanism of cross stimulation. *Amer. J. Physiol.*, 175: 363—374.

Keeler, R. (1974) Natriuresis after unilateral stimulation of carotid receptors in unanesthetized rats. *Amer. J. Physiol.*, 226: 507—511.

Kezdi, P. (1953) Sinoaortic regulatory system. Role in pathogenesis of essential and malignant hypertension. *Arch. intern. Med.*, 91: 26—34.

Kezdi, P. (1960) Persistent hypertension in the dog following disruption of the carotid sinus nerves and subsequent unilateral renal artery constriction. *Circulat. Res.*, 8: 934—940.

Kezdi, P., Spickler, J.W. and Kordenat, R.K. (1972) Alteration of baroreceptor function in hypertension. In *Proc. Symp. Clinical Application of Carotid Sinus Nerve Stimulation in Hypertension*, Medtronic Inc., The Netherlands, p. 13.

Kirchheim, H.R. (1976) Systemic arterial baroreceptor reflexes. *Physiol. Rev.*, 56: 100—176.

Korner, P.I., Oliver, J.R., Sleight, P., Robinson, J.S. and Chalmers, J.P. (1975) Assessment of cardiac autonomic excitability in renal hypertensive rabbits using clonidine-induced resetting of the baroreceptor-heart rate reflex. *Europ. J. Pharmacol.*, 33: 353—362.

Koushnapour, E. and Kelso, D.M. (1972) Partition of the carotid sinus baroreceptor response in dogs between the mechanical properties of the wall and the receptor elements. *Circulat. Res.*, 31: 831—845.

Krieger, E.M. (1970) Time course of baroreceptor resetting in acute hypertension. *Amer. J. Physiol.*, 218: 486—490.

Krieger, E.M. and Marseillan, R.F. (1966) Neural control in experimental hypertension. The role of baroreceptor and splanchnic fibers. *Acta physiol. lat.-amer.*, 16: 343—352.

Kylstra, P.H. and Lisander, B. (1970) Differentiated interaction between the hypothalamic defence area and baroreceptor reflexes. II. Effects on aortic blood flow as related to work load on the left ventricle. *Acta physiol. scand.*, 78: 386—392.

Landgren, S. (1952) On the excitation mechanism of the carotid baroreceptors. *Acta physiol. scand.*, 26: 1—35.

Lawrence, J.R. and Dickinson, C.J. (1964) Synergistic effect of carotid sinus denervation on renal hypertension in the rabbit. *Clin. Sci.*, 27: 381—384.

Liard, J.-F., Cowley, A.W., McCaa, R.E., McCaa, C.S. and Guyton, A.C. (1974) Renin, aldosterone, body fluid volumes, and the baroreceptor reflex in the development and reversal of Goldblatt hypertension in conscious dogs. *Circulat. Res.*, 34: 549—560.

Little, R., Wennergren, G. and Öberg, B. (1975) Aspects of the central integration of arterial baroreceptor and cardiac ventricular receptor reflexes in the cat. *Acta physiol. scand.*, 93: 85—96.

Littler, W.A., West, M.J., Honour, A.J. and Sleight, P. (1976) The variability of arterial pressure. Submitted for publication.

Louis, W.J., Doyle, A.E. and Anavekar, S. (1973) Plasma norepinephrine levels in essential hypertension. *New Engl. J. Med.*, 288: 599—601.

Lowe, R.D. (1961) Ischaemia of the brain as a cause of chronic hypertension in man. *Clin. Sci.*, 21: 403—407.

Malliani, A., Lombardi, F., Pagani, M., Recordati, G. and Schwartz, P.J. (1975) Spinal sympathetic reflexes in the cat and the pathogenesis of arterial hypertension. *Clin. Sci. molec. Med.*, 48: 259S-260S.

Mancia, G., Romero, J.C. and Shepherd, J.T. (1975a) Continuous inhibition of renin release in dogs by vagally innervated receptors in the cardiopulmonary region. *Circulat. Res.*, 36: 529—535.

Mancia, G., Shepherd, J.T. and Donald, D.E. (1975b) Role of cardiac, pulmonary, and carotid mechanoreceptors in the control of hind-limb and renal circulation in dogs. *Circulat. Res.*, 37: 200—208.

McCubbin, J.W., Green, J.H. and Page, I.H. (1956) Baroreceptor function in chronic renal hypertension. *Circulat. Res.*, 4: 205—210.

Moruzzi, G. (1940) Paleocerebellar inhibition of vasomotor and respiratory carotid sinus reflexes. *J. Neurophysiol.*, 3: 20—32.

Ninomiya, I., Nisimaru, N. and Irisawa, H. (1971) Sympathetic nerve activity to the spleen, kidney, and heart in response to baroreceptor input. *Amer. J. Physiol.*, 221: 1346—1351.

Nosaka, S. and Wang, S.C. (1972) Baroreceptor reflex functions in the spontaneously hypertensive rat. In *Spontaneous Hypertension. Its Pathogenesis and Complications*, K. Okamoto (Ed.), Igaku Shoin, Tokyo, pp. 79—82.

Pickering, T.G., Gribbin, B. and Oliver, D.O. (1972) Baroreflex sensitivity in patients on long-term haemodialysis. *Clin. Sci.*, 43: 645—657.

Pickering, T.G., Brucker, B., Dworkin, B.R., Frankel, H.L., Mathias, C.J. and Miller, N.E. (1976) Mechanisms of learned voluntary blood pressure control in patients with generalised bodily paralysis. In *NATO Symposium on Biofeedback*, In press.

Rees, P.M., Sleight, P. and Robinson, J.L. (1976) Histology and ultrastructure of the carotid sinus in experimental renal hypertension. Submitted for publication.

Reis, D.J. and Cuénod, M. (1965) Central neural regulation of carotid baroreceptor reflexes in the cat. *Amer. J. Physiol.*, 209: 1267—1279.

Salgado, H.C. and Krieger, E.M. (1973) Reversibility of baroreceptor adaptation in chronic hypertension. *Clin. Sci. molec. Med.*, 45: 123S—126S.

Sleight, P. and West, M.J. (1975) The effects of clonidine on the baroreflex arc in man. In *Control Action of Drugs in the Regulation of Blood Pressure*, D.S. Davis and J.L. Reid (Eds.), Pitman, London, pp. 291—299.

Sleight, P., Robinson, J.L., Brooks, D.E. and Rees, P.M. (1975) Carotid baroreceptor re-setting in the hypertensive dog. *Clin. Sci. molec. Med.*, 48: 261S—263S.

Sleight, P., Robinson, J.L. and Brooks D.E. (1976) Characteristics of carotid sinus baroreceptor nerve activity in normotensive and renal hypertensive dogs. Submitted for publication.

Smyth, H.S., Sleight, P. and Pickering, G.W. (1969) Reflex regulation of arterial pressure during sleep in man; a quantitative method of assessing baroreflex sensitivity. *Circulat. Res.*, 24: 109—121.

Stone, R.A., Gunnels, J.C., Robinson, R.R., Schanberg, S.M. and Kirshner, N. (1974) Dopamine-beta-hydroxylase in primary and secondary hypertension. *Circulat. Res.*, 34—35, Suppl. 1: 47—56.

Szekely, J.I., Koo, E. and Adam, G. (1963) Carotid afferentation and higher nervous activity. III. Experimental neurosis in rats deprived of their carotid innervation. *Acta physiol. Acad. Sci. hung.*, 23: 343—346.

Takeshita, A., Tanaka, S., Kuroiwa, A. and Nakamura, M. (1975) Reduced baroreceptor sensitivity in borderline hypertension. *Circulat. Res.*, 51: 738—742.

Tobian, L., Olson, R. and Chesley, G. (1969) Water content of arteriolar wall in renovascular hypertension. *Amer. J. Physiol.*, 216: 22—24.

Wallin, G., Delius, W. and Hagbarth, K.E. (1973) Comparison of sympathetic nerve activity in normo- and hypertensive subjects. *Circulat. Res.*, 33: 9—21.

Wennergren, G., Lisander, B. and Öberg, B. (1976) Interaction between the hypothalamic defence reaction and cardiac ventricular receptor reflexes. *Acta physiol. scand.*, 96: 532—547.

Wilson, M.F., Ninomiya, I., Judy, W.V. and Franz, G.N. (1971) Hypothalamic stimulation and baroreceptor reflex interaction on renal nerve activity. *Amer. J. Physiol.*, 221: 1768—1773.

Wolinsky, H. (1970) Response of the rat aortic media to hypertension. *Circulat. Res.*, 26: 507—552.

Zanchetti, A., Guazzi, M. and Baccelli, G. (1967) Role of sino-aortic reflexes in the regulation of experimental renal hypertension during natural sleep. In *Baroreceptors and Hypertension*, P. Kezdi (Ed.), Pergamon, Oxford, pp. 387—400.

Brain Stem Vasomotor Circuits Involved in the Genesis and Entrainment of Sympathetic Nervous Rhythms

GERARD L. GEBBER and SUSAN M. BARMAN

Department of Pharmacology, Michigan State University, East Lansing, Mich. 48824 (U.S.A.)

INTRODUCTION

This paper constitutes a review of those experiments performed in our laboratory on the organization of brain stem circuits responsible for the genesis of naturally occurring (i.e., tonic) discharges in sympathetic vasoconstrictor nerves. We have worked under the assumption that one of the keys to this problem is understanding the bases for the rhythms or periodicities which appear in the tonic discharges of sympathetic nerve bundles. More specifically, we have entertained the question of whether the periodic components in sympathetic nerve discharge are imposed upon central networks by external afferent input or whether they are representative of rhythm generating mechanisms intrinsic to the brain stem. Each of these alternative explanations for the genesis of rhythmic activity has its own special implication. Rhythmicity solely of extrinsic origin would imply a primitively organized central vasomotor network lacking internal oscillating circuits. Rhythms intrinsic to the brain stem, on the other hand, would imply the existence of well organized central networks containing positive and/or negative feedback loops. In this case, the periodic components in sympathetic nerve discharge would be representative of the fundamental organization of those brain stem circuits which generate tonic activity in pre- and postganglionic nerves.

The experiments to be described were performed on cats anesthetized with a mixture of diallylbarbiturate and urethane (Gebber, 1976). Electrical discharges of the postganglionic sympathetic external carotid or renal nerve were monitored with standard recording techniques (Gebber et al., 1973; Taylor and Gebber, 1975). Most, if not all of the efferent fibers of these nerves are thought to subserve vasoconstrictor function (Gebber et al., 1973; Hukuhara and Takeda, 1975). Thus, their discharge patterns can be viewed as indicators of central vasomotor organization. As shown in Fig. 1, periodicities related temporally to the cardiac and respiratory cycles are prominent in naturally occurring sympathetic nerve discharge. Discharges of the external carotid and renal sympathetic nerves are synchronized into bursts (recorded as slow waves with a preamplifier bandpass of 1—1000 Hz) which are locked in a 1:1 relation to the cardiac cycle. In addition, the amplitude of the cardiac-related slow wave waxes and wanes with the period of the central respiratory cycle (monitored by

62

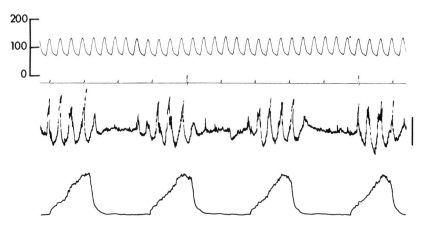

Fig. 1. Rhythmic components in sympathetic nerve discharge of a vagotomized cat. Top trace is blood pressure (mm Hg). Middle trace shows tonic discharges of external carotid postganglionic sympathetic nerve (negativity recorded as an upward deflection in this and in subsequent figures; preamplifier bandpass was 1—1000 Hz). Bottom trace shows RC integrated (time constant 0.05 sec) phrenic nerve discharge (inspiration recorded as an upward deflection in this and in subsequent figures). Time base (below blood pressure) is 1 sec/division and applies to all traces. Vertical calibration is 40 μV and applies to sympathetic nerve discharge.

RC integrated phrenic nerve discharge in the vagotomized, paralyzed and artificially ventilated cat). The rapid and slow rhythms will be referred to respectively as the cardiac-related periodicity and the respiratory-related periodicity. These terms are used solely to describe patterns of temporal relationship.

Our studies on the cardiac-related and respiratory-related periodicities contradict the traditional view of a primitively organized central vasomotor network whose output patterns are primarily determined by periodic external afferent input. Rather, the experiments to be described demonstrate that brain stem networks are inherently capable of synchronizing the discharges of sympathetic nerves both on a fast and on a slow time scale. It is our contention that internal oscillators rather than external afferent sources are the principle determinants of the cardiac-related and respiratory-related periodicities in sympathetic nerve discharge.

CARDIAC-RELATED PERIODICITY

As already noted, the tonic discharges of sympathetic nerve bundles usually are synchronized into bursts which are locked in a 1:1 relation to the cardiac cycle (Fig. 1). This relationship traditionally is considered to result as the simple consequence of the baroreceptor reflexes (Adrian et al., 1932; Heymans and Neil, 1958; Green and Heffron, 1968; Cohen and Gootman, 1970). That is, increased baroreceptor nerve discharge during systole supposedly causes a delayed inhibition of sympathetic nerve discharge, while the removal of inhibition during diastole supposedly leads to an increase in sympathetic nerve

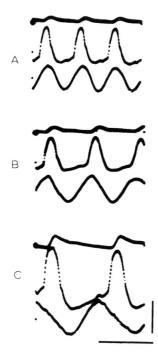

Fig. 2. Shifts in phase relations between carotid sinus and renal sympathetic nerve discharges during stimulation of peripheral end of sectioned right cervical vagus nerve. Traces represent sum of 64 R wave-triggered trials. Top tracings: arterial pulse. Middle tracings: afferent carotid sinus nerve discharge. Bottom tracings: renal sympathetic nerve discharge. A: control; mean blood pressure was 145 mm Hg. B: vagus stimulation (3 Hz); blood pressure was 140 mm Hg. C: vagus stimulation (5 Hz); blood pressure was 140 mm Hg.
Horizontal calibration, 500 msec; vertical calibration, 534 μV (for nerve recordings).

discharge. A number of observations made in our laboratory, however, do not support this view (Gebber et al., 1975; Taylor and Gebber, 1975; Gebber, 1976).

It was possible to produce dramatic shifts in the phase relations between baroreceptor and sympathetic nerve discharges by slowing the heart rate. The R wave-triggered computer-summed traces in Fig. 2 illustrate this point. The vagus and aortic depressor nerves were sectioned bilaterally in this experiment. As shown in panel A, the decay of renal sympathetic nerve discharge began approximately 75 msec after the start of the pulse-synchronous component of carotid sinus nerve discharge when heart rate was 3 beats/sec. This interval generally is considered to represent the central delay of sympathoinhibition of baroreceptor reflex origin. Note, however, that the beginning of the decay of sympathetic nerve discharge was shifted to a position which actually preceded the start of the pulse-synchronous component of carotid sinus nerve activity when heart rate was decreased by stimulation of the distal end of the sectioned right cervical vagus (panel C). This observation indicates that the decay of sympathetic nerve discharge cannot be directly related to delayed inhibition of baroreceptor reflex origin. That is, the cardiac-related periodicity in sympathetic nerve discharge cannot be explained as a direct result of the

64

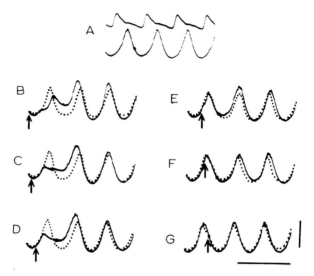

Fig. 3. Effect of single shock (10 V; 0.5 msec) applied to paramedian reticular nucleus on cardiac-related bursts of renal nerve discharge. A: R wave-triggered computer-summed traces (64 sweeps) of arterial pulse (top) and renal nerve discharge (bottom). Mean blood pressure was 135 mm Hg. B—G: comparison of computer-summed trace of sympathetic nerve discharge shown in A (dotted line) with those (solid line) summed following paramedian stimulation at selected points in cardiac cycle. Single shock stimulation of paramedian nucleus was delayed as follows with respect to the R wave. B: 0 msec; C: 50 msec; D: 120 msec; E: 150 msec; F: 200 msec; G: 250 msec. Arrows show point of application of single shock. Horizontal calibration is 500 msec. Vertical calibration is 267 μV (Taylor and Gebber, 1975).

waxing and waning of baroreceptor nerve activity during each heart beat. Rather, shifts in the phase relations between carotid sinus and sympathetic nerve discharges suggest that the sympathetic slow wave is representative of a vasomotor rhythm of central origin which is entrained to the cardiac cycle by the baroreceptor reflexes. This contention is further supported by the results presented in Fig. 3.

Fig. 3 illustrates the effect of a single shock (10 V; 0.5 msec) applied to the paramedian reticular nucleus on the cardiac-related periodic component of renal sympathetic nerve discharge. The paramedian nucleus of the medullary depressor region receives primary and secondary projections from the carotid sinus nerve (Humphrey, 1967; Miura and Reis, 1969). The computer-summed records in panel A show locking of the slow wave of renal nerve activity to the arterial pulse. Panels B—G compare the cardiac-related slow waves of sympathetic nerve discharge shown in panel A with those oscillations which were summed when a single shock was applied to the paramedian nucleus at selected points (indicated by arrows) in the cardiac cycle. Two observations in Fig. 3 indicate that generation of the sympathetic slow wave essentially is an "all or none" phenomenon. First, an oscillation of sympathetic nerve activity was extinguished (panel C) or prematurely aborted (panel D) when the shock was applied just before or at its beginning. Thus, one complete oscillation could be eliminated by a stimulus delivered to a synaptic station within the

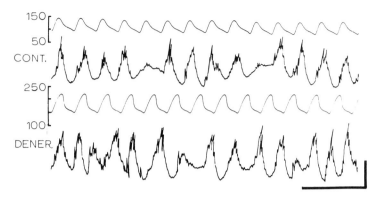

Fig. 4. Persistence of synchronized sympathetic nerve discharge after baroreceptor nerve section. Oscillographic records show synchronized bursts (slow waves) of renal nerve discharge before and after bilateral section of carotid sinus, aortic depressor and vagus nerves. Top traces are blood pressure (mm Hg). Bottom traces are sympathetic nerve discharge. Horizontal calibration is 1 sec. Vertical calibration is 50 μV for nerve recordings.

baroreceptor reflex arc during a time span which accounted for less than 1% of the duration of the cardiac cycle. Second, stimulation of the paramedian nucleus during the greater proportion of the cardiac cycle failed to affect the slow wave of sympathetic nerve activity. For instance, no effect was observed when the stimulus was delivered as little as 50 msec after the onset of the oscillation (panel E).

Significantly, it was also demonstrated that bilateral section of the carotid sinus, aortic depressor and vagus nerves did not desynchronize sympathetic nerve discharge (Fig. 4). Rather, baroreceptor nerve section simply unlocked the phase relations between the slow wave of sympathetic nerve discharge and the cardiac cycle. Disruption of the phase relations between sympathetic nerve discharge and the cardiac cycle was indicated by two observations. First, the number of slow waves per cardiac cycle on the average was greater than one after baroreceptor denervation (Fig. 4). Thus, section of the baroreceptor nerves increased the frequency of occurrence of sympathetic nerve oscillations relative to the heart rate. This effect presumably played a role in the hypertension which accompanied baroreceptor denervation. Second, using computer summation techniques, Taylor and Gebber (1975) demonstrated the complete loss of the R wave time-locked component of sympathetic nerve discharge in those experiments in which a 3—5 c/sec periodicity persisted after baroreceptor nerve section.

The results presented in Figs. 2—4 have led us to conclude that the cardiac-related periodicity in sympathetic nerve discharge is representative of a vasomotor rhythm of central origin. The rhythm (3—5 c/sec periodicity) is generated in the brain stem since it could not be demonstrated in residual sympathetic nerve discharge after transection of the spinal cord at the first cervical segment (McCall and Gebber, 1975), and because it persisted after midcollicular transection (Taylor and Gebber, 1975). The 3—5 c/sec periodic component in sympathetic nerve discharge normally is entrained to the cardiac cycle by the baroreceptor reflexes, the purpose for which is discussed below.

66

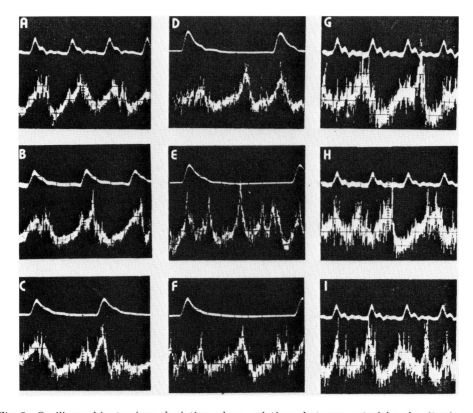

Fig. 5. Oscillographic tracings depicting phase relations between arterial pulse (top) and naturally occurring external carotid postganglionic sympathetic nerve discharge (bottom). A: control. B—F: during stimulation of distal end of right vagus nerve. B: 3 Hz; C: 5 Hz; D: 10 Hz; E: 15 Hz; F: 20 Hz. G—I: after bilateral section of carotid sinus nerves (vagus and aortic depressor nerves previously cut). Changes in mean blood pressure are not depicted in records. Blood pressure was 150 mm Hg before (A) and 185 mm Hg after (G) section of carotid sinus nerves. Horizontal calibration, 200 msec; vertical calibration, 20 μV (Gebber, 1976).

Fig. 5A—F depicts the relationship between the arterial pulse and external carotid postganglionic sympathetic nerve activity at different heart rates in the same cat. The distal end of the cut right vagus nerve was stimulated (2—20 Hz) to slow heart rate. Bursts of sympathetic nerve discharge were locked in a 1:1 relation to the cardiac cycle at heart rates above 1.5 beats/sec (panels A—C). This relationship was disrupted, however, when heart rate was further lowered (panels D—F). Bursts of sympathetic nerve discharge occurred irregularly at frequencies ranging from 3 to 5 c/sec when heart rate was less than 1.5 beats/sec. On the average, the periodicity in sympathetic nerve discharge rose from a control value of about 3 c/sec (panel A) to approximately 4 c/sec. This change was duplicated (panels G—I) when the carotid sinus nerves were sectioned (vagus and aortic depressor nerves previously cut). These observations indicate that the purpose of 1:1 locking of synchronized bursts of sympathetic nerve discharge to the cardiac cycle by the baroreceptor reflexes is to limit sympathetic periodicity below the maximum output frequency (5 c/sec) of the brain stem rhythmogenic mechanism. This control system, however, is disrupted when heart rate is decreased below 1.5 beats/sec.

RESPIRATORY-RELATED PERIODICITY

As previously noted (Fig. 1), the naturally occurring discharges of sympathetic nerve bundles in the vagotomized, paralyzed and artificially ventilated cat exhibit a slow rhythmic component with the period of the respiratory cycle. The synchronization of sympathetic and phrenic nerve discharges generally is assumed to result as a consequence of direct coupling between phase-locked (Koizumi et al., 1971; Preiss et al., 1975) or phase-spanning (Cohen and Gootman, 1970; Gootman and Cohen, 1974) neurons of the brain stem respiratory oscillator and central vasomotor networks. The interaction is thought to occur in the brain stem since the discharges of medullary vasomotor neurons have been shown to exhibit a respiratory periodicity (Gootman et al., 1975; Hukuhara and Takeda, 1975). A number of observations made in our laboratory, however, contradict the view of direct coupling between brain stem respiratory and vasomotor neurons. Rather, our results support the hypothesis that the slow periodic components of sympathetic and phrenic nerve discharges are generated by independent brain stem oscillators which normally are entrained to each other by a common phase switching mechanism.

First, it was possible to demonstrate that the phase relations between sympathetic and phrenic nerve discharges in vagotomized cats were dependent upon respiratory rate (Fig. 6). The pattern of phase relations between external carotid postganglionic sympathetic and phrenic nerve discharges could be described as inspiratory when the respiratory rate was 31 c/min (panel A). That is, sympathetic nerve discharge began to increase near the beginning of inspiration, reached a maximum near the peak of inspiration, and then decayed in time with phrenic nerve discharge. This relationship was changed to an expiratory-inspiratory phase-spanning pattern when the respiratory rate spontaneously decreased to 24 c/min (panel B). That is, sympathetic nerve discharge began to increase from a minimum in early expiration and reached a maximum during inspiration. The shift in phase relations was associated with an increase in the durations of expiration and of the excitatory phase of the cycle of sympathetic nerve activity. These results make it difficult to accept the notion that the respiratory-related periodicity in sympathetic nerve discharge results from direct coupling between one of the components of the brain stem respiratory oscillator and central vasomotor networks. If such was the case, then the phase relations between sympathetic and phrenic nerve discharges should have been independent of respiratory rate.

Second, the slow oscillations of sympathetic and phrenic nerve activity were not always locked in a 1:1 relation. As shown in Fig. 7, the slow rhythmic component of sympathetic nerve discharge occasionally occurred at a frequency greater than (panel A) or less than (panel B) the respiratory rate. This observation also suggested that the slow rhythms in phrenic and sympathetic nerve discharges were generated by independent oscillators.

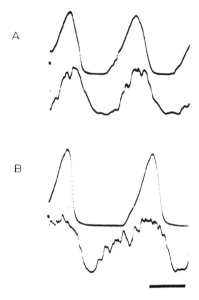

Fig. 6. Shift in phase relations between phrenic and external carotid postganglionic sympathetic nerve discharges accompanying decrease in respiratory rate in vagotomized cat. Each panel shows computer-summed records (32 trials) of RC integrated (time constant 0.05 sec) phrenic (top traces) and sympathetic (bottom traces) nerve activity. Increased nerve discharge is shown as an upward deflection. The sweep of the computer was triggered by a timing pulse derived near the beginning of the inspiratory phase of the phrenic nerve discharge cycle. Respiratory rate was 31 c/min in A and 24 c/min in B. Horizontal calibration is 1 sec.

The independent oscillator hypothesis is further supported by the observation that the slow periodic component of sympathetic nerve discharge often persisted when the rhythmic discharges of the phrenic nerve disappeared during hypocapnia. Hyperventilation to the point of phrenic nerve quiescence was accomplished by increasing the respirator pump rate. Contrary to the results reported by others (Cohen, 1968; Koizumi et al., 1971; Preiss et al., 1975), the slow sympathetic rhythm persisted in 11 of 18 experiments when the rhythmic discharge of the phrenic nerve ceased. A typical experiment is shown in Fig. 8A. Note that the form and frequency of the slow sympathetic oscillations were not markedly changed during hyperventilation. The slow rhythmic component of sympathetic nerve discharge was eliminated during hyperventilation in the remaining 7 experiments (Fig. 8B).

Persistence of the slow rhythmic component in sympathetic nerve discharge during hyperventilation is pertinent when viewed in the light of experiments performed by Cohen (1968). He reported that hypocapnia in the vagotomized cat led to disappearance of the rhythmic discharge patterns of brain stem respiratory neurons. The discharges of expiratory neurons as a general rule became continuous while those of inspiratory neurons became sporadic and eventually ceased when arterial pCO_2 was lowered to the point at which the phrenic nerve lost its rhythmic discharge pattern. Thus, phrenic nerve quiescence produced by hyperventilation in our experiments presumably was associated with disappearance of the rhythmic discharges in those mutually

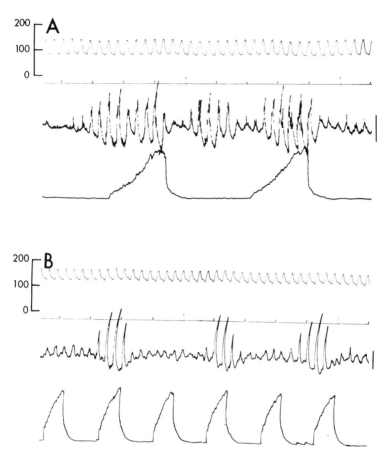

Fig. 7. Dissociation of 1:1 relation between slow rhythmic components of sympathetic and phrenic nerve discharges in 2 vagotomized cats (A and B). Sequence of traces in each panel is as described in Fig. 1. Vertical calibrations are 40 μV. Time base is 1 sec/division.

inhibitory neuronal pairs which comprise the central respiratory oscillator (Cohen, 1970, 1974; Hukuhara, 1974). If this assumption is accepted, then it would be impossible to attribute the persistence of the slow rhythmic component of sympathetic nerve discharge to a direct connection between the brain stem respiratory oscillator and central vasomotor networks. Rather, the slow rhythmic components of sympathetic and phrenic nerve discharges would have been generated by independent brain stem oscillators normally entrained to each other by a common phase switching mechanism. It would also follow that the neuronal types which constitute the slow sympathetic oscillator most often are less apt to lose their rhythmic discharge pattern during hyperventilation than are those neurons which comprise the brain stem respiratory oscillator.

Since the functional state of the central respiratory oscillator in our experiments was inferred from the discharges of the phrenic nerve rather than from brain stem units, it was important to establish that descending inspiratory pathways and spinal inspiratory motoneurons remained excitable when

70

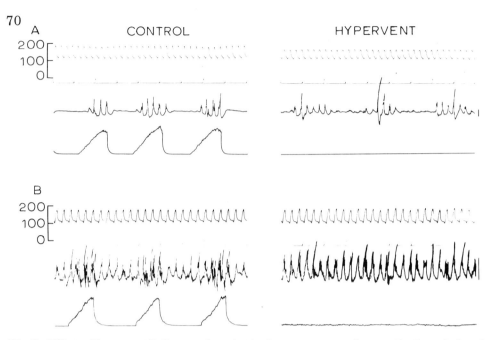

Fig. 8. Effect of hyperventilation on slow rhythmic components of sympathetic and phrenic nerve discharges in 2 vagotomized cats (A and B). Sequence of traces in each panel is as described in Fig. 1. Vertical calibrations are 40 μV. Time base is 1 sec/division.

rhythmic phrenic nerve activity ceased during hyperventilation. Thus, discharges evoked in the phrenic nerve by single shocks (10 V; 0.5 msec) applied to inspiratory-facilitatory sites located in the dorsolateral pontine reticular formation (P 3, L 3.5, H $-$3 to H $-$6) were compared in the normocapnic and hyperventilated states. A typical experiment is shown in Fig. 9. Significantly,

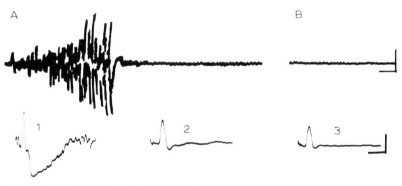

Fig. 9. Effect of hyperventilation on phrenic nerve response evoked by single shock stimulation (10 V; 0.5 msec) of an inspiratory-facilitatory site in dorsolateral pontine reticular formation. Top traces show phrenic neurogram before (A) and during (B) hyperventilation. Bottom traces (records 1—3) are computer-summed phrenic nerve action potentials (32 trials) evoked by pontine stimulation. Record 1: phrenic discharge elicited by shock applied during inspiration. Record 2: response evoked by shock applied during expiration. Record 3: response evoked by shock applied once every 4 sec after disappearance of spontaneously occurring phrenic nerve activity during hyperventilation. Vertical calibrations are 20 μV for phrenic neurogram and 66 μV for computer-summed evoked potentials. Horizontal calibrations are 200 msec for phrenic neurogram and 10 msec for evoked responses.

the phrenic nerve response evoked by pontine stimulation during hyper-ventilation (B3) was only slightly smaller than the discharges elicited previously during inspiration (A1) or early expiration (A2) in the normocapnic state. Thus, disappearance of rhythmic phrenic nerve activity during hyperventilation could be attributed to upset within the brain stem respiratory oscillator.

MODEL OF BRAIN STEM VASOMOTOR CIRCUITS INVOLVED IN GENERATION OF SYMPATHETIC NERVE DISCHARGE

A model of those neuronal circuits presumed to be responsible for the genesis of rhythmic discharges in vasoconstrictor nerve bundles is presented in Fig. 10. The model admittedly is oversimplified and, in part, hypothetical. However, it is intended to provide a reasonable basis for future investigation.

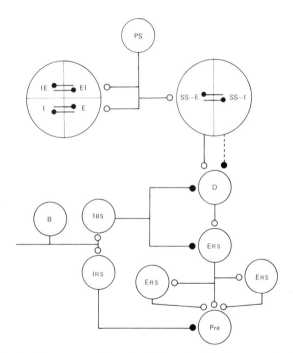

Fig. 10. Model of brain stem vasomotor circuits involved in the genesis of rhythmic activity in sympathetic nerve discharge. Unfilled circles: excitatory connections. Filled circles: inhibitory connections. Slow sympathetic oscillator (top, right) is comprised of mutually inhibitory half-centers, slow sympathetic excitatory (SS-E) and slow sympathetic inhibitory (SS-I). Respiratory oscillator (top, left) is comprised of 2 pairs of mutually inhibitory neurons, inspiratory (I) and expiratory (E) medullary units; and expiratory-inspiratory (EI) and inspiratory-expiratory (IE) pontine phase-spanning units (after Cohen, 1970, 1974). PS (top, center): phase-switching inputs responsible for synchronization of slow rhythmic components in phrenic and sympathetic nerve discharges. Circuit responsible for genesis and entrainment of 3—5 c/sec periodicity is shown in lower half of figure. B, baroreceptor afferent; D, driver mechanism; ERS, interconnected population of excitatory pontomedullary reticulospinal neurons; IBS, inhibitory brain stem interneuron; IRS, inhibitory reticulospinal tract; Pre, preganglionic sympathetic neurons.

(A) Circuit responsible for 3—5 c/sec periodicity

Synchronization of sympathetic nerve discharge into 3—5 c/sec oscillations in baroreceptor denervated cats suggests the existence of extensive inter-connections between groups of functionally similar brain stem neurons. Concerning this point, axon collaterals connecting large numbers of pontomedullary reticulospinal neurons have been described (Brodal, 1957; Scheibel and Scheibel, 1958, 1967). Thus, the 3—5 c/sec oscillations of sympathetic nerve discharge would arise from "avalanche excitation" trans-mitted through an interconnected population of brain stem reticulospinal neurons (ERS). The ERS network presumably is triggered at a frequency varying between 3 and 5 c/sec in baroreceptor denervated preparations by a presently unidentified "driver" mechanism (D).

(B) Circuit responsible for entrainment of 3—5 c/sec periodicity

As already discussed, brain stem inhibition (IBS) of baroreceptor afferent (B) origin functions to entrain bursts of sympathetic nerve discharge in a 1:1 relation to the cardiac cycle. The purpose of entrainment is to limit sympathetic periodicity below the maximum output frequency (5 c/sec) of circuit A. Entrainment is most easily explained by inhibitory-phasing. That is, waves of "avalanche excitation" through the ERS network would be triggered when baroreceptor nerve activity drops below some critical level during each cardiac cycle. In Fig. 2A, for example, the decay of carotid sinus nerve activity in the first cardiac cycle would trigger the formation of the synchronized burst of sympathetic nerve discharge occurring during the succeeding cardiac cycle. This explanation (Gebber, 1976) for the phase relations between baroreceptor and sympathetic nerve discharges is quite different from the classic view which relates the decay of sympathetic nerve discharge to the development of inhibition associated with the pulse-synchronous component of baroreceptor nerve activity occurring in the same cardiac cycle. The inhibitory-phasing hypothesis would explain shifts in the phase relations between baroreceptor and sympathetic nerve discharges produced by slowing the heart (Fig. 2). Stimulation of cardiac vagal efferents would prolong the interval between heart beats without significantly changing the interval between the start of a given cardiac cycle and the point on the decaying curve of baroreceptor nerve discharge at which the synchronized burst of sympathetic activity is generated.

Brain stem inhibition (IBS) is depicted as occurring either on D or on the more rostral elements of the ERS network. Positioning inhibition at either of these locales would explain why oscillations of sympathetic nerve discharge could be terminated only when the paramedian nucleus was stimulated early in the cycle (Fig. 3). That is, once "avalanche excitation" reaches a certain point in the ERS network, formation of the oscillation of sympathetic nerve discharge no longer is influenced by the brain stem component of baro-receptor-induced inhibition. A spinal component (IRS) of inhibition of baroreceptor origin also is included in the wiring diagram. The role played by this system in the control of sympathetic nerve discharge has been discussed in previous reports from this laboratory (Taylor and Gebber, 1975; Gebber, 1976).

(C) Circuit responsible for respiratory-related periodicity

It is postulated that a brain stem oscillator distinct from that responsible for the rhythmic discharges of the phrenic nerve is involved in generating the slow periodic component of sympathetic nerve discharge. This oscillator is presumed to be comprised of mutually inhibitory half-centers which are labeled slow sympathetic-excitatory (SS-E) and slow sympathetic-inhibitory (SS-I). The slow sympathetic rhythm is manifested by the waxing and waning of the amplitude of the cardiac-related bursts of sympathetic nerve discharge. Thus, the output of the slow sympathetic oscillator is directed to the brain stem network responsible for generation of the 3—5 c/sec periodicity (i.e., circuit A).

(D) Circuit responsible for entrainment of slow sympathetic and respiratory oscillators

Cohen (1968, 1970, 1974) has suggested that mechanisms exist to shift the respiratory oscillator between the inspiratory and expiratory states, since otherwise it would remain indefinitely in one of the two states. He postulated that such mechanisms are provided by tonic inputs to medullary expiratory (E) neurons and pontine expiratory-inspiratory (EI) phase-spanning neurons since it is these elements of the brain stem respiratory oscillator (top, left in Fig. 10) which usually discharge uninterruptedly when rhythmic phrenic activity is lost during hypocapnia. We propose that the same inputs (PS) act to switch the phase of the slow sympathetic oscillator. A phase-switching mechanism common to both oscillators would explain why the slow rhythmic components of phrenic and sympathetic nerve discharges usually are synchronized in a 1:1 relation. Such a mechanism might be important in coordinating cardiovascular and respiratory responses to a variety of environmental conditions in the unanesthetized state. The results in Fig. 8B support the view that PS inputs are distributed to SS-E neurons of the slow sympathetic oscillator. As already mentioned, the slow sympathetic rhythm was lost during hyperventilation in 7 of 18 experiments. In such instances, the amplitude of the cardiac-related bursts of sympathetic nerve discharge was relatively constant, reaching a level comparable to that observed during the peak excitatory phase of the slow cycle of activity in the normocapnic state. This observation suggests that disappearance of the slow sympathetic rhythm was associated with uninterrupted activation of SS-E neurons by PS.

SUMMARY

These studies have demonstrated that brain stem vasomotor networks are inherently capable of producing rhythmic activity in sympathetic nerve bundles. The more rapid periodicity (3—5 c/sec) in sympathetic nerve discharge is thought to be representative of the fundamental organization of an interconnected population of pontomedullary reticulospinal neurons. The baroreceptor reflexes function to entrain oscillations of sympathetic nerve activity in a 1:1 relation to the cardiac cycle so as to limit the periodicity in sympathetic discharge below the maximum output frequency (5 c/sec) of the brain stem rhythmogenic mechanism. A slower sympathetic rhythm (with the period of the cycle of phrenic nerve activity) is thought to be representative of the fundamental organization of a brain stem oscillator distinct from the respiratory oscillator. A common phase switching mechanism is proposed to synchronize the slow sympathetic and respiratory oscillators, presumably for the purpose of coordinating cardiovascular and respiratory responses. These studies have prompted us to formulate a model of brain stem vasomotor circuits which generate naturally occurring discharges in sympathetic nerve bundles.

ACKNOWLEDGEMENT

This research was supported by Public Health Service Grant HL-13187.

REFERENCES

Adrian, E.D., Bronk, D.W. and Phillips, G. (1932) Discharges in mammalian sympathetic nerves. *J. Physiol. (Lond.)*, 74: 115—133.

Brodal, A. (1957) *The Reticular Formation of the Brain Stem. Anatomical Aspects and Functional Correlations*, Oliver and Boyd, London, pp. 1—87.

Cohen, M.I. (1968) Discharge patterns of brain-stem respiratory neurons in relation to carbon dioxide tension. *J. Neurophysiol.*, 31: 142—165.

Cohen, M.I. (1970) How respiratory rhythm originates: evidence from discharge patterns of brain stem respiratory neurones. In *Ciba Foundation Hering—Breuer Centenary Symposium; Breathing*, R. Porter (Ed.), Churchill, London, pp. 125—150.

Cohen, M.I. (1974) The genesis of respiratory rhythmicity. In *Central Rhythmic and Regulation*, W. Umbach and H.P. Koepchen (Eds.), Hippokrates, Stuttgart, pp. 15—35.

Cohen, M.I. and Gootman, P.M. (1970) Periodicities of efferent discharges of splanchnic nerve of the cat. *Amer. J. Physiol.*, 218: 1092—1101.

Gebber, G.L. (1976) Basis for phase relations between baroreceptor and sympathetic nervous discharge. *Amer. J. Physiol.*, 230: 263—270.

Gebber, G.L., Taylor, D.G. and Weaver, L.C. (1973) Electrophysiological studies on organization of central vasopressor pathways. *Amer. J. Physiol.*, 224: 470—481.

Gebber, G.L., Taylor, D.G. and McCall, R.B. (1975) Organization of central vasomotor system. *Proc. 6th int. Congr. Pharmacol.*, 4: 49—58.

Gootman, P.M. and Cohen, M.I. (1974) The interrelationships between sympathetic discharge and central respiratory drive. In *Central Rhythmic and Regulation*, W. Umbach and H.P. Koepchen (Eds.), Hippokrates, Stuttgart, pp. 195—209.

Gootman, P.M., Cohen, M.I., Piercey, M.P. and Wolotsky, P. (1975) A search for medullary neurons with activity patterns similar to those in sympathetic nerves, *Brain Res.*, 87: 395—406.

Green, J.H. and Heffron, P.F. (1968) Studies upon the relationship between baroreceptor and sympathetic activity. *Quart. J. exp. Physiol.*, 53: 23—32.

Heymans, C. and Neil, W. (1958) *Reflexogenic Areas of the Cardiovascular System*, Little, Brown and Co., Boston, Mass., pp. 1—271.

Hukuhara, T. (1974) Functional organization of brain stem respiratory neurons and rhythmogenesis. In *Central Rhythmic and Regulation*, W. Umbach and H.P. Koepchen (Eds.), Hippokrates, Stuttgart, pp. 35—49.

Hukuhara, T. and Takeda, R. (1975) Neuronal organization of central vasomotor control mechanisms in the brain stem of the cat. *Brain Res.*, 87: 419—429.

Humphrey, D.R. (1967) Neuronal activity in the medulla oblongata of cat evoked by stimulation of the carotid sinus nerve. In *Baroreceptors and Hypertension*, P. Kezdi (Ed.), Pergamon, New York, pp. 131—167.

Koizumi, K., Seller, H., Kaufman, A. and Brooks, C. McC. (1971) Pattern of sympathetic discharges and their relation to baroreceptor and respiratory activities. *Brain Res.*, 27: 281—294.

McCall, R.B. and Gebber, G.L. (1975) Brain stem and spinal synchronization of sympathetic nervous discharge. *Brain Res.*, 88: 139—143.

Miura, M. and Reis, D.J. (1969) Termination and secondary projections of carotid sinus nerve in the cat brain stem. *Amer. J. Physiol.*, 217: 142—153.

Preiss, G., Kirchner, F. and Polosa, C. (1975) Patterning of sympathetic preganglionic neuron firing by the central respiratory drive. *Brain Res.*, 87: 363—374.

Scheibel, M.E. and Scheibel, A.B. (1958) Structural substrates for integrative patterns in the brain stem reticular core. In *Reticular Formation of the Brain*, H.H. Jasper, L.D. Proctor, R.S. Knighton, W.C. Noshay and R.T. Costello (Eds.), Little, Brown and Co., Boston, Mass., pp. 31—55.

Scheibel, M.E. and Scheibel, A.B. (1967) Anatomical basis of attention mechanisms in vertebrate brains. In *The Neurosciences, A Study Program*, G.C. Quarton, T. Melnechuk and F.O. Schmitt (Eds.), Rockefeller Univ. Press, New York, pp. 577—602.

Taylor, D.G. and Gebber, G.L. (1975) Baroreceptor mechanisms controlling sympathetic nervous rhythms of central origin. *Amer. J. Physiol.*, 228: 1002—1013.

Supramedullary Organization of Vasomotor Control

S.M. HILTON

*Department of Physiology, The Medical School, Vincent Drive,
Birmingham B15 2TJ (Great Britain)*

The main advantage of studying the supramedullary control of the heart and circulation is that such control is then seen immediately in the context of a set of basic biological response patterns. From the work of pioneers in the field, most notably Bard, Cannon and Hess, it was already clear that these parts of the rostral brain stem were concerned with the integration of alimentary, sexual and defence behavior, as well as temperature regulation, and that this integration includes all their components, hormonal and visceral. More recent work has not only confirmed and extended these earlier conclusions, it has also shown that the medulla contains regions with similar integrative functions as well as being the place of origin of some important efferent pathways and of termination of relevant afferent inputs (cf., Coote et al., 1973; Hilton, 1975). So complex is the detailed organisation, even as presently known, that it is clearly misleading to continue to talk of pressor areas or pathways, or of areas or pathways for any single variable, except perhaps in the case of certain specific cranial nuclei, such as the nucleus ambiguus where the vagal output to the heart originates in the cat (McAllen and Spyer, 1976).

Most is known, at present, of the topographical organisation of the areas integrating the defence (or arousal) reaction, in the hypothalamus, midbrain and medulla (Hilton, 1975). These regions are part of what was once known as the ascending, reticular activating system and, hence, are excited by the polysynaptic, extralemniscal input. Transmission through this input is so depressed or distorted by most anaesthetics used in animal experiments that the defence reaction pattern cannot then be obtained in response to appropriate stimuli. Abrahams et al. (1960) could only demonstrate it as a reflex response to peripheral nerve stimulation in the high decerebrate preparation. More interesting perhaps is the later finding that chemoreceptor stimulation could do the same (Bizzi et al., 1961; Hilton and Joels, 1964).

The cardiovascular component of the defence response is readily interpreted as a preparation for muscular exercise, as it consists of constriction of veins, inotropic and chronotropic stimulation of the heart, all leading to an increase of cardiac output which is distributed chiefly to skeletal muscles; for these exhibit vasodilatation, while there is vasoconstriction in the skin, gastro-intestinal tract and kidney. As shown in some recent experiments of ours (Hilton and Marshall, unpublished observations), this response can be obtained reflexly in animals lightly anaesthetised with the steroid anaesthetic, althesin (Glaxo). The muscle vasodilatation is then found to be due in part to reduction of on-going vasoconstrictor activity, in part to circulating adrenaline and in part to activation of cholinergic vasodilator fibres, the actual contribution of each component varying somewhat from animal to animal.

Althesin is proving to be a most useful anaesthetic agent in the investigation of rostral brain stem function in the cat; for only under this anaesthetic can stimulation in the amygdala elicit the full pattern of cardiovascular response characteristic of the defence reaction. Zbrożyna and I had to use conscious cats with implanted electrodes in order to map the region of the amygdala concerned with the defence reaction (Hilton and Zbrożyna, 1963). We could identify the amygdalo-fugal pathway, entering the hypothalamus ventrally after passing just dorsal to the optic tract. The amygdaloid region itself was activated from the septal area, via the stria terminalis. The point I wish to emphasize is that whereas such mapping would have been impossible in animals anaesthetized with chloralose or barbiturates because of failure of transmission, the hypothalamic connexions from higher parts of the brain seem to be functioning normally under althesin; for not only are full defence responses obtained, but the map is identical with that we had previously worked out so laboriously in conscious animals (Timms, unpublished observations).

We took advantage of the properties of althesin in order to re-investigate the question of whether stimulation of the motor cortex can elicit the cardio-vascular pattern of response typical of the defence response, or at least muscle vasodilatation, via the sympathetic system, as reported by Eliasson et al. (1952) and Zwirn and Corriol (1962). In our experiments, there was never any vasodilatation in skeletal muscle unless the muscle contracted. The vasodilatation was resistant to guanethidine (3–4 mg/kg, i.v.) and to atropine (0.4–0.8 mg/kg, i.v.), unless the latter reduced the contraction: it was abolished by gallamine triethiodide (3–4 mg/kg, i.v.) or by cordotomy at the level of L_4-L_5. The vasodilatation, therefore, was secondary to muscle contraction — in reality an example of functional hyperaemia (Hilton et al., 1975). This might have been missed by earlier workers, because the muscle contractions are relatively weak and, in our experience, are best assessed by registering electromyographic activity from the whole limb. We have not yet found any way of eliciting the pattern of cardiovascular response characteristic of the defence reaction from higher parts of the brain except by stimulation of the stria terminalis–amygdala system. We have preliminary evidence, however, of cortical inhibition of conduction from the amygdala to the hypothalamus, chiefly from a small area between the premotor and motor cortex.

Significant features of the cardiovascular response in the defence reaction are an increase in mean blood pressure and pulse pressure together with a large tachycardia. As it seemed hardly likely, therefore, that the baroreceptor reflex was functioning normally, I tested its efficacy some time ago and found that it could be virtually completely suppressed (Hilton, 1963).

It seems appropriate to designate the system which the baroreceptor inputs bring intó play as a "deactivating system". We now know much about the topographical organisation of this "deactivating system". As in the case of the arousal system, it also extends through the length of the brain stem, from the hypothalamus to medulla (Hilton and Spyer, 1971; Hilton, 1975). The "deactivating system" elicits a pattern of cardiovascular response almost exactly opposite to the alerting system and, under the right conditions, it can suppress it (Bartorelli et al., 1960). These systems thus appear to be mutually inhibitory and it is a challenging reflection that one is brought into action by baroreceptor afferents and the other by chemoreceptor afferents.

There is already a report of activation of single neurones in the medial hypothalamus on sinus nerve stimulation, presumably of chemoreceptor fibres (Thomas and Calaresu, 1972). In the case of inhibition by the alerting system of the deactivating system, moreover, we now have good evidence that conduction can be blocked in the baroreceptor afferent pathway (McAllen, 1976).

Accordingly, it has been natural to suggest that, if an individual were subject to prolonged arousal, verging on fear, the cardiovascular adjustments necessarily entailed might initiate real hypertension (Hilton, 1965). With the passage of time, however, this idea has become difficult to sustain. Hypertensive subjects show good responses to baroreceptor stimulation, to such an extent that electrical stimulation of the sinus nerve is currently in use as a means of therapeutic control. Even more telling, however, has been the finding that subjects suffering from chronic anxiety states show all the cardiovascular features of the defence response, including a large increase in muscle blood flow (Kelly and Walker, 1968). Indeed, a return of muscle blood flow towards normal may be the best early indication of successful therapy. If there were a real connexion between long-term defence responses and hypertension, it should show up in these patients. Yet, as far as I know, no one has reported it.

To return, finally, to my main theme, there is no need to emphasize the long-known fact that the anterior hypothalamus plays a major role in temperature regulation. Recent work has been more concerned with the elucidation of the patterns of cardiovascular response in the reaction to heating or cooling, notably that by Simon and his co-workers (Kullmann et al., 1970; Riedel et al., 1972). Muscle blood flow changes in the same direction as skin blood flow though to a lesser extent, but splanchnic blood flow changes in the opposite direction, thus keeping the balance of total peripheral resistance much the same. This pattern, like that in the arousal reaction, is organised centrally in the nervous system and does not require the intervention of the baroreceptor reflex.

In conclusion, therefore, the deactivating system and the baroreceptor input to it do not seem to be so important for short-term homoeostasis. Perhaps we should concentrate more on the long-term setting of equilibrium levels to understand the part played by this system, in interaction mainly with the arousal system, in normal as well as abnormal physiology.

SUMMARY

The defence (or arousal) reaction and the baroreceptor (or deactivating) response are in constant interplay in daily life: each has its own characteristic pattern of cardiovascular response. The topographical organisation of the brain stem regions integrating each pattern of response is longitudinally distributed through the length of the brain stem, from hypothalamus to medulla. Higher parts of the brain can excite the defence response via specific regions of the amygdala: the motor cortex is not involved, indeed the only cortical influence detected so far has been inhibitory. This influence could be exerted through the deactivating system; for strong activation of either system can suppress the other. The neurophysiological basis of this mutual inhibition is being studied. Present evidence suggests, however, that this is not a mechanism underlying hypertension. It is concluded that the deactivating system and the baroreceptor input to it are not so important for short-term homoeostasis as has been thought hitherto.

REFERENCES

Abrahams, V.C., Hilton, S.M. and Zbrożyna, A.W. (1960) Active muscle vasodilatation produced by stimulation of the brain stem: its significance in the defence reaction. *J. Physiol. (Lond.)*, 154: 491—513.

Bartorelli, C., Bizzi, E., Libretti, A. and Zanchetti, A. (1960) Inhibitory control of sinocarotid pressoceptive afferents on hypothalamic autonomic activity and sham-rage behaviour. *Arch. ital. Biol.*, 98: 308—326.

Bizzi, E., Libretti, A., Malliani, A. and Zanchetti, A. (1961) Reflex chemoceptive excitation of diencephalic sham-rage behaviour. *Amer. J. Physiol.*, 200: 923—926.

Coote, J.H., Hilton, S.M. and Zbrożyna, A.W. (1973) The ponto-medullary area integrating the defence reaction in the cat and its influence on muscle blood flow. *J. Physiol. (Lond.)*, 229: 257—274.

Eliasson, S., Lindgren, P. and Uvnäs, B. (1952) Representation in the hypothalamic and the motor cortex in the dog of the sympathetic vasodilator outflow to the skeletal muscles. *Acta physiol. scand.*, 27: 18—37.

Hilton, S.M. (1963) Inhibition of baroreceptor reflexes on hypothalamic stimulation. *J. Physiol. (Lond.)*, 165: 56—57P.

Hilton, S.M. (1965) Hypothalamic control of the cardiovascular responses in fear and rage. *Sci. Basis Med. Ann. Rev.*: 217—238.

Hilton, S.M. (1975) Ways of viewing the central nervous control of the circulation — old and new. *Brain Res.*, 87: 213—219.

Hilton, S.M. and Joels, N. (1964) Facilitation of chemoreceptor reflexes during the defence reaction. *J. Physiol. (Lond.)*, 176: 20—22P.

Hilton, S.M. and Spyer, K.M. (1971) Participation of the anterior hypothalamus in the baroreceptor reflex. *J. Physiol. (Lond.)*, 218: 271—293.

Hilton, S.M. and Zbrożyna, A.W. (1963) Amygdaloid region for defence reactions and its efferent pathway to the brain stem. *J. Physiol. (Lond.)*, 165: 160—173.

Hilton, S.M., Spyer, K.M. and Timms, R.J. (1975) Hind limb vasodilatation evoked by stimulation of the motor cortex. *J. Physiol. (Lond.)*, 252: 22—23P.

Kelly, D.H.W. and Walter, C.J.S. (1968) The relationship between clinical diagnosis and anxiety, assessed by forearm blood flow and other measurements. *Brit. J. Psychiat.*, 114: 611—626.

Kullman, R., Schonung, W. and Simon, E. (1970) Antagonistic changes of blood flow and sympathetic activity in different vascular beds following central thermal stimulation. 1. Blood flow in skin, muscle and intestine during spinal cord heating and cooling in anaesthetized dogs. *Pflügers Arch. ges. Physiol.*, 319: 146—161.

McAllen, R.M. (1976) Inhibition of the baroreceptor input to the medulla by stimulation of the hypothalamic defence area. *J. Physiol. (Lond.)*, 257: 45P.

McAllen, R.M. and Spyer, K.M. (1976) The location of cardial preganglionic motoneurones in the medulla of the cat. *J. Physiol. (Lond.)*, 258: 187—204.

Riedel, W., Iriki, M. and Simon, E. (1972) Regional differentiation of sympathetic activity during peripheral heating and cooling in anaesthetized rabbits. *Pflügers Arch. ges. Physiol.*, 332: 239—247.

Thomas, M.R. and Calaresu, F.R. (1972) Responses of single units in the medial hypothalamus to electrical stimulation of the sinus nerve in the cat. *Brain Res.*, 44: 49—62.

Zwirn, P. et Corriol, J. (1962) Fibres corticopyramidales dilatatrices des membres. *Arch. Sci. physiol.*, 16: 325—345.

SESSION II

NEUROTRANSMISSION IN RELATION TO CARDIOVASCULAR CONTROL

Chairmen: J.P. Chalmers (Adelaide)
D.H.G. Versteeg (Utrecht)

The Role of Central Catecholamines in the Control of Blood Pressure through the Baroreceptor Reflex and the Nasopharyngeal Reflex in the Rabbit

J.P. CHALMERS, S.W. WHITE, J.B. GEFFEN and R. RUSH

Departments of Medicine and Physiology, Flinders Medical Centre, Bedford Park, Adelaide, South Australia 5042 (Australia)

INTRODUCTION

There is now a great deal of evidence that central catecholaminergic neurones participate in the regulation of arterial blood pressure, both in normal animals and in animals with experimental hypertension (Chalmers, 1975). In particular there is good evidence for participation of these neurones in baroreflex control of blood pressure and in the development of neurogenic hypertension (Chalmers and Wurtman, 1971; Chalmers and Reid, 1972; Doba and Reis, 1974; Chalmers, 1975). In this paper we will briefly review the role of central catecholamines in baroreceptor control of pressure and then describe more recent experiments from our laboratory on the role of central catecholaminergic nerves in the control of blood pressure through the nasopharyngeal reflex.

CENTRAL CATECHOLAMINERGIC NERVES AND ARTERIAL BARORECEPTOR REFLEXES

The arterial baroreceptor reflex is illustrated schematically in Fig. 1. The reflex functions as a homoeostatic mechanism regulating arterial pressure through a negative feedback loop which acts to minimise any change in pressure and return arterial pressure back towards its set-point (Korner, 1971). This negative feedback mechanism depends upon the presence of inhibitory neurones between the afferent and efferent limbs of the reflex (Fig. 1). The afferent neurones arise from the carotid sinus and aortic arch and make their primary synapse in the nucleus of the tractus solitarii (NTS). The efferent limb effectively begins with bulbospinal neurones having their cell bodies in the brain stem in various "vasomotor" areas (VMC) and terminating in the intermediolateral cell columns of the spinal cord. Here, the bulbospinal neurones synapse either directly, or indirectly through short interneurones, with the sympathetic preganglionic neurones which pass out in the thoracolumbar outflow of the peripheral autonomic system (Fig. 1). The pathway between NTS and the vasopressor areas (or VMC) is polysynaptic, and it is within this polysynaptic pathway that the inhibitory neurones are located. For

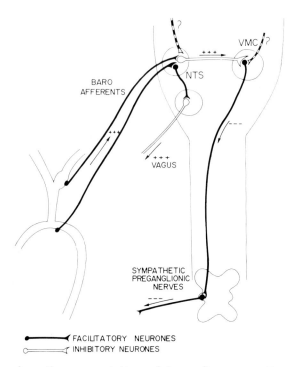

Fig. 1. Simplified schematic representation of baroreflex connections showing afferent nerves from arterial baroreceptors making their primary synapse in the nucleus of the tractus solitarii (NTS), inhibitory neurones from the NTS to the vasomotor centre (VMC), descending facilitatory bulbospinal vasomotor neurones and sympathetic preganglionic nerves. Connections from the NTS to the vagal nuclei and efferent vagal fibres are also shown. Facilitatory neurones are black and inhibitory neurones are white. The half black-half white neurones connecting with the NTS and the VMC represent suprabulbar fibres which could be either inhibitory or facilitatory. The plus and minus signs indicate the reciprocal relationship between afferent traffic and efferent sympathetic activity. The pluses indicate an increase in activity and the minuses a decrease (Chalmers, 1975).

the sake of schematic simplicity this is drawn to show one inhibitory neurone only in Fig. 1. There is increasing evidence for modulation of baroreceptor reflex function from connections with higher centres, both ascending and descending (Korner, 1971; Doba and Reis, 1974). Activity in afferent fibres from arterial baroreceptors, stimulated by a rise in pressure, provides a major source of inhibition of central vasomotor tone and hence of peripheral sympathetic vasomotor activity. Deafferentation of the arterial baroreceptors eliminates this inhibition and hence causes an increase in sympathetic activity and an increase in pressure, accompanied by tachycardia (Heymans and Neil, 1958; De Quattro et al., 1969; Korner, 1971).

The pathways followed by central catecholaminergic nerves are similar to those of neurones subserving central cardiovascular control (Chalmers, 1975), and it would seem reasonable to suggest that the neurones participating in central cardiovascular control do in fact utilise catecholamines as neurotransmitters. This concept is supported by experiments in rabbits which show that sinoaortic denervation produces a selective increase in noradrenaline turnover in the hypothalamus and the thoracolumbar cord, measured by the rate of disappearance of intracisternally administered tritiated noradrenaline (Chalmers and Wurtman, 1971). The increase in hypothalamic noradrenaline turnover in this situation is consistent with the concept that baroreflex function is not mediated only at medullary level, but in fact utilises neural loops involving higher centres. The selective increase in noradrenaline turnover in the thoracolumbar cord (there was no significant change in turnover rate in cervical or lumbar segments) is consistent with an increase in the activity of bulbospinal noradrenergic nerves terminating in the lateral sympathetic horn. It should be noted that there are no monoaminergic cell bodies in the spinal cord (Dahlström and Fuxe, 1965) so that changes in noradrenaline metabolism in this region reflect changes in activity in nerve endings of descending bulbospinal noradrenergic tracts. The observation that sinoaortic denervation accelerates noradrenaline turnover in the thoracolumbar cord has been supported by the finding that the activity of tyrosine hydroxylase, the rate limiting enzyme in catecholamine biosynthesis, is also selectively increased in this region (Chalmers and Wurtman, 1971).

On the basis of these experiments it was suggested that bulbospinal catecholaminergic nerves mediate baroreceptor reflexes, and that bulbospinal vasomotor neurones utilise catecholamines as neurotransmitters. This suggestion has been strengthened by the finding that destruction of central catecholaminergic nerves, by intracisternal administration of 6-hydroxy-dopamine (6-OHDA), does in fact prevent and reverse the hypertension produced by sinoaortic denervation in the rabbit (Chalmers and Reid, 1972). Doba and Reis (1973, 1974) have made similar observations in a different model of neurogenic hypertension, produced by central deafferentation of the baroreflexes using stereotactic lesions of the NTS in the rat. These workers have found that intracisternal 6-OHDA prevents the increase in pressure seen after this mode of baroreceptor deafferentation.

It has also been shown that destruction of catecholaminergic nerves in the NTS, by local stereotactic injection of 6-OHDA into this nucleus, produces an increase in blood pressure lasting about 10 days (Doba and Reis, 1974). These authors have therefore suggested that, whereas bulbospinal noradrenergic nervous activity facilitates an increase in pressure, the activity of catechol-aminergic nerves synapsing in the NTS depresses arterial pressure. This suggestion is further supported by experiments in which local injection of noradrenaline into the NTS decreased arterial pressure in rats (De Jong, 1974). The simplest explanation for this phenomenon might be that there are catecholaminergic nerves terminating in the NTS (originating either from higher centres such as the hypothalamus, or from within the brain stem) synapsing with the inhibitory neurones drawn in Fig. 1.

CENTRAL CATECHOLAMINERGIC NERVES AND THE NASOPHARYNGEAL REFLEX

In more recent experiments, we have looked in greater depth at the mechanism whereby central administration of 6-OHDA affects arterial pressure and sought to delineate in more detail some of the peripheral autonomic mechanisms mediated by reflex activation of central catecholaminergic neurones. In these experiments, we have used a different model, namely the rabbit exposed to vaporous stimuli, which when present in the inspired air, stimulate nasopharyngeal receptors to produce marked reflex activation of peripheral sympathetic vasoconstrictor fibres. The nasopharyngeal reflex produces a response in terrestial animals such as the rabbit, which is in many ways analogous to that seen in the diving response in marine animals (White et al., 1974, 1975). In brief, the reflex response consists of apnoea in expiration, bradycardia, little change or a rise in blood pressure and widespread peripheral vasoconstriction (White et al., 1974, 1975). Trigeminal nerve afferents originating in the nares are responsible for the apnoea, the duration of which is influenced by arterial chemoreceptor activity; the circulatory response is again mainly evoked by trigeminal afferents with a contribution from arterial baroreceptor reflexes (White et al., 1975). The cardiovascular elements of the reflex appear to be integrated mainly at bulbospinal sites with some modulation from suprabulbar areas.

In the present experiments, we used intracisternal 6-OHDA (600 μg/kg) to examine the role of central catecholaminergic mechanisms in this reflex. In order to facilitate the analysis of the cardiovascular responses, the experiments were carried out both with and without intravenous sodium pentobarbitone (30 mg/kg), which is known to interfere centrally with resting and reflex vagal activity (Crocker et al., 1967). Cigarette smoke and ammonia were used to evoke the nasopharyngeal reflex in the rabbit. Arterial pressure and heart rate were recorded through a cannula in the ear artery of the rabbit and flow was measured in the hindlimb by chronically implanted Doppler flow probes placed around the lower abdominal aorta, immediately above the bifurcation (White et al., 1974).

The effects of intracisternal 6-OHDA and intravenous sodium pento-barbitone on resting cardiovascular parameters are shown in Fig. 2. In 6 rabbits the mean heart rate was 247 ± 10.0 (S.E.M.) bpm and this fell to 199 ± 21.5 (S.E.M.) bpm one week after 6-OHDA ($P_{\text{diff}} < 0.001$). In the same rabbits intravenous sodium pentobarbitone caused a rise in heart rate from 247 ± 10.0 (S.E.M.) bpm to 297 ± 15.2 (S.E.M.) bpm ($P_{\text{diff}} < 0.001$). When intravenous sodium pentobarbitone was given to animals previously treated with 6-OHDA, the resting heart rate rose from 199 ± 21.5 to 249 ± 20.2 ($P_{\text{diff}} < 0.001$). The resting mean arterial pressure, hindlimb flow and hindlimb conductance were not significantly altered by either 6-OHDA i.c. or sodium pentobarbitone i.v. (Fig. 2). The restoration of the resting heart rate to 249 bpm by the injection of sodium pentobarbitone in animals pretreated with 6-OHDA suggests that the resting bradycardia induced by 6-OHDA is due in large part to centrally mediated reduction of resting cardiac sympathetic activity; if the activity of cardiac sympathetic nerves was normal in these animals, then central suppression of vagal activity with sodium pentobarbitone might have been expected to elevate heart rate, towards the levels seen in normal animals given this anaesthetic, viz. about 300 bpm. These results are consistent with previous experiments which suggested that the resting bradycardia induced by 6-OHDA was in part due to decreased cardiac sympathetic activity and also in part due

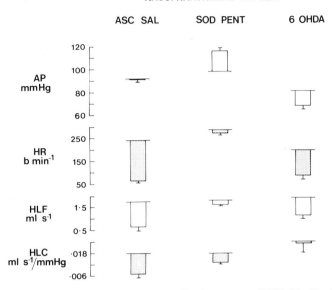

Fig. 2. Peak changes in mean arterial pressure (AP), heart rate (HR), hindlimb flow (HLF), and hindlimb conductance (HLC) following exposure to smoke in 6 rabbits which were sequentially tested (1) one week after intracisternal injection of 0.9% saline containing ascorbic acid (ASC SAL), (2) while anaesthetised with sodium pentobarbitone (SOD PENT, 30 mg/kg) and (3) one week after intracisternal injection of 6-hydroxydopamine (6-OHDA, 600 μg/kg). Values are means plus the standard error of the mean change as determined by analysis of variance.

to destruction of central noradrenergic tracts that normally inhibit the vagus (vagal disinhibition) (Chalmers and Reid, 1972). The results of these two studies (i.e., the present studies and those of Chalmers and Reid, 1972) clearly imply that the resting bradycardia produced by 6-OHDA has a complex mechanism originating both from destruction of noradrenergic bulbospinal fibres facilitating cardiac sympathetic activity, and from destruction of central noradrenergic neurones inhibiting cardiac vagal activity.

When animals inhaled cigarette smoke through the nose there was apnoea, little change in mean arterial pressure, a marked bradycardia, and a marked reduction in hindlimb blood flow and conductance (Fig. 2; left panels). Following intravenous sodium pentobarbitone the same stimulus caused transient slowing of respiration, and the reflex bradycardia was almost abolished but there was a substantial rise in arterial pressure and a significant fall in hindlimb conductance indicating that while reflex cardiac vagal activity was almost abolished, the peripheral sympathetic vasoconstrictor mechanism was still largely intact (Fig. 2; middle panels).

One week after intracisternal 6-OHDA, nasopharyngeal stimulation evoked apnoea and bradycardia. However, in contrast to the experiments described above (middle and left panels of Fig. 2), arterial blood pressure fell and the fall in hindlimb conductance was significantly attenuated (Fig. 2; right panels). These results suggest that 6-OHDA has a selective effect on central noradrenergic neurones subserving sympathetic vasoconstrictor mechanisms. In addition

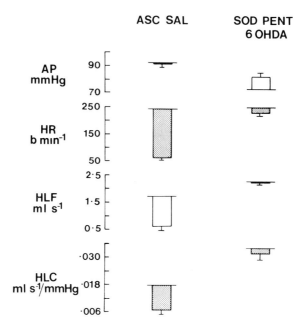

ASC SAL   SOD PENT
                 6 OHDA

AP mmHg

HR b min⁻¹

HLF ml s⁻¹

HLC ml s⁻¹/mmHg

Fig. 3. Peak changes in the same 6 rabbits shown in Fig. 2 following exposure to cigarette smoke (1) one week after intracisternal injection of 0.9% saline containing ascorbic acid (left panels), and (2) during anaesthesia with sodium pentobarbitone (30 mg/kg) one week after intracisternal injection of 6-hydroxydopamine (600 μg/kg). Notation is as in Fig. 2.

it seems likely that the vagal elements of the reflex are largely intact, since although the absolute magnitude of the bradycardia is less, this has to be interpreted in the presence of a fall in pressure in these animals (evoking a different baroreceptor response) compared to a maintenance of pressure in normal animals (Fig. 2).

In an extension of these experiments, intravenous sodium pentobarbitone was given to animals previously treated with 6-OHDA. Following naso-pharyngeal stimulation in these experiments, apnoea still occurred and there was a small rise in arterial pressure and a slight fall in hindlimb conductance (Fig. 3). In other words, the cardiovascular disturbance of nasopharyngeal stimulation can be virtually eliminated by the selective attenuation of the two major autonomic components of the response, namely, the vagal mechanism by sodium pentobarbitone and the sympathetic vasoconstrictor mechanism by 6-OHDA.

At the end of the experiments the animals were sacrificed, and the brains removed and dissected over ice into 5 regions — medulla-pons, midbrain, cerebellum, hypothalamus and telencephalon — and brain noradrenaline was extracted and assayed as previously described (Chalmers and Wurtman, 1971). The noradrenaline concentration in these brain regions was reduced to about 50% of control in the 6-OHDA treated animals, as previously reported in this species (Chalmers and Reid, 1972). Dopamine-beta-hydroxylase (DBH) activity and phenylethanolamine-N-methyl-transferase (PNMT) activity were also

TABLE I

DBH AND PNMT ACTIVITIES IN BRAIN REGIONS

	DBH (p moles/mg/hr)		PNMT (p moles/mg/hr)	
	Control animals (n = 6)	6-OHDA treated animals (n = 6)	Control animals (n = 6)	6-OHDA treated animals (n = 6)
Telencephalon	156.9 ± 21.1	70.0 ± 14.6	1.11 ± 0.17	0.95 ± 0.20
Midbrain	171.1 ± 24.2	106.7 ± 23.6	0.691 ± 0.05	0.633 ± 0.12
Medulla-pons	474.6 ± 64.0	210.4 ± 13.7	0.478 ± 0.05	0.465 ± 0.08
Cerebellum	141.2 ± 11.1	71.7 ± 16.5	0.653 ± 0.10	0.665 ± 0.09
Spinal cord	76.0 ± 9.6	15.4 ± 3.7	1.001 ± 0.11	0.961 ± 0.12

Values are means ± S.E.M.

assayed in these 5 brain regions using the assays described by Deguchi and Barchas (1971) and Kato et al. (1974).

The data from preliminary experiments (Table 1) revealed that the activity of DBH was reduced to about 50% of control in all regions, whereas the activity of PNMT was virtually unchanged. This confirms the suggestion of Reid (1975), that central neurones using the putative neurotransmitter, adrenaline, are relatively resistant to the actions of 6-OHDA, compared to noradrenergic nerves. It also suggests that the central catecholaminergic nerves contributing to the nasopharyngeal reflex utilise noradrenaline rather than adrenaline as a neurotransmitter.

CONCLUSIONS

Experiments on the role of central catecholaminergic nerves in neurogenic hypertension and in baroreflex control of arterial pressure have previously demonstrated that bulbospinal catecholaminergic neurones participate in the central regulation of blood pressure and form an integral component of the baroreceptor reflex arc. The present experiments, using the nasopharyngeal reflex to study cardiovascular control, further suggest that the regulation of arterial pressure involves the participation of central catecholaminergic neurones mediating peripheral sympathetic vasoconstrictor activity. Furthermore the data on DBH and PNMT activity suggest that these central catecholaminergic nerves utilise noradrenaline as a neurotransmitter. It seems possible that noradrenergic bulbospinal nerves form an essential link in the central control of blood pressure in a number of cardiovascular reflexes.

SUMMARY

There is good evidence that central monoaminergic nerves participate in baroreflex control of the circulation. In particular, there is evidence that bulbospinal catecholaminergic fibres terminating in the lateral horns of the spinal cord form an essential element in the baroreflex arc and mediate changes in efferent sympathetic activity. Catecholaminergic nerves also appear to play a part in a brain stem depressor mechanism involving the nucleus tractus solitarii, the site of primary synapse for afferent fibres from the arterial baroreceptors.

We have recently examined the role of central catecholamines in another cardiovascular reflex — the "smoke reflex". This is a trigeminal nerve reflex that produces a pronounced sympathetic vasoconstriction and a vagally mediated bradycardia in response to cigarette smoke stimulation of the nasopharynx of the rabbit. Following intracisternal 6-hydroxydopamine (6-OHDA), the vasoconstrictor component of the response was inactivated, but the bradycardia appeared to be unaffected. At the end of experiments, measurements were made of regional brain noradrenaline concentration, dopamine-beta-hydroxylase (DBH) activity and phenylethanolamine-N-methyl-transferase (PNMT) activity. In animals receiving 6-OHDA, noradrenaline concentration and DBH activity were reduced to about 50% of control, but PNMT activity was unchanged. These data suggest that central pathways mediating vasoconstriction in response to nasopharyngeal stimulation, utilise noradrenaline rather than adrenaline as a neurotransmitter.

ACKNOWLEDGEMENTS

This work was supported by a grant from the National Health and Medical Research Council of Australia.

We would like to thank Mrs. Soi Yen Lewis and Mrs. Lorraine Rosenberg for their expert technical assistance.

REFERENCES

Chalmers, J.P. (1975) Brain amines and models of experimental hypertension. *Circulat. Res.*, 36: 469—480.

Chalmers, J.P. and Reid, J.L. (1972) Participation of central noradrenergic neurones in arterial baroreceptor reflexes in the rabbit: a study with intracisternally administered 6-hydroxydopamine. *Circulat. Res.*, 31: 789—804.

Chalmers, J.P. and Wurtman, R.J. (1971) Participation of central noradrenergic neurones in arterial baroreceptor reflexes in the rabbit. *Circulat. Res.*, 28: 480—491.

Crocker, E.F., Johnson, R.O., Korner, P.I., Uther, J.B. and White, S.W. (1968) Effects of hyperventilation on the circulatory response of the rabbit to arterial hypoxia. *J. Physiol. (Lond.)*, 199: 267—282.

Dahlström, A. and Fuxe, K. (1965) Evidence for the existence of monoamine neurones in the central nervous system. II. Experimentally induced changes in the intraneuronal amine levels of bulbospinal neurone systems. *Acta physiol. scand.*, 64, Suppl. 247: 1—37.

Deguchi, T. and Barchas, J. (1971) Inhibition of transmethylation of biogenic amines by S-adenosylhomocysteine. *J. biol. Chem.*, 246: 3175—3181.

De Jong, W. (1974) Noradrenaline: central inhibitory control of blood pressure and heart rate. *Europ. J. Pharmacol.*, 29: 179—181.

De Quattro, V., Nagatsu, T., Maronde, R. and Alexander, N. (1969) Catecholamine synthesis in rabbits with neurogenic hypertension. *Circulat. Res.*, 24: 545—555.

Doba, N. and Reis, D.J. (1973) Acute fulminating neurogenic hypertension produced by brainstem lesions in the rat. *Circulat. Res.*, 32: 584—593.

Doba, N. and Reis, D.J. (1974) Role of central and peripheral adrenergic mechanisms in neurogenic hypertension produced by brainstem lesion in rats. *Circulat. Res.*, 34: 293—301.

Heymans, C. and Neil, E. (1958) *Reflexogenic Areas of the Cardiovascular System*, Churchill, London.

Kato, T., Kuzuya, H. and Nagatsu, T. (1974) A simple and sensitive assay for dopamine-β-hydroxylase activity by dual wavelength spectrophotometry. *Biochem. Med.*, 10: 320—328.

Korner, P.I. (1971) Integrative neural cardiovascular control. *Physiol. Rev.*, 51: 312—367.

Reid, J.L. (1975) Discussion remark. In *Central Action of Drugs in Blood Pressure Regulation*, D.S. Davies and J.L. Reid (Eds.), Pitman Medical, London, p. 35.

White, S.W., McRitchie, R.J. and Franklin, D.L. (1974) Autonomic cardiovascular effects of nasal inhalation of cigarette smoke in the rabbit. *Aust. J. exp. Biol. med. Sci.*, 52: 111—126.

White, S.W., McRitchie, R.J. and Korner, P.I. (1975) Central nervous system control of cardiorespiratory nasopharyngeal reflexes in the rabbit. *Amer. J. Physiol.*, 228: 404—409.

Neuronal Mechanisms Influencing Transmission in the Baroreceptor Reflex Arc

GUENTHER HAEUSLER

Pharmaceutical Research Department,
F. Hoffmann-La Roche and Co., Ltd., Basel (Switzerland)

THE BARORECEPTOR REFLEX AND CENTRAL ADRENERGIC NEURONES

Anatomical studies on the course of baroreceptor reflex fibres in various species have located the major part of the terminations of the primary afferents from baroreceptors contained in the vagal and glossopharyngeal nerves within the divisions of the nucleus of the solitary tract (Torvik, 1956; Kerr, 1962; Cottle, 1964; Rhoton et al., 1966). These morphological findings have been supported on the whole by several electrophysiological investigations (Hellner and von Baumgarten, 1961; Calaresu and Pearce, 1965; Crill and Reis, 1968; Miura and Reis, 1969; Seller and Illert, 1969; Miura and Reis, 1972). Although projections of the nucleus of the solitary tract to the nucleus ambiguus, the paramedian reticular nucleus, the nucleus intercalatus and the intermediate nucleus have been described in the cat (Cottle and Calaresu, 1975), the further course of the baroreceptor reflex arc and the localization of its second synapse is not known. Similarly, the neurotransmitters operating within the baroreceptor reflex arc have not yet been identified. In this respect attention has been focussed recently on central adrenergic neurones.

In various types of experimental or genetic hypertension, alterations of the turnover of noradrenaline have been found in the hypothalamus, the medulla oblongata or the spinal cord (Chalmers and Wurtman, 1971; Nakamura et al., 1971a, b; Chalmers and Reid, 1972). Sinoaortic denervation in rabbits caused an increase in the turnover of noradrenaline and in the activity of tyrosine hydroxylase in the thoracolumbar segments of the spinal cord (Chalmers and Wurtman, 1971). On this basis, it has been postulated that section of the buffer nerves augments the activity of descending bulbospinal adrenergic neurones by releasing them from baroreceptor inhibition and this increased activity in turn mediates the rise in arterial blood pressure (Chalmers and Wurtman, 1971; Chalmers and Reid, 1972; Chalmers, 1975). In a recent review, Chalmers (1975) defined the role of central adrenergic neurones with regard to peripheral sympathetic nervous activity as inhibitory on the bulbar level, and as excitatory on the spinal level. The latter conclusion is supported by a study of Neumayr et al. (1974) in which drug-induced stimulation of spinal α-adrenoceptors was found to facilitate excitatory transmission to the preganglionic sympathetic neurone.

96

Evidence for a relationship between central adrenergic neurones and the baroreceptor reflex function stems also from another source. It was suggested that the action of clonidine, a hypotensive drug which reduces sympathetic nervous activity (Kobinger and Walland, 1967; Schmitt et al., 1968; Schmitt and Schmitt, 1969; Haeusler, 1973, 1974a, c), resembles an activation of the central part of the baroreceptor reflex (Haeusler, 1973, 1974a, 1975). Among several pieces of evidence, it was shown that the reduction of spontaneous sympathetic nervous activity in response to bilateral electrical stimulation of the carotid sinus nerves was augmented by clonidine (Fig. 1), resulting in a shift of the frequency-response curve of sinus nerve stimulation to lower frequencies (Fig. 2). Since the sympatho-inhibitory effect of clonidine is related to a

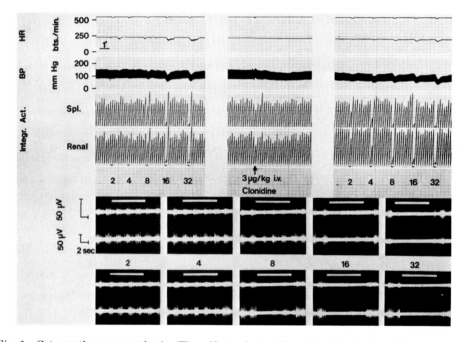

Fig. 1. Cat, urethane anaesthesia. The effect of clonidine (3 µg/kg i.v.) on the response to bilateral carotid sinus nerve stimulation of heart rate, blood pressure and spontaneous sympathetic nerve activity. The 4 channels of the pen record show from top to bottom: heart rate, blood pressure and the integrated electrical activity of the right sympathetic preganglionic splanchnic and a sympathetic postganglionic renal nerve in arbitrary units. The left panel of the pen record presents the effects of bilateral sinus nerve stimulation with increasing frequencies (2, 4, 8, 16 and 32 Hz) under control conditions, the middle panel the absence of a major effect of clonidine (3 µg/kg i.v.) on the parameters recorded and the right panel the facilitation of the depressor baroreceptor reflex after clonidine. The original oscilloscope recordings below the pen records show the effect of a 10 sec bilateral sinus nerve stimulation on the spontaneous activity in the splanchnic (upper trace) and a renal sympathetic nerve (lower trace) before (upper row of photographs) and after (lower row of photographs) the injection of clonidine. The photographs correspond to the respective events on the pen record. The white horizontal bars in the oscilloscope recordings indicate the duration of bilateral sinus nerve stimulation. The calibrations are given on the left side of the left panel. The time between left and middle panel was 10 min, between middle and right panel 25 min. (Reprinted from Haeusler (1974a) with permission.)

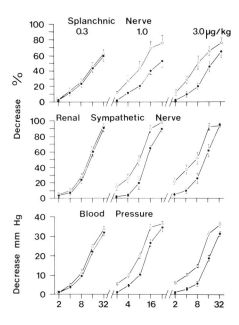

Fig. 2. The effect of 3 doses of clonidine (0.3, 1 and 3 μg/kg i.v.) on the response to a 10 sec bilateral sinus nerve stimulation (2, 4, 8, 16 and 32 Hz). The upper and the middle panel show the percent decrease in spontaneous activity of the splanchnic and renal sympathetic nerves, respectively; the lower panel shows the decrease in blood pressure (mm Hg). The numbers beneath the lower panel give the rate of stimulation in Hz. The frequency-response curves with the filled circles represent the response to sinus nerve stimulation before and those with the open circles 30 min after the i.v. injection of the respective doses of clonidine indicated on the top of the upper panel. For each frequency-response curve the mean values (± S.E.M. as vertical bars) of 6 experiments are shown. Only one dose of clonidine was given to each cat. (Reprinted from Haeusler (1974a) with permission.)

stimulation of central α-adrenoceptors (Schmitt and Schmitt, 1970; Schmitt et al., 1971; Haeusler, 1973), it seemed conceivable that central adrenergic neurones participate in the transmission of signals through the baroreceptor reflex arc. Such a function was suggested by Coote and Macleod (1974) for descending bulbospinal adrenergic neurones which, contrary to the postulates of Neumayr et al. (1974) and Chalmers (1975), would then inhibit the activity of the preganglionic sympathetic neurone.

Several experiments in our laboratory dealt with the question of whether central adrenergic neurones form an integral link within the baroreceptor reflex arc. Partial destruction of central adrenergic neurones by injection of 6-hydroxydopamine into a lateral brain ventricle of rats had no influence on the falls in blood pressure produced by bilateral electrical stimulation of the sinus nerves (Haeusler and Lewis, 1975). Similarly, pretreatment of rabbits with intraventricular injections of 6-hydroxydopamine virtually did not change the relationship between drug-induced rises of blood pressure and the resulting bradycardia (Haeusler and Lewis, 1975). These results militate against a participation of central adrenergic neurones in the baroreceptor reflex

TABLE I

NORADRENALINE CONTENT OF SEVERAL BRAIN
REGIONS AND OF THE SPINAL CORD IN CONTROL
CATS AND AFTER PRETREATMENT FOR
SUPPRESSION OF SYNTHESIS AND STORAGE OF
NORADRENALINE

Pretreatment consisted of i.p. injections of reserpine
(5 mg/kg) and the methylester of α-methyl-p-tyrosine
(2 x 300 mg/kg). Noradrenaline content was determined
fluorimetrically 15 hr after reserpine and the first dose of
α-methyl-p-tyrosine and 2 hr after the second dose. Given
are the mean values ± S.E.M. of 5 cats.

	Noradrenaline content	
Region of the CNS	Controls (ng/g)	Pretreated cats (ng/g)
Tele-diencephalon	210 ± 18	<5
Mesencephalon	347 ± 21	<5
Cerebellum	147 ± 15	<5
Pons	295 ± 24	<5
Medulla oblongata	223 ± 39	<5
Spinal cord	185 ± 19	<5

function. However, destruction of central adrenergic neurones by intraventricular 6-hydroxydopamine is known to be incomplete and transmission through the reflex arc may have been maintained in these experiments by residual adrenergic neurones.

A very marked depletion of central and peripheral stores of noradrenaline was achieved in another series of experiments by pretreatment of cats with a high dose of reserpine (5 mg/kg, i.p.). In addition, the biosynthesis of noradrenaline was inhibited in these animals by two i.p. doses of 300 mg/kg α-methyl-p-tyrosine. This combined treatment reduced the noradrenaline content of various parts of the brain and the spinal cord to very low levels (< 5 ng/g tissue) (Table I). The spontaneous sympathetic nervous activity of these animals as recorded from the preganglionic splanchnic and a postganglionic renal nerve was much higher than in controls and did not show the characteristic discharge pattern synchronous with respiration. The high discharge rate of the sympathetic nerves apparently resulted from the low blood pressure of noradrenaline-depleted animals, since the elevation of blood pressure by an infusion of angiotensin or noradrenaline caused a prompt reduction of sympathetic nervous activity. This observation indicates a functional integrity of the baroreceptor reflex even after marked noradrenaline depletion. In order to evaluate more precisely the function of the reflex under these conditions, the reflex was activated by bilateral electrical stimulation of the carotid sinus nerves with various frequencies; Fig. 3 shows that the stimulation produced percentagewise a very similar reduction of preganglionic and postganglionic sympathetic nervous activity in controls and depleted animals (Haeusler, 1974b; Haeusler and Lewis, 1975). This finding seems to

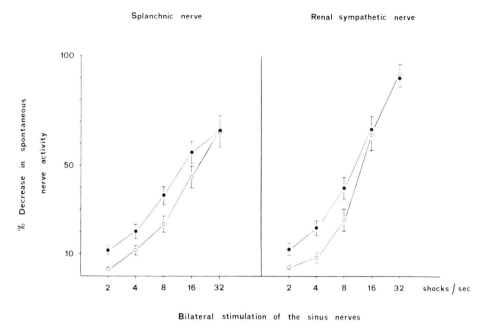

Fig. 3. The effect of noradrenaline depletion (see text and Table I) on the decrease in spontaneous activity of the sympathetic preganglionic splanchnic and a sympathetic postganglionic renal nerve produced by bilateral stimulation of the carotid sinus nerves. Controls ($\circ$———$\circ$), cats pretreated with reserpine and α-methyl-p-tyrosine ($\bullet$———$\bullet$). Given are the mean values ± S.E.M. (as vertical bars) of 8 cats.

exclude the possibility that descending bulbospinal adrenergic neurones are an integral part of the baroreceptor reflex arc. However, another possibility still exists, namely that central adrenergic neurones project onto the baroreceptor reflex arc and modulate impulse transmission through the reflex. In this context it is interesting to note that noradrenaline depletion prevented neither the sympatho-inhibitory effect of clonidine (Haeusler, 1974c) nor the clonidine-induced and vagally mediated reduction of heart rate in response to rises in blood pressure (Kobinger and Pichler, 1975).

REGULATION OF SYMPATHETIC NERVOUS ACTIVITY THROUGH THE BARORECEPTOR REFLEX AT THE SPINAL LEVEL

Alexander (1946) proposed that the medullary depressor area is capable of reducing vasomotor outflow from the spinal cord independently of supraspinal mechanisms. Since this suggestion, an increasing amount of evidence has been accumulated indicating that the regulation of the activity of sympathetic neurones can occur even at the level of the spinal cord. Recently, Illert and Seller (1969), Illert and Gabriel (1970, 1972) and Coote and Macleod (1972, 1974, 1975) have located sympatho-inhibitory tracts within the dorsolateral funiculus and the ventrolateral and ventral funiculi of the spinal cord. It was concluded that these pathways descend from three regions of the medulla oblongata, two of which contain bulbospinal monoamine neurones originating in the ventrolateral reticular formation and the midline caudal raphe nuclei, and the other lying in the ventromedial reticular formation (Coote and Macleod, 1974).

Recently, Gebber et al. (1973) provided evidence that in the cat vasopressor outflow from the brain to the external carotid postganglionic sympathetic nerve is organized into two pathways. Postganglionic potentials evoked from the first pathway have a long latency (> 50 msec) and are susceptible to blockade upon baroreceptor reflex activation. Postganglionic potentials evoked from the second pathway are not inhibited by baroreceptor reflex activation and have shorter latencies. There are also two distinct sympatho-inhibitory systems which can be activated from the depressor region of the medial medulla oblongata (Snyder and Gebber, 1973). The first mimics the baroreceptor reflexes and inhibits the long-latency vasopressor response at a spinal level (see above). The second does not belong to the baroreceptor reflex system and inhibits at a supraspinal level transmission in the pressor pathway with short-latency sympathetic nerve responses (see above).

Recent experiments from our laboratory suggest that descending fibres of the baroreceptor reflex system affect transmission of sympatho-excitatory impulses at the spinal level. Cats anaesthetized with urethane were used for the studies. In the first series of experiments it was studied how a generalized excitation of the sympathetic nervous system produced by electrical stimulation of the posterior hypothalamus is influenced by a simultaneous activation of the baroreceptor reflex induced by bilateral electrical stimulation of the carotid sinus nerves. Stimulation of the posterior hypothalamus for 10 sec evoked a marked increase in the activities of sympathetic nerves as recorded from the preganglionic splanchnic nerve, from a branch to the adrenal glands and from a postganglionic renal nerve (Fig. 4). Furthermore, hypothalamic stimulation produced a rise in blood pressure and contractions of the nictitating membranes (Fig. 4). Although simultaneous stimulation of the carotid sinus nerves reduced responses to hypothalamic stimulation of blood pressure and sympathetic nerve activity, contractions of the nictitating membranes were left unaffected (Fig. 4). Similarly, pupillary dilatation and inhibition of jejunal peristalsis in response to hypothalamic stimulation (not shown in Fig. 4) were not diminished by simultaneous activation of the baroreceptor reflex. It is generally accepted that splanchnic discharges predominantly represent the activity of vasomotor fibres, although non-vascular structures such as intestinal smooth muscle are also innervated by the splanchnic nerve. This assumption is based within certain limits on the linear relationship between splanchnic discharge and blood pressure. The postganglionic renal nerve also follows such a relationship. There is no doubt concerning the importance of the adrenal medulla for the maintenance of cardiovascular homoeostasis. It would then follow that baroreceptor fibres interact with the sympatho-excitatory tracts descending from the hypothalamus in such a way that increased impulse flow to the cardiovascular organs is selectively suppressed by activation of the reflex. The stimulation-induced increase in sympathetic outflow to non-cardiovascular organs apparently remains uninfluenced by the baroreceptor reflex. This conclusion agrees with findings that

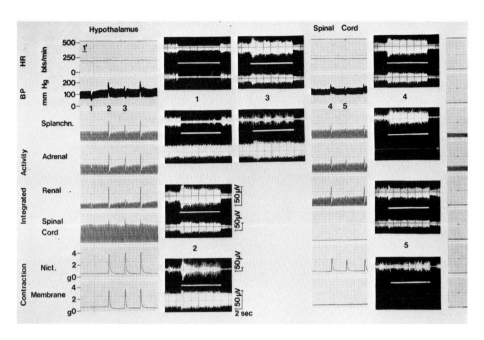

Fig. 4. Cat, urethane anaesthesia. The effect of an activation of the baroreceptor reflex produced by bilateral electrical stimulation of the carotid sinus nerves on the responses to electrical stimulation of the posterior hypothalamus (left panel of the pen record) or to electrical stimulation of a descending sympatho-excitatory tract in the right dorsolateral funiculus of the spinal cord at the level of C_4 (middle panel of the pen record). The 8 channels of the pen record show from top to bottom: heart rate, blood pressure, the integrated electrical activity in arbitrary units of a right sympathetic preganglionic splanchnic nerve, of a nerve to the right adrenal gland, of a right sympathetic postganglionic renal nerve and of a descending sympatho-excitatory tract in the right dorsolateral funiculus of the spinal cord at the level of C_4, contractile state of the right and left nictitating membranes. During that part of the experiment which is depicted on the middle panel, the electrode in the dorsolateral funiculus of the spinal cord was used for stimulation. Parameters of the stimulation with monophasic rectangular pulses were for the carotid sinus nerves 5 V, 2 msec, 16 Hz, for the posterior hypothalamus 10 V, 0.1 msec, 80 Hz and for the spinal cord 15 V, 0.1 msec, 80 Hz. The numbers in the second channel of the pen record correspond to the numbers of the oscilloscope recordings and show at which time in the course of the experiment the photographs were taken from the oscilloscope screen. Two photographs of the oscilloscope recordings separated by the aforementioned numbers present the same event. The respective upper photograph shows the electrical activity of the right splanchnic nerve (upper trace) and of a right adrenal nerve branch (lower trace), the respective lower photograph the electrical activity of a right sympathetic renal nerve (upper trace) and of the right dorsolateral funiculus of the spinal cord (lower trace). The white horizontal bars in the oscilloscope recordings indicate the duration (10 sec) of hypothalamic or spinal stimulation. The integrators which accumulated the input voltage from each nerve were reset to zero at 10 sec intervals. 1, the effect of bilateral electrical stimulation of the carotid sinus nerve; 2, the effect of electrical stimulation of the right posterior hypothalamus; 3, the effect of simultaneous stimulation of the posterior hypothalamus and the carotid sinus nerves; 4, the effect of electrical stimulation of a descending sympatho-excitatory tract in the right dorsolateral funiculus of the spinal cord at the level of C_4; 5, the effect of simultaneous stimulation of the spinal cord and the carotid sinus nerves. At the end of the experiment, the integrated activity of the nerve records after sacrifice of the animal was determined (right panel of the pen record). This part of the integrated activity is due to amplifier noise and other disturbances. All calibrations are given in the figure.

sympathetic gastric nerve activity contains approximately 80% of baroreceptor-independent components (Nisimaru, 1971) and that the major part of sympathetic skin nerve activity is not controlled by the baroreceptor reflex (Ninomiya et al., 1973).

It must be emphasized that in the present experiments a selective influence of the carotid sinus baroreceptor reflex was found on sympathetic discharges, elevated by hypothalamic stimulation. It is not clear whether such a selectivity would also hold when other sympatho-excitatory areas in the central nervous system are stimulated. Different effects of baroreceptor reflex activation on the discharge rate in various sympathetic nerves is suggestive of a segmental spinal organization of the baroreceptor reflex. The following are two observations which support this concept.

A descending sympatho-excitatory pathway was localized in the dorsolateral funiculus of the spinal cord by Illert and Gabriel (1972) in cats and by Barman and Wurster (1975) in dogs. When we explored this part of the spinal cord in cats at the level of C_4, we were able to record within the dorsolateral funiculus an increase in activity during hypothalamic stimulation (Fig. 4). Activation of the baroreceptor reflex by electrical stimulation of the carotid sinus nerves had no influence either on the basal activity recorded from the dorsolateral funiculus or on the increased activity during hypothalamic stimulation (Fig. 4). This observation indicates that an interaction between the baroreceptor reflex fibres and the sympatho-excitatory tracts descending from the hypothalamus does not occur to any major degree at a supraspinal level.

When the recording electrode in the dorsolateral funiculus was used as the stimulating electrode, the effects of stimulation on sympathetic nerve activity, blood pressure and contractile state of the nictitating membranes were qualitatively similar to those of hypothalamic stimulation with the exception that only the ipsilateral nictitating membrane responded (Fig. 4). Electrical stimulation of the carotid sinus nerves reduced the increases in sympathetic nerve activity and blood pressure in response to spinal cord stimulation but did not alter the contraction of the ipsilateral nictitating membranes (Fig. 4). Thus, the increase in activity of the sympathetic nervous system evoked by electrical stimulation of the dorsolateral funiculus of the spinal cord at the level of C_4 was influenced by the activation of the baroreceptor reflex in the same selective way as that produced by hypothalamic stimulation. The most probable explanation is that an interaction occurred between the descending baroreceptor reflex and the sympatho-excitatory fibres at segmental spinal levels. It remains to be determined whether this interaction takes place at the cell body of the sympathetic preganglionic neurone or whether interneurones are involved.

MODULATION OF SYMPATHETIC NERVOUS ACTIVITY THROUGH SPINAL α-ADRENERGIC AND SEROTONERGIC MECHANISMS

As indicated in the first chapter of this paper, it appears highly improbable that descending bulbospinal adrenergic neurones represent and integral link of the baroreceptor reflex arc (Haeusler, 1974b; Haeusler and Lewis, 1975).

However, they may well modulate transmission through the reflex. Since descending bulbospinal adrenergic and serotonergic neurones terminate in the intermediolateral cell columns between the first thoracic and second lumbar segments (Dahlström and Fuxe, 1965), which is the site of origin of the preganglionic sympathetic neurones, it is possible that such a modulation occurs at the spinal level.

The kind of influence which bulbospinal adrenergic and serotonergic neurones exert on the function of the sympathetic preganglionic neurone is a matter of controversy. Coote and Macleod (1974) postulated that sympathetic preganglionic neurones are inhibited by a bulbospinal pathway which utilizes noradrenaline as a transmitter. The opposite view is held by Chalmers and his coworkers, who studied the turnover of central noradrenaline and the effects of 6-hydroxydopamine-induced destruction of central adrenergic neurones in hypertensive animals (Chalmers and Wurtman, 1971; Chalmers and Reid, 1972; Chalmers, 1975). They interpret bulbospinal adrenergic neurones as having an excitatory influence on the function of the sympathetic preganglionic neurone. Neumayr et al. (1974) arrived at the same conclusion on the basis of pharmacological manipulation of sympathetic discharges evoked by medullary or spinal stimulation. In addition, these authors claimed that a bulbospinal serotonergic pathway has an inhibitory influence on the function of the preganglionic sympathetic neurone.

Studies in the author's laboratory also dealt with the problem of how bulbospinal adrenergic and serotonergic pathways modulate transmission to the sympathetic preganglionic neurone. The experiments were carried out in spinal cats by stimulating a sympatho-excitatory tract in the dorsolateral funiculus of the spinal cord at the level of C_4 and recording the evoked discharges from the sympathetic preganglionic splanchnic nerve and a sympathetic postganglionic renal nerve. The influence of the evoked discharges was attempted using pharmacological manipulations. For this type of experiment, the use of spinal cats has several advantages compared to employing animals with an intact neuraxis. Firstly, the sympathetic discharges are not evoked by stimulation of afferent spinal pathways and mediation of supraspinal centres. Therefore, drug-induced alterations of evoked sympathetic preganglionic discharges must have occurred in the spinal cord. Secondly, in spinal cats the bulbospinal adrenergic and serotonergic pathways are interrrupted and cannot propagate impulses. Therefore, drug-induced changes in evoked sympathetic discharges cannot be the result of an altered release of noradrenaline or serotonin from the respective nerve endings of the two pathways, the latter action arising from an activation of presynaptic receptors by the drugs employed. Thirdly, the cats were prepared for stimulation and recording and were made spinal under ether anaesthesia, and subsequently, the anaesthesia was terminated. Hence, the function of spinal neurones was not affected by an anaesthetic agent.

The electrical stimulation of the dorsolateral funiculus of the spinal cord for 10 sec with frequencies between 10 and 80 Hz resulted in frequency-dependent increases in preganglionic and postganglionic sympathetic nerve activity (Fig. 5). The stimulation-induced preganglionic discharges were virtually not affected by i.v. administration of the a-adrenoceptor blocking agents, phenoxybenzamine (Fig. 5) and phentolamine and by the β-adrenoceptor

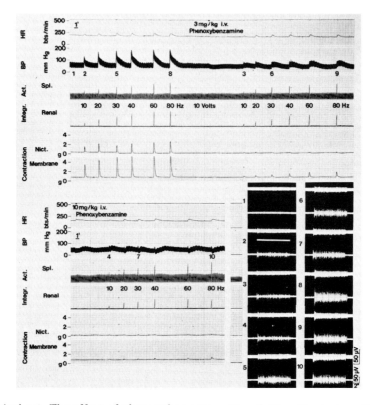

Fig. 5. Spinal cat. The effect of phenoxybenzamine (3 and 10 mg/kg i.v.) on the responses of heart rate, blood pressure, sympathetic preganglionic splanchnic nerve activity, sympathetic postganglionic renal nerve activity and of the right and left nictitating membranes to electrical stimulation with various frequencies of a descending sympatho-excitatory tract in the left dorsolateral funiculus of the spinal cord at the level of C_4. The oscilloscope recordings show the activity in the splanchnic (upper trace) and renal sympathetic nerve (lower trace). For explanation of all further details see legend to Fig. 4.

blocking agent propranolol. After high doses of the α-adrenergic blockers (10 mg/kg i.v. phenoxybenzamine, 30 mg/kg i.v. phentolamine) they were slightly augmented (Fig. 5). This observation indicates that the sympatho-excitatory pathway stimulated in the dorsolateral funiculus is non-adrenergic; in particular this finding seems to exclude stimulation of bulbospinal adrenergic pathways which are located near the site of stimulation used (Dahlström and Fuxe, 1965) and which are supposed to be sympatho-excitatory (Neumayr et al., 1974; Chalmers, 1975).

The α-adrenoceptor stimulating agent clonidine (10 and 30 μg/kg i.v.) reduced the preganglionic sympathetic discharges produced by stimulation of the dorsolateral funiculus of the spinal cord. This effect was maximal with 10 μg/kg i.v. clonidine. Sympathetic discharges in response to cord stimulation with 10 or 30 Hz were more susceptible to clonidine-induced inhibition than those in response to 60 or 80 Hz. The inhibition was reversed by the α-adrenergic blockers phentolamine (30 mg/kg i.v.) or piperoxan (1 mg/kg i.v.).

D,L-α-Methyldopa (30 and 100 mg/kg i.v.) also produced an inhibition of sympathetic discharges in response to cord stimulation and this inhibition was antagonized by phentolamine or piperoxan (Fig. 6). While the onset of the inhibitory action of clonidine was immediate, it took 90 min until the maximal effect of D,L-α-methyldopa was obtained (Fig. 6). This gradual increase in inhibition by D,L-α-methyldopa is best explained by a progressive formation of α-methylnoradrenaline from the amino acid within the spinal cord. After both clonidine and D,L-α-methyldopa, inhibition of transmission of sympatho-excitatory impulses to the sympathetic preganglionic neurone was not complete. Maximal inhibition of the sympathetic discharges produced by cord stimulation with 10 or 30 Hz was about 40% for both drugs.

5-Hydroxy-L-tryptophan ethyl ester (200 mg/kg i.v.) increased sympathetic discharges in the preganglionic splanchnic nerve in response to cord stimulation and this increase was reversed by methysergide (1—3 mg/kg i.v.).

The present results indicate the existence of spinal α-adrenergic and serotonergic receptors which inhibit and facilitate, respectively, the transmission of sympatho-excitatory impulses to the sympathetic preganglionic

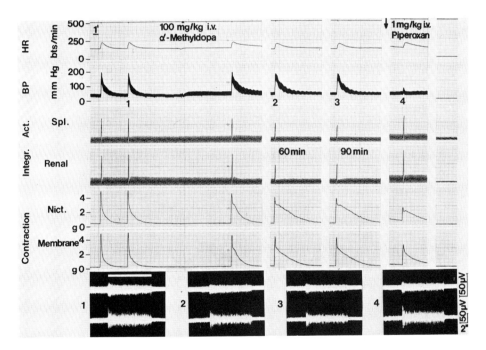

Fig. 6. Spinal cat. The effect of D,L-α-methyldopa (100 mg/kg i.v.) on the responses of heart rate, blood pressure, sympathetic preganglionic splanchnic nerve activity, sympathetic postganglionic renal nerve activity and of the right and left nictitating membranes to electrical stimulation (15 V, 0.1 msec, 80 Hz) of a descending sympatho-excitatory tract in the dorsolateral funiculus of the spinal cord at the level of C₄. The oscilloscope recordings show the activity in the splanchnic (upper trace) and renal sympathetic nerve (lower trace). The inhibitory effect of D,L-α-methyldopa on stimulation-induced sympathetic discharges was maximal at 90 min after its i.v. injection (third panel of the pen record) and was completely reversed by the α-adrenoceptor blocking agent piperoxan (1 mg/kg i.v.) (fourth panel of the pen record). For explanation of all further details see legend to Fig. 4.

106

neurone. The experiments provide no information about the localization of these receptors within the spinal cord. In view of the high density of catecholamine and serotonin nerve terminals in the sympathetic intermedio-lateral cell columns it seems, however, conceivable that cell bodies of the sympathetic preganglionic neurones bear such receptors. From the effects of the stimulation of the two receptor types, I am inclined to conclude that bulbospinal adrenergic and serotonergic neurones modulate transmission of excitation to the sympathetic preganglionic neurone in an inhibitory and facilitatory way, respectively.

The results reported here are just opposite to those of Neumayr et al. (1974) which were obtained in the same species with a similar technique. For the moment, I cannot envisage any reasonable explanation for the discrepancy. As far as the influence of bulbospinal adrenergic neurones on the function of the sympathetic preganglionic system is concerned, the present conclusion of an adrenergic inhibition is in good agreement with the postulate of Coote and Macleod (1974). Furthermore, the present conclusions are in line with results reported by De Groat and Ryall (1967) and by Ryall (1967). These authors found that iontophoretic application of noradrenaline inhibited, whereas serotonin excited, those spinal neurones which had been identified by antidromic activation as sympathetic preganglionic.

SUMMARY

In cats anaesthetized with urethane, a general increase in the activity of the sympathetic nervous system was produced by electrical stimulation of the posterior hypothalamus. Simultaneous activation of the baroreceptor reflex reduced this elevation of sympathetic outflow to the cardiovascular system, but not to some non-cardiovascular organs. Furthermore, the increase in activity recorded during hypothalamic stimulation from a descending sym-patho-excitatory pathway in the dorsolateral funiculus of the spinal cord was not diminished by baroreceptor reflex activation. These findings are compatible with the assumption that descending baroreceptor reflex fibres influence sympathetic activity at segmental spinal levels. Bulbospinal adrenergic neurones would be candidates for such descending fibres. However, the virtually complete depletion of noradrenaline with reserpine plus the inhibition of noradrenaline biosynthesis with α-methyl-p-tyrosine did not inactivate the baroreceptor reflex, excluding the possibility that central adrenergic neurones are integral to the baroreceptor reflex arc. In spinal cats, a descending sympatho-excitatory tract in the dorsolateral funiculus of the spinal cord was stimulated at the level of C_4 and induced electrical discharges were recorded from the preganglionic splanchnic nerve. Under these conditions, evoked discharges were reduced by clonidine and D,L-α-methyldopa (reversal by α-adrenoceptor blocking agents) and augmented by 5-hydroxy-L-tryptophan ethyl ester (reversal by methysergide). The results suggest the existence of spinal α-adrenergic and serotonin receptors inhibiting and facilitating respectively transmission to the preganglionic sympathetic neurone.

ACKNOWLEDGEMENT

I thank Mr. R. Osterwalder for skilful and reliable technical assistance.

REFERENCES

Alexander, R.S. (1946) Tonic and reflex functions of medullary sympathetic cardiovascular centres. *J. Neurophysiol.*, 9: 205—217.

Barman, S.M. and Wurster, R.D. (1975) Visceromotor organization within descending spinal sympathetic pathways in the dog. *Circulat. Res.*, 37: 209—214.

Calaresu, F.R. and Pearce, J.W. (1965) Electrical activity of efferent vagal fibres and dorsal nucleus of the vagus during reflex bradycardia in the cat. *J. Physiol. (Lond.)*, 176: 228—240.

Chalmers, J.P. (1975) Brain amines and models of experimental hypertension. *Circulat. Res.*, 36: 469—480.

Chalmers, J.P. and Reid, J.L. (1972) Participation of central noradrenergic neurons in arterial baroreceptor reflexes in the rabbit. A study with intracisternally administered 6-hydroxydopamine. *Circulat. Res.*, 31: 789—804.

Chalmers, J.P. and Wurtman, R.J. (1971) Participation of central noradrenergic neurons in arterial baroreceptor reflexes in the rabbit. *Circulat. Res.*, 28: 480—491.

Coote, J.H. and Macleod, V.H. (1972) The possibility that noradrenaline is a sympatho-inhibitory transmitter in the spinal cord. *J. Physiol. (Lond.)*, 225: 44—46P.

Coote, J.H. and Macleod, V.H. (1974) The influence of bulbospinal monoaminergic pathways on sympathetic nerve activity. *J. Physiol. (Lond.)*, 241: 453—475.

Coote, J.H. and Macleod, V.H. (1975) The spinal route of sympatho-inhibitory pathways descending from the medulla oblongata. *Pflügers Arch. ges. Physiol.*, 359: 335—347.

Cottle, M.K. (1964) Degeneration studies of primary afferents of IXth and Xth cranial nerves in the cat. *J. comp. Neurol.*, 122: 329—345.

Cottle, M.K. and Calaresu, F.R. (1975) Projections from the nucleus and tractus solitarius in the cat. *J. comp. Neurol.*, 161: 143—158.

Crill, W.E. and Reis, D.J. (1968) Distribution of carotid sinus and depressor nerves in cat brain stem. *Amer. J. Physiol.*, 214: 269—276.

Dahlström, A. and Fuxe, K. (1965) Evidence for the existence of monoamine neurones in the central nervous system. II. Experimentally induced changes in the intraneuronal amine levels of bulbospinal neurone systems. *Acta physiol. scand.*, 64, Suppl. 247: 1—36.

De Groat, W.C. and Ryall, R.W. (1967) Excitatory action of 5-hydroxytryptamine on sympathetic preganglionic neurones in the spinal cord. *Exp. Brain Res.*, 3: 299—305.

Gebber, G.L., Taylor, D.G. and Weaver, L.C. (1973) Electrophysiological studies on organization of central vasopressor pathways. *Amer. J. Physiol.*, 224: 470—481.

Haeusler, G. (1973) Activation of the central pathway of the baroreceptor reflex, a possible mechanism of the hypotensive action of clonidine. *Naunyn-Schmiedeberg's Arch. exp. Path. Pharmak.*, 285: 1—14.

Haeusler, G. (1974a) Further similarities between the action of clonidine and a central activation of the depressor baroreceptor reflex. *Naunyn-Schmiedeberg's Arch. exp. Path. Pharmak.*, 285: 1—14.

Haeusler, G. (1974b) Organization of central cardiovascular pathways in the cat and the question of an involvement of adrenergic neurones. *Naunyn-Schmiedeberg's Arch. exp. Path. Pharmak.*, 285: R28.

Haeusler, G. (1974c) Clonidine-induced inhibition of sympathetic nerve activity: no indication for a central presynaptic or an indirect sympathomimetic mode of action. *Naunyn-Schmiedeberg's Arch. exp. Path. Pharmak.*, 286: 97—111.

Haeusler, G. (1975) Cardiovascular regulation of central adrenergic mechanisms and its alteration by hypotensive drugs. *Circulat. Res.*, 36 and 37, Suppl. I: 223—232.

Haeusler, G. and Lewis, P. (1975) The baroreceptor reflex and its relations to central adrenergic mechanisms. In *Recent Advances in Hypertension*, Vol. 2, P. Milliez and M. Safar (Eds.), Laboratoires Boehringer Ingelheim, Reims, pp. 17—26.

Hellner, K. and von Baumgarten, R. (1961) Ueber ein Endigungsgebiet afferenter, kardiovaskulärer Fasern des Nervus vagus im Rautenhirn der Katze. *Pflügers Arch. ges. Physiol.*, 273: 223—234.

Illert, M. and Gabriel, M. (1970) Mapping the cord of the spinal cat for sympathetic and blood pressure responses. *Brain Res.*, 23: 274—276.

Illert, M. and Gabriel, M. (1972) Descending pathways in the cervical cord of cats affecting blood pressure and sympathetic activity. *Pflügers Arch. ges. Physiol.*, 335: 109—124.

Illert, M. and Seller, H. (1969) A descending sympatho-inhibitory tract in the ventrolateral column of the cat. *Pflügers Arch. ges. Physiol.*, 313: 343—360.

Kerr, F.W.L. (1962) Facial, vagal and glossopharyngeal nerves in the cat: afferent connections. *Arch. Neurol. (Chic.)*, 6: 264—281.

Kobinger, W. and Pichler, L. (1975) The central modulatory effect of clonidine on the cardiodepressor reflex after suppression of synthesis and storage of noradrenaline. *Europ. J. Pharmacol.*, 30: 56—62.

Kobinger, W. and Walland, A. (1967) Investigations into the mechanism of the hypotensive effect of 2-(2,6-dichlorophenyl-amino)-2-imidazoline-HCl. *Europ. J. Pharmacol.*, 2: 9—13.

Miura, M. and Reis, D.J. (1969) Termination and secondary projections of carotid sinus nerve in the cat brain stem. *Amer. J. Physiol.*, 217: 142—153.

Miura, M. and Reis, D.J. (1972) The role of the solitary and paramedian reticular nuclei in mediating cardiovascular reflex responses from carotid baro- and chemoreceptors. *J. Physiol. (Lond.)*, 223: 525—548.

Nakamura, G., Gerold, M. and Thoenen, H. (1971a) Experimental hypertension of the rat: reciprocal changes of norepinephrine turnover in heart and brainstem. *Naunyn-Schmiedeberg's Arch. exp. Path. Pharmak.*, 268: 125—139.

Nakamura, K., Gerold, M. and Thoenen, H. (1971b) Genetically hypertensive rats: relationship between the development of hypertension and the changes in norepinephrine turnover of peripheral and central adrenergic neurons. *Naunyn-Schmiedeberg's Arch. exp. Path. Pharmak.*, 271: 157—169.

Neumayr, R.J., Hare, B.D. and Franz, D.N. (1974) Evidence for bulbospinal control of sympathetic preganglionic neurons by monoaminergic pathways. *Life Sci.*, 14: 793—806.

Ninomiya, I., Irisawa, A. and Nisimaru, N. (1973) Nonuniformity of sympathetic nerve activity to the skin and kidney. *Amer. J. Physiol.*, 224: 256—264.

Nisimaru, N. (1971) Comparison of gastric and renal nerve activity. *Amer. J. Physiol.*, 220: 1303—1308.

Rhoton, A.L., O'Leary, J.L. and Ferguson, J.P. (1966) The trigeminal, facial, vagal, and glossopharyngeal nerves in the monkey. *Arch. Neurol. (Chic.)*, 14: 530—540.

Ryall, R.W. (1967) Effect of monoamines upon sympathetic preganglionic neurons. *Circulat. Res.*, 20 and 21, Suppl. III: 83—87.

Schmitt, H. and Schmitt, H. (1969) Localization of the hypotensive effect of 2-(2,6-dichlorophenylamino)-2-imidazoline hydrochloride (St 155, Catapresan). *Europ. J. Pharmacol.*, 6: 8—12.

Schmitt, H. and Schmitt, H. (1970) Interactions between 2-(2,6-dichlorophenyl-amino)-2-imidazoline hydrochloride (St 155, Catapresan ®) and α-adrenergic blocking drugs. *Europ. J. Pharmacol.*, 9: 7—13.

Schmitt, H., Schmitt, H., Boissier, J.R., Giudicelli, J.F. and Fichelle, J. (1968) Cardiovascular effects of 2-(2.6-dichlorophenylamino)-2-imidazoline hydrochloride (St 155). II. Central sympathetic structures. *Europ. J. Pharmacol.*, 2: 340—346.

Schmitt, H., Schmitt, H. and Fenard, S. (1971) Evidence for an α-sympathomimetic component in the effects of Catapresan on vasomotor centres: antagonism by piperoxan. *Europ. J. Pharmacol.*, 14: 98—100.

Seller, H. and Illert, M. (1969) The localization of the first synapse in the carotid sinus baroreceptor reflex pathway and its alteration of the afferent input. *Pflügers Arch. ges. Physiol.*, 306: 1—19.

Snyder, D.W. and Gebber, G.L. (1973) Relationships between medullary depressor region and central vasopressor pathways. *Amer. J. Physiol.*, 225: 1129—1137.

Torvik, A. (1956) Afferent connections to the sensory trigeminal nuclei, the nucleus of the solitary tract and adjacent structures. An experimental study in the rat. *J. comp. Neurol.*, 106: 51—141.

The Spontaneously Hypertensive Rat: Catecholamine Levels in Individual Brain Regions

DIRK H.G. VERSTEEG, MIKLÓS PALKOVITS*, JAN VAN DER GUGTEN, HENK J.L.M. WIJNEN, GERARD W.M. SMEETS and WYBREN DE JONG

Rudolf Magnus Institute for Pharmacology, Medical Faculty, University of Utrecht, Utrecht (The Netherlands)

The spontaneously hypertensive rat (SH-rat), established as an inbred strain by Okamoto and associates at the University of Kyoto, Japan, in 1962 (see Okamoto et al., 1971), has been the subject of extensive studies in the past decade. In experiments on the possible relation between the elevated blood pressure levels in these rats and changes in central and/or peripheral catecholamine metabolism, however, the choice of controls has remained a problem. Initially, rats of normotensive Wistar strains were generally used as controls. Comparisons based on such controls showed lower noradrenaline levels, decreased aromatic amino acid decarboxylase activity (Yamori et al., 1970) and decreased noradrenaline synthesis (Louis et al., 1970) in the brain stem of SH-rats. These findings were not corroborated in later studies in which rats of the genetically related Wistar/Kyoto strain (W/K-rats) were used as controls (Sjoerdsma, 1971; Yamabe et al., 1973; Lovenberg et al., 1973). The latter studies do not support the existence of correlates between changes in brain catecholamine metabolism and the elevated blood pressure level of the SH-rats. An obvious possibility, however, is that changes in small brain areas had escaped detection in these studies. In our laboratory it was found that noradrenaline levels were slightly elevated in the pons-medulla of recent generation SH-rats, 7 and 10 weeks after birth, compared to W/K-rats of the same age (De Jong et al., 1975a).

This communication summarizes the results of a study comparing catecholamine levels in punched regions from the brains of 16-week-old SH- and W/K-rats (Versteeg et al., 1976a). We used a sensitive radiometric method for the simultaneous assay of noradrenaline, dopamine and adrenaline (Van der Gugten et al., 1976). The assay involves the conversion of the catecholamines to their respective tritiated methoxy derivatives by incubating them for 60 min at 37°C with S-adenosyl-l-[methyl-^{3}H]-methionine in the presence of the enzyme catechol-O-methyltransferase. Subsequently, the labeled methoxy derivatives are extracted and separated by descending paper chromatography. The assay is linear up to 2 ng; the sensitivity is approximately 10 pg for all three catecholamines. Cross-interference is less than 1% and is corrected for

*1st Department of Anatomy, Semmelweis University Medical School, Budapest, Hungary.

(for details of the method see Van der Gugten et al., 1976). In the present experiments the interference was: 0.38% of noradrenaline in dopamine; 0.27% of noradrenaline in adrenaline; 0.36% of dopamine in noradrenaline; 0.90% of dopamine in adrenaline.

Adult male SH-rats (body weight: 288 ± 3 g; systolic blood pressure: 196 ± 2 mm Hg; heart rate: 450 ± 9 bpm; n = 18) and W/K-rats (body weight: 324 ± 4 g; systolic blood pressure: 125 ± 1 mm Hg; heart rate: 375 ± 9 bpm; n = 18) were used at an age of 16 weeks. SH-rats were of SHR-NIH Cpb (F32) and the W/K-rats were of W/K-NIH Cpb (F6) (for genealogy see De Jong et al., 1975a). Systolic blood pressure was measured in conscious trained rats during the last two weeks before decapitation using a tail plethysmographic method (Leenen and De Jong, 1971). A total of 27 regions were punched (Palkovits, 1973) from frozen sections of 300 μm with hollow needles from telencephalon, diencephalon, mesencephalon, pons and medulla oblongata (for details and references see Versteeg et al., 1976b). Regions from three rats were pooled. After homogenization in 100 μl 0.1 N HClO$_4$, samples were taken for assay of the protein content (Lowry et al., 1951). The homogenates were then centrifuged and catecholamines were assayed in 20 μl samples of the supernatants. Data are expressed as pg catecholamine/μg protein $\pm$ S.E.M.

No significant alterations were observed in the noradrenaline levels of the telencephalic and diencephalic regions of the SH-rats. Dopamine concentrations, however, were elevated in the frontal cortex (143%) and the nucleus interstitialis striae terminalis (88%; NIST) of the SH-rats (Table I). This finding is in agreement with the small but significant elevation in telencephalic dopamine concentration observed in the study of Yamabe et al. (1973). Dopamine in the frontal cortex and also in the NIST only occurs in nerve terminals. Their perikarya are located in the A9—A10 catecholaminergic cell groups in the mesencephalon. Dopamine concentrations in the A9—A10 regions from SH-rats were similar to those of the control animals. The fact that the dopamine level of the NIST of SH-rats is elevated is particularly interesting, since it has been shown that electrical stimulation of cells in this relay nucleus, which connects the hypothalamus with the amygdala, resulted in a decrease in blood pressure and bradycardia (Hilton and Spyer, 1971). No changes were observed in catecholamine concentrations of either the septal and amygdaloid nuclei investigated or of the other limbic areas (hippocampus, mammillary body, habenula).

No differences were found in noradrenaline and dopamine levels in the hypothalamic nuclei (Table I). Recent studies (Koslow and Schlumpf, 1974; Van der Gugten et al., 1976) have shown that the hypothalamus is relatively rich in adrenaline. Cells containing this amine are located in the lower brain stem (Hökfelt et al., 1974), whereas adrenaline containing terminals are concentrated in the hypothalamus. All the hypothalamic regions which were investigated showed a higher adrenaline level in the SH-rat than in the control animals, but a significant elevation was observed only in the nucleus paraventricularis (Table II).

Several regions in the brain stem have been implicated in the control of arterial blood pressure. An important area in this respect is that of the nucleus tractus solitarii complex (NTS), which contains the primary synapses of the

TABLE I

NORADRENALINE AND DOPAMINE LEVELS IN BRAIN NUCLEI FROM W/K- AND SH-RATS

Data are expressed in pg/μg protein ±S.E.M. (n = 5—6).

	Noradrenaline (pg/μg protein)		Dopamine (pg/μg protein)	
	W/K	SH	W/K	SH
Telencephalon				
Frontal cortex	5.5 ± 0.4	6.2 ± 0.7	2.1 ± 0.2	5.0 ± 1.0**
Cingulate cortex	4.6 ± 0.5	4.7 ± 1.3	1.3 ± 0.2	1.2 ± 0.3
Hippocampus	7.1 ± 1.1	7.1 ± 0.5	1.1 ± 0.2	1.5 ± 0.2
Caudate nucleus	0.5 ± 0.06	0.6 ± 0.1	75.2 ± 11.4	95.3 ± 11.0
Dorsal septal nucl.	15.1 ± 1.3	11.4 ± 1.3	8.8 ± 1.4	6.3 ± 0.4
Lateral septal nucl.	19.4 ± 1.8	18.8 ± 1.3	17.3 ± 3.3	18.3 ± 1.8
Medial septal nucl.	20.4 ± 1.6	23.3 ± 2.7	2.8 ± 0.3	3.0 ± 0.3
Nucl. interst. striae term.	21.9 ± 4.8	25.7 ± 2.5	6.7 ± 1.0	12.7 ± 2.2*
Medial amygd. nucl.	10.6 ± 1.0	9.4 ± 0.4	0.8 ± 0.1	0.6 ± 0.2
Central amygd. nucl.	14.2 ± 1.6	11.4 ± 2.2	4.5 ± 0.9	4.6 ± 1.0
Diencephalon				
Paraventricular nucl.	55.0 ± 4.7	65.0 ± 8.1	5.9 ± 0.3	6.9 ± 0.8
Arcuate nucl.	27.6 ± 3.1	24.4 ± 2.7	7.5 ± 1.4	6.5 ± 0.5
Median eminence	22.5 ± 2.5	26.8 ± 0.7	53.2 ± 5.7	54.6 ± 10.7
Medial forebr. bundle	32.1 ± 2.6	29.5 ± 2.8	3.0 ± 0.3	3.9 ± 0.6
Mammillary body	15.7 ± 2.2	15.4 ± 2.5	1.9 ± 0.4	1.4 ± 0.4
Habenula	6.0 ± 1.1	7.3 ± 0.2	1.3 ± 0.2	1.4 ± 0.1
Brain stem				
Substantia nigra	5.0 ± 0.4	5.9 ± 1.1	22.1 ± 2.1	24.1 ± 4.6
A10-region	12.6 ± 3.2	13.7 ± 2.4	14.1 ± 3.9	16.1 ± 5.3
A7-region	4.3 ± 0.7	8.0 ± 0.4***	1.7 ± 0.4	1.7 ± 0.3
Locus coeruleus	19.0 ± 3.6	22.3 ± 4.5	7.6 ± 1.2	7.4 ± 2.0
A5-region	4.3 ± 0.5	6.6 ± 0.6**	0.9 ± 0.1	1.0 ± 0.1
Nucl. raphe magnus	6.0 ± 0.7	10.4 ± 1.6*	1.1 ± 0.2	1.3 ± 0.2
Reticular formation	4.4 ± 0.4	7.2 ± 0.7**	0.6 ± 0.1	0.8 ± 0.1
A1-region	5.1 ± 0.7	8.1 ± 0.8*	1.1 ± 0.2	1.4 ± 0.3
Rostral NTS	15.2 ± 1.0	17.3 ± 2.8	2.9 ± 0.5	3.3 ± 0.3
A2-region	18.0 ± 3.0	33.7 ± 5.2*	4.7 ± 0.8	8.7 ± 1.3*
Inferior olive	5.6 ± 0.8	7.3 ± 0.9	1.5 ± 0.2	1.9 ± 0.1

*P < 0.05.
**P < 0.02.
***P < 0.001.

afferents of the arterial baroreceptors (see Palkovits and Záborszky, 1977). This complex nucleus (rostral NTS, caudal NTS and nucleus commissuralis) contains catecholaminergic cell bodies which are mainly concentrated in the A2 region (caudal part of the NTS at the level of the posterior part of the area postrema and the rostral part of the nucleus commissuralis). The A1 region of the medulla and the hypothalamus are intimately involved in cardiovascular control as well (see Hilton and Spyer, 1971; De Jong et al., 1975b; Palkovits and Záborszky, 1977).

Major differences in brain noradrenaline concentrations between SH- and W/K-rats were found in the brain stem regions (Table I). In all noradrenergic cell body regions except for the locus coeruleus, the noradrenaline concentrations were found to be elevated (A1, A2, A5 and A7 region). In addition to this, elevated noradrenaline levels were measured in the reticular formation and in the nucleus raphe magnus. It is of interest to note that no changes were apparent in the rostral NTS. The fact that elevations in noradrenaline levels are restricted to a limited number of brain stem nuclei can explain why no changes had previously been detected in the whole brain stem (Yamabe et al., 1973), and only a slightly elevated noradrenaline concentration had been found in the pons-medulla (De Jong et al., 1975a).

Dopamine occurs in relatively low concentrations in the lower brain stem regions where the highest levels were measured in the A2 region (Versteeg et al., 1976b). In the SH-rats this region showed an elevated dopamine concentration (Table I). No data are available concerning the origin of dopamine in this area. On the basis of histofluorescence studies, Fuxe (1965) suggested that, in the NTS and the dorsal vagal nucleus, dopamine occurs in nerve terminals. Immunohistofluorescence studies have indicated that PNMT containing cell bodies are present in the brain stem in regions which mostly correspond with the A1 and A2 regions (Hökfelt et al., 1974). In agreement with this, it has been reported that PNMT activity is high in these regions (Saavedra et al., 1974), and that adrenaline is measurable only in a moderately high concentration in the A2 region and not in the A1 region (Van der Gugten et al., 1976). These data may indicate that the A1 region contains mainly adrenaline cell bodies with a low density of terminals and that the A2 region contains a relatively high number of both adrenaline containing perikarya and terminals. Saavedra et al. (1976) recently have reported that in the A1 and A2 regions of SH-rats PNMT acitivity is significantly higher than in these regions of W/K-rats. In the present study, we found a markedly elevated adrenaline concentration in the A2 region of the SH-rats (Table II).

TABLE II

ADRENALINE LEVELS IN BRAIN NUCLEI FROM W/K- AND SH-RATS

Data are expressed in pg/μg protein ±S.E.M. (n = 5—6).

	Adrenaline (pg/μg protein)	
	W/K	SH
Paraventricular nucl.	2.04 ± 0.16	3.40 ± 0.40**
Arcuate nucl.	0.97 ± 0.13	1.23 ± 0.19
Median eminence	0.95 ± 0.18	1.18 ± 0.14
Medial forebr. bundle	0.72 ± 0.07	0.89 ± 0.08
Rostral NTS	0.38 ± 0.06	0.35 ± 0.10
A2-region	0.43 ± 0.13	0.92 ± 0.14*
Inferior olive	0.10 ± 0.02	0.10 ± 0.02

*$P < 0.05$.
**$P < 0.005$.

Although the concentration of all three catecholamines was elevated in the A2 region of the SH-rats, the observed changes indicate a high degree of specificity of the alterations. An elevation of dopamine concentration was only observed in the two other regions, viz. the frontal cortex and the NIST. Similarly, an increased adrenaline concentration occurred only in the paraventricular nucleus. Most cell body regions of the lower brain stem had an increased noradrenaline concentration. These increases, however, were not accompanied by alterations in the level of the two other catecholamines, except in the A2 region.

Obviously, further experiments are needed to analyze the changes in regional catecholamine metabolism in the brain of the SH-rat. Possible goals for further investigation are the assessment of the activity of the enzymes involved in catecholamine synthesis and breakdown as well as the measurement of catecholamine synthesis and turnover in key areas. Another prerequisite is that the relationship of changes in brain catecholamine metabolism to the evolution of hypertension in genetic and other forms of hypertension be settled.

SUMMARY

The concentration of noradrenaline, dopamine and adrenaline was measured in 27 brain regions of adult spontaneously hypertensive rats (SH-rats) with established hypertension and normotensive Wistar/Kyoto rats (W/K-rats). Selectively elevated catecholamine levels were found in a restricted number of these regions from the SH-rats. Most differences (elevated noradrenaline) occurred in cell body regions of the medulla oblongata. In the A2 region of the NTS complex, increased levels of all three catecholamines were observed. In some supramedullary regions implicated in the control of blood pressure, elevated dopamine or adrenaline levels were found as well.

ACKNOWLEDGEMENTS

The skilful assistance of Miss Kitty Gielens and Mr. Henk Spierenburg is gratefully acknowledged.

This study was supported in part by the Foundation for Medical Research (FUNGO), which is subsidized by the Netherlands Organisation for the Advancement of Pure Research (ZWO).

REFERENCES

De Jong, W., Nijkamp, F.P. and Bohus, B. (1975a) Role of noradrenaline and serotonin in the central control of blood pressure in normotensive and spontaneously hypertensive rats. *Arch. int. Pharmacodyn.*, 213: 272—284.

De Jong, W., Zandberg, P. and Bohus, B. (1975b) Central inhibitory noradrenergic cardiovascular control. In *Hormones, Homeostasis and the Brain, Progress in Brain Res., Vol. 42*, W.H. Gispen, Tj.B. van Wimersma Greidanus, B. Bohus and D. De Wied (Eds.), Elsevier, Amsterdam, pp. 285—298.

116

Fuxe, K. (1965) Evidence for the existence of monoamine neurons in the central nervous system. IV. Distribution of monoamine nerve terminals in the central nervous system. *Acta physiol. scand.*, 64, Suppl. 247: 39—85.

Hilton, S.M. and Spyer, K.M. (1971) Participation of the anterior hypothalamus in the baroreceptor reflex. *J. Physiol. (Lond.)*, 218: 271—293.

Hökfelt, T., Fuxe, K., Goldstein, M. and Johansson, O. (1974) Immunohistochemical evidence for the existence of adrenaline neurons in the rat brain. *Brain Res.*, 66: 235—251.

Koslow, S.H. and Schlumpf, M. (1974) Quantitation of adrenaline in rat brain nuclei and areas by mass fragmentography. *Nature (Lond.)*, 251: 530—531.

Leenen, F.H.H. and De Jong, W. (1971) A solid silver clip for induction of predictable levels of renal hypertension in the rat. *J. appl. Physiol.*, 31: 142—144.

Louis, W.J., Krauss, K.R., Kopin, I.J. and Sjoerdsma, A. (1970) Catecholamine metabolism in hypertensive rats. *Circulat. Res.*, 27: 589—594.

Lovenberg, W., Yamabe, H., Jong, W. De and Hansen, C.T. (1973) Genetic variation of the catecholamine biosynthetic enzyme activities in various strains of rats including the spontaneously hypertensive rat. In *Frontiers in Catecholamine Research*, E. Usdin and S. Snyder (Eds.), Pergamon Press, Oxford, pp. 891—895.

Lowry, O.H., Rosebrough, N.J., Farr, A.L. and Randall, R.J. (1951) Protein measurement with Folin phenol reagent. *J. biol. Chem.*, 193: 265—275.

Okamoto, K., Yamori, Y., Ooshima, A., Park, C., Haebara, H., Matsumoto, M., Tanaka, T., Okuda, T., Hazama, F. and Kyogoku, M. (1971) Establishment of the inbred strain of the spontaneously hypertensive rat and genetic factors involved in hypertension. In *Spontaneous Hypertension: its Pathogenetics and Complication*, K. Okamoto (Ed.), Igaku Shoin, Tokyo, pp. 1—8.

Palkovits, M. (1973) Isolated removal of hypothalamic or other brain nuclei of the rat. *Brain Res.*, 59: 449—450.

Palkovits, M. and Záborszky, L. (1977) The neuroanatomy of central cardiovascular control: the nucleus tractus solitarii; afferent and efferent neuronal connections in relation to the baroreceptor reflex arc. In *Hypertension and Brain Mechanisms, Progr. in Brain Res., Vol. 47*, W. De Jong, A.P. Provoost and A.P. Shapiro (Eds.), Elsevier, Amsterdam, pp. 9—34.

Saavedra, J.M., Palkovits, M., Brownstein, M.J. and Axelrod, J. (1974) Localisation of phenylethanolamine N-methyltransferase in rat brain nuclei. *Nature (Lond.)*, 248: 695—696.

Saavedra, J.M., Grobecker, H. and Axelrod, J. (1976) Adrenaline-forming enzyme in brainstem: elevation in genetic and experimental hypertension. *Science*, 191: 483—484.

Sjoerdsma, A. (1971) Catecholamine metabolism in the spontaneously hypertensive rat. In *Spontaneous Hypertension: its Pathogenetics and Complication*, K. Okamoto (Ed.), Igaku Shoin, Tokyo, pp. 27—30.

Van der Gugten, J., Palkovits, M., Wijnen, H.J.L.M. and Versteeg, D.H.G. (1976) Regional distribution of adrenaline in rat brain. *Brain Res.*, 107: 171—175.

Versteeg, D.H.G., Palkovits, M., Van der Gugten, J., Wijnen, H.J.L.M., Smeets, G.W.M. and De Jong, W. (1976a) Catecholamine content of individual brain regions of spontaneously hypertensive rats (SH-rats). *Brain Res.*, 112: 429—434.

Versteeg, D.H.G., Van der Gugten, J., De Jong, W. and Palkovits, M. (1976b) Regional concentrations of noradrenaline and dopamine in rat brain. *Brain Res.*, 113: 563—574.

Yamabe, H., De Jong, W. and Lovenberg, W. (1973) Further studies on catecholamine synthesis in the spontaneously hypertensive rat: catecholamine synthesis in the central nervous system. *Europ. J. Pharmacol.*, 22: 91—98.

Yamori Y., Lovenberg, W. and Sjoerdsma, A. (1970) Norepinephrine metabolism in brainstem of spontaneously hypertensive rats. *Science*, 170: 544—546.

Localization of Catecholaminergic Receptor Sites in the Nucleus Tractus Solitarii involved in the Regulation of Arterial Blood Pressure

PIETER ZANDBERG and WYBREN DE JONG

Rudolf Magnus Institute for Pharmacology, Medical Faculty, University of Utrecht, Utrecht (The Netherlands)

α-Methyldopa has a potent hypotensive action which may be centrally mediated. The central formation of α-methylnoradrenaline (α-MNA) is an essential requirement for the hypotensive action of α-methyldopa (Nijkamp and De Jong, 1975, 1977). A noradrenergic inhibitory effect in the lower brain stem has been proposed as the mechanism by which α-methyldopa, after its conversion, exerts its central hypotensive action (Van Zwieten, 1975). Several authors have postulated that this drug, like L-DOPA, mimics baroreceptor activation through direct noradrenergic receptor stimulation in the brain. Recent studies indicate that the nucleus tractus solitarii (NTS) of the medulla oblongata, a primary site of termination of afferent carotid sinus baroreceptor fibers, plays an important role (De Jong et al., 1975a, b). For example, ablation of the area of the NTS produces acute hypertension in conscious rats (Doba and Reis, 1973; De Jong et al., 1975b) and electrical stimulation of the mediocaudal part of the NTS causes hypotension and bradycardia (De Jong et al., 1975a, b). This area has been shown by fluorescent histochemistry to be heavily innervated by catecholaminergic terminals (Dahlström and Fuxe, 1964; it also contains catecholaminergic cell bodies (Fuxe, 1965). Bilateral local application of noradrenaline and α-MNA in this area causes hypotension (De Jong, 1974; Nijkamp and De Jong, 1975). In addition, prior administration at the same site of the α-adrenergic blocking agent, phentolamine, prevents the central inhibitory action of the two catecholamines and may even reverse the effect on blood pressure.

Thus, these data suggest that the area of the NTS may be a site of action for central hypotensive drugs which act by adrenergic receptor stimulation in the brain. However, due to limitations of the technique, the injection studies did not allow a conclusion to be reached about the precise localization of these active sites within the rather elongated NTS. In these studies a volume of 0.6—1.0 μl had been administered bilaterally via a stainless steel needle with an outer diameter of 200 μm. Therefore, the presence of active sites in the nuclei surrounding the NTS could not be excluded.

Myers (1966) has examined the extent of diffusion into the tissue when minute quantities of 4 dye solutions were injected. Calculating the average of all injections of the different dyes, he found that 0.5 μl had a diffusion area of approx. 1 mm; 1 μl one of 1.9 mm and 2 μl one of 2.4 mm. He has also shown that volumes such as 1 μl or more injected in a short time could produce lesions along the cannula track. Therefore, in the present experiments we used glass needles with an outer diameter of 60 μm. The injection volume was 0.4 μl and the injection time 10 sec. To ensure as accurate a microscopic localization as possible, microinjections were given unilaterally, and only one injection was given to each rat.

Male Wistar rats weighing 200—250 g were used and anesthetized with urethane. Blood pressure was recorded via an indwelling cannula in the femoral artery. Implantation of the cannula in the medulla oblongata was carried out with a stereotaxic apparatus following exposure of the lower brain stem by a limited occipital craniotomy. The head of the rat was flexed to 45° and the caudal tip of the area postrema in the midline was used as a rostrocaudal zero. Preliminary work indicated that an injection of 0.4 μl methylene blue into the NTS just medial of the tractus solitarius was distributed along the NTS. The rostral-caudal diffusion was about 1200 μm, while the dorsal-ventral and lateral diffusion was about 500 μm. The same distribution pattern was also found with [^{14}C] clonidine. This peculiar pattern of distribution probably results from the structure of the NTS which consists mainly of nuclei with only one major tractus laterally. The adjacent structures are more compact both with nuclei and especially fibers, and therefore distribution along the NTS and tractus may be easier.

The results indicate that a decrease in blood pressure of 30—40 mm Hg can be induced by 20 nmoles α-MNA when this is injected unilaterally in the mediocaudal part of the NTS. The maximal fall in blood pressure was reached within 5—10 min. The blood pressure returned to control value in 30—45 min. The (plus) stereoisomer of α-MNA was ineffective even when administered in a 10 times higher dose, indicating the stereospecificity of the response (De Jong et al., 1976). Injection in the tractus or medial of the tractus in the NTS causes a depressor response. There was no difference in hypotensive response from 500 μm rostral to 400 μm caudal of the zero level. However, injections at the transition of the NTS with the intercalate nucleus and the dorsal located nuclei were less effective (20—25 mm Hg). In the areas dorsal, ventral and lateral to the NTS and the tractus no effect was observed with α-MNA (Zandberg and De Jong, 1976). With higher and lower doses of α-MNA, the same effective localization was found. The minimal effective dose when given unilaterally was 0.3 nmoles. Bilateral injections were more effective than were unilateral ones, with the minimal effective dose ranging between 20 and 80 pmoles.

The hypotensive response to unilateral injections in the more rostral and caudal part of the NTS (Fig. 1) was diminished and was furthermore absent when the injection sites were more than 1300 μm rostral of the zero plane. At 800—1200 μm caudal of the zero plane the decrease in blood pressure was significantly less. Local injection of 20 nmoles α-MNA or higher doses caused a short lasting initial pressor response followed by a fall in blood pressure. Prior local administration of the α-adrenergic blocking agent, phentolamine, blocked the decrease in blood pressure and potentiated the initial pressor response (De Jong et al., 1975a).

The results of De Jong and Nijkamp (1976) indicated that in addition to the noradrenergic mechanism, a cholinergic one may be involved in the central cardiovascular effects of α-MNA since systemic administration of atropine

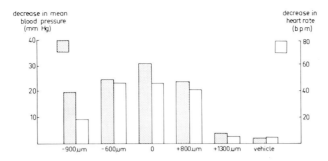

Fig 1. Effect of a unilateral injection of (−) α-methylnoradrenaline (20 nmoles) on mean blood pressure and heart rate at different caudal (−) and rostral (+) sites in the nucleus tractus solitarii of rats anesthetized with urethane. 0 is zero plane (caudal tip of the area postrema). Data from at least 4 rats are given.

combined with vagotomy potentiated the inhibitory effects of α-MNA. Intravenous (Varagić and Krstić, 1966) or intracerebroventricular injections (Brezenoff, 1973) of the cholinesterase inhibitor, physostigmine, can produce a blood pressure rise both in unanesthetized rats and in rats anesthetized with urethane. The pressor response is a consequence of increased sympathetic activity (Varagić and Vojvodić, 1962) probably resulting from an action of the drug in the lower brain stem (Brezenoff and Jenden, 1970) and may involve the active participation of brain acetylcholine (Brezenoff and Rusin, 1974). Bilateral injection of 1–5 μg physostigmine in the NTS at zero level elicits a dose dependent increase in blood pressure of 39–60 mm Hg. A representative example is given in Fig. 2.

A subsequent experiment was designed to localize the area where physostigmine elicits a pressor response. Bilateral injections of 1 μg in the most effective area for α-MNA caused a rise in blood pressure, but injections in the intercalate nucleus were also effective (Fig. 3). When the injection points were more than 500 μm rostral or caudal of the zero plane, physostigmine was ineffective. The blood pressure rise following the injection in the NTS area was

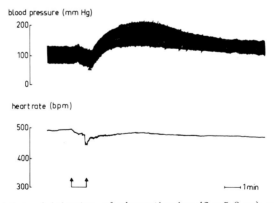

Fig. 2. Effect of a bilateral injection of physostigmine (2 × 5.0 μg) on blood pressure and heart rate of a rat anesthetized with urethane after a local injection in the area of the nucleus tractus solitarii.

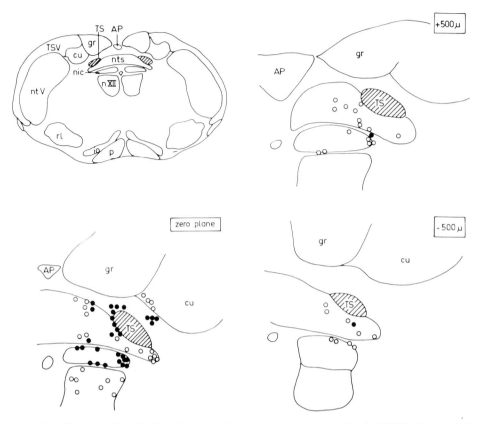

Fig. 3. Distribution of effective sites in the nucleus tractus solitarii (NTS) from which pressor responses were evoked by physostigmine. The influence of a bilateral application of physostigmine (2 × 1.0 μg) in the caudal part of the medulla oblongata on blood pressure of individual rats is shown. A transverse section at the level of the caudal tip of the area postrema (zero plane) is shown in the upper left part of the figure. This zero plane corresponds to P 7.4 mm of the atlas of Palkovits and Jacobowitz (1974). This area of the NTS is shown enlarged at different rostral caudal levels. ●, Sites where there was an increase of 20 mm Hg or more. ○, Sites where the response was less than 20 mm Hg. AP, area postrema; cu, nucleus cuneatus; gr, nucleus gracilis; io, nucleus olivaris inferior; nic, nucleus intercalatus; nts, nucleus tractus solitarii; nt V, nucleus tractus spinalis nervi trigemini; n XII, nucleus orginis nervi hypoglossi; P, tractus corticospinalis; rl, nucleus reticularis lateralis; TS, tractus solitarius; TSV, tractus spinalis nervi trigemini. Abbreviations according to Palkovits and Jacobowitz (1974).

greater than after injection into the nucleus intercalatus; a marked reduction in heart rate was only seen with the injection into the NTS. With intravenous injection, a dose of 200 μg/kg was needed to cause a similar increase of blood pressure. Therefore, we can conclude that in the area where α-MNA causes a decrease in blood pressure, an increase in blood pressure can be evoked by physostigmine. An i.p. injection of up to 15 mg/kg of atropine 20 min before the local injection of physostigmine could not block the pressor response. In contrast, Brezenoff (1973) was able to block the pressor response elicited by an intravenous or intracerebroventricular injection of physostigmine with an i.v. injection of 1 mg/kg atropine.

In conclusion, the most effective area for α-MNA appears to be from 500 μm rostral to 400 μm caudal of the zero level. This part of the NTS corresponds to the A2 region which contains catecholaminergic cell bodies· and is innervated by catecholaminergic terminals. It is just caudal to the area where bilateral lesion of the NTS evokes an acute elevation of blood pressure (De Jong et al., 1977). In the A2 region a pressor response could be evoked by bilateral administration of physostigmine. Our results suggest that catecholaminergic receptor sites are located in the A2 region of the NTS and may modulate tonic inhibitory control and reflex regulation of cardiovascular function.

SUMMARY

Data are presented for the localization of catecholaminergic receptor sites in the mediocaudal part of the nucleus tractus solitarii (A2 region). This region may be a site for hypotensive drugs which act by adrenergic receptor stimulation. The minimum effective dose of α-methylnoradrenaline in this region causing a hypotensive response after bilateral local application was 80 pmoles.

In contrast, an injection of physostigmine in the same region elicited a hypertensive response.

REFERENCES

Brezenoff, H.E. (1973) Centrally induced pressor responses to intravenous and intraventricular physostigmine evoked via different pathways. *Europ. J. Pharmacol.*, 23: 290—292.

Brezenoff, H.E. and Jenden, D.J. (1970) Changes in arterial blood pressure after microinjections of carbachol into the medulla and IVth ventricle of the rat brain. *Neuropharmacology*, 9: 341—348.

Brezenoff, H.E. and Rusin, J. (1974) Brain acetylcholine mediates the hypertensive response to physostigmine in the rat. *Europ. J. Pharmacol.*, 29: 262—266.

Dahlström, A. and Fuxe, K. (1964) Evidence for the existence of monoamine containing neurones in the central nervous system. I. Demonstration of monoamines in the cell bodies of brain stem neurons. *Acta physiol. scand.*, 62, Suppl. 232: 1—55.

De Jong, W. (1974) Noradrenaline; central inhibitory control of blood pressure and heart rate. *Europ. J. Pharmacol.*, 29: 179—181.

De Jong, W. and Nijkamp, F.P. (1976) Centrally induced hypotension by α-methyldopa and α-methylnoradrenaline in normotensive and renal hypertensive rats. *Brit. J. Pharmacol.*, 58: 593—598.

De Jong, W., Nijkamp, F.P. and Bohus, B. (1975a) Role of noradrenaline and serotonin in the central control of blood pressure in normotensive and spontaneously hypertensive rats. *Arch. int. Pharmacodyn.*, 213: 272—284.

De Jong, W., Zandberg, P. and Bohus, B. (1975b) Central inhibitory noradrenergic cardiovascular control. In *Hormones, Homeostasis and the Brain, Progr. Brain Res.*, Vol. 42, W.H. Gispen, Tj.B. van Wimersma Greidanus, B. Bohus and D. De Wied (Eds.), Elsevier, Amsterdam, pp. 285—298.

De Jong, W., Zandberg, P. and Versteeg, D.H.G. (1977) Brainstem structures and catecholamines in the control of arterial blood pressure in the rat. *Clin. Sci. molec. Med.*, in press.

De Jong, W., Zandberg, P., Palkovits, M. and Bohus, B. (1977) Acute and chronic

122

hypertension after lesions and transections of the rat brainstem. In *Hypertension and Brain Mechanisms, Progr. Brain Res., Vol. 47*, W. De Jong, A.P. Provoost and A.P. Shapiro (Eds.), Elsevier, Amsterdam, pp. 189—197.

Doba, N. and Reis, D.J. (1973) Acute fulminating neurogenic hypertension produced by brainstem lesions in the rat. *Circulat. Res.*, 32: 584—593.

Fuxe, K. (1965) Evidence for the existence of monoamine neurons in the central nervous system. IV. Distribution of monoamine nerve terminals in the central nervous system. *Acta physiol. scand.*, 64, Suppl. 247: 37—85.

Myers, R.D. (1966) Injection of solutions into cerebral tissue: relation between volume and diffusion. *Physiol. Behav.*, 1: 171—174.

Nijkamp, F.P. and De Jong, W. (1975) α-Methylnoradrenaline induced hypotension, and bradycardia after administration into the area of the nucleus tractus solitarii. *Europ. J. Pharmacol.*, 32: 361—364.

Nijkamp, F.P. and De Jong, W. (1977) Centrally induced hypotension by α-methyldopa and α-methylnoradrenaline in normotensive and renal hypertensive rats. In *Hypertension and Brain Mechanisms, Progr. Brain Res., Vol. 47*, W. De Jong, A.P. Provoost and A.P. Shapiro (Eds.), Elsevier, Amsterdam, pp. 349—368.

Palkovits, M. and Jacobowitz, D.M. (1974) Topographic atlas of catecholamine and acetylcholinesterase containing neurons in the rat brain. II. Hindbrain (mesencephalon, rhombencephalon). *J. comp. Neurol.*, 157: 29—42.

Varagić, V. and Krstić, M. (1966) Adrenergic activation by anti-cholinesterases. *Pharmacol. Rev.*, 18: 799—800.

Varagić, V. and Vojvodić, N. (1962) Effect of guanethidine, hemicholinum and mebutamate on the hypertensive response to eserine and catecholamines. *Brit. J. Pharmacol.*, 19: 451—457.

Zandberg, P. and De Jong, W. (1977) α-Methylnoradrenaline induced hypotension in the nucleus tractus solitarii of the rat: a localization study. *Neuropharmacology*, in press.

Van Zwieten, P.A. (1975) Antihypertensive drugs with a central action. *Progr. Pharmacol.*, 1: 1—63.

Role of Central Cholinoceptors in Cardiovascular Regulation

K.K. TANGRI*, I.P. JAIN and K.P. BHARGAVA

Department of Pharmacology, K.G. Medical College, Lucknow 226003 (India)

INTRODUCTION

Since acetylcholine (ACh), along with choline acetylase and cholinesterase, the enzymes concerned in its synthesis and degradation (Feldberg and Vogt, 1948; De Robertis et al., 1962) and cholinergic pathways (Shute and Lewis, 1967) are present in different regions of brain, a neurotransmitter role has been suggested for ACh in the CNS. ACh may therefore be concerned with the regulation of a number of physiological functions. Intracerebroventricular injection of cholinomimetic drugs has been shown to evoke excitatory cardiovascular responses in dogs (Sinha et al., 1967; Lang and Rush, 1973) and variable effects — excitatory, inhibitory and biphasic — in cats (Armitage and Hall, 1967; Armitage et al., 1967). Brezenoff (1972) and Brezenoff and Jenden (1970) also observed biphasic cardiovascular responses after intrahypothalamic and intramedullary injections of cholinomimetic agents in rats. Thus, neither the role of central cholinoceptors in cardiovascular regulation nor their nature is clear. Therefore, the present study was planned to determine the cardiovascular effects of superfusion of cholinergic drugs into the posterior hypothalamus and the "pressor" area of the lateral medullary reticular formation in cats.

METHODS

Cats (3.5 kg) of either sex were anaesthetized with pentobarbitone sodium (30 mg/kg i.p.), bilaterally vagotomized and maintained on positive pressure artificial respiration. The arterial blood pressure was measured from the femoral artery through an indwelling polyethylene catheter filled with heparin—saline and connected to a Statham P23Dc pressure transducer. The arterial pressure recordings were done on a Grass Model P5 polygraph. The heart rate was determined from lead 2 of ECG recorded on another channel of

*Fellow of Commonwealth Universities Association, Department of Clinical Pharmacology, Royal Postgraduate Medical School, Ducane Road, London W12 OHS, Great Britain.

the polygraph. The animals were routinely pretreated with atropine methylnitrate (1 mg/kg i.v.) to eliminate peripheral effects of centrally superfused cholinergic drugs due to their leakage in the peripheral circulation.

Superfusion technique

The cholinomimetic drugs were superfused into the posterior hypothalamus (PH) and "pressor" area in the lateral medullary reticular formation (LMPA) according to the technique of Phillipu et al. (1973) using a concentric double barrel push-pull cannula. The superfusion of the PH and LMPA was carried out with artificial cerebrospinal fluid (CSF) at pH 7.2 (Merlis, 1940) at the rate of 0.1 ml/min. The placement of the cannula in the PH and LMPA was done stereotaxically (PH = AP 10 mm, L 2 mm, V−2 to −4 mm; LMPA = AP −9 mm, L 2−4 mm, V −8 mm). The correct placement of cannula was checked by elicitation of pressor responses to electrical stimulation of these areas with square wave pulses (frequency, 30−100 Hz; pulse duration, 2−5 msec; 1−5 V) delivered from a Grass Model S4 stimulator, the outer tube of the cannula serving as monopolar electrode. The drugs were dissolved in artificial CSF and superfused for 10 min.

Drugs used

Acetylcholine hydrochloride (E. Merck), carbachol chloride (BDH), oxotremorine sesque fumarate (Sandoz), physostigmine salicylate (E. Merck), nicotine hydrogen tartrate (BDH), chlorisondamine salicylate (Ciba), ethybenztropine bromide (Sandoz) and atropine methylnitrate. All drug concentrations used in this study refer to their salts.

RESULTS

Superfusion of cholinergic drugs in the "pressor" area in the lateral medullary reticular formation (LMPA)

The cardiovascular effects of superfusion of both nicotinic and muscarinic agents, viz., nicotine, carbachol, acetylcholine and oxotremorine, were investigated and the results are shown in Table I. Carbachol superfusion (500 μg/ml) evoked a biphasic response consisting of an initial pressor response associated with tachycardia followed by a delayed depressor phase and bradycardia in 5 cats. The excitatory cardiovascular response appeared immediately, reaching its maximum in 2 min and lasting for 10−15 mins. The maximum increase in blood pressure was 23 mm Hg with a tachycardia of 12 bpm. On the other hand, the delayed depressor response (25 mm Hg) and bradycardia (41 bpm) lasted for 30−40 min.

Similarly, acetylcholine (500 μg/ml) superfusion in the LMPA evoked a biphasic cardiovascular response in 4 cats pretreated with local superfusion of physostigmine (1 mg/ml) lasting for 30−40 min. The initial pressor phase and tachycardia were 36 mm Hg and 40 bpm respectively followed by a depressor response and bradycardia of 34 mm Hg and 10 bpm, respectively. Nicotine (250 µg/ml) superfusion in the LMPA also evoked a biphasic cardiovascular response of greater magnitude in 4 cats. On the other hand, oxotremorine (200 µg/ml) evoked only a depressor response (28 mm Hg) and bradycardia (42 bpm) after superfusion in the LMPA in 5 cats. The peak effects of oxotremorine were observed in 5—10 min and lasted for 25—30 min.

Cardiovascular effects of cholinomimetic drugs after pretreatment with superfusion of cholinergic blocking agents in the LMPA

Pretreatment consisting of local superfusion of the nicotinic and muscarinic blocking agents chlorisondamine and ethybenztropine affected the cardiovascular actions of carbachol superfusion in the LMPA as shown in Fig. 1B. Following chlorisondamine (2 mg/ml), the initial pressor response and tachycardia evoked by carbachol (500 µg/ml) superfusion was completely blocked in 3 cats and only a depressor phase (26 ± 3 mm Hg) with bradycardia (53 ± 9 bpm) could be observed. On the other hand, when chlorisondamine and ethybenztropine (2 mg/ml each) were superfused together in the LMPA prior to carbachol superfusion, carbachol failed to evoke any cardiovascular response. A similar blockade of the excitatory cardiovascular effects of

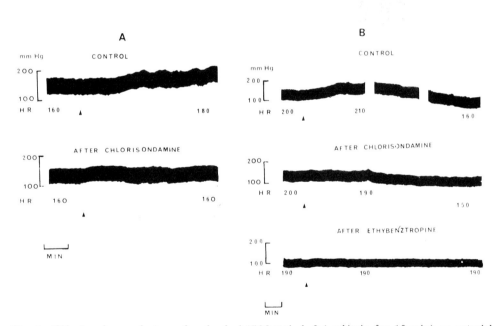

Fig. 1. Effects of superfusion of carbachol (500 µg/ml, 0.1 ml/min for 10 min) on arterial blood pressure and heart rate (HR) into (A) posterior hypothalamus (PH). Blockade of hypertension and tachycardia response of carbachol by chlorisondamine (2 mg/ml, 0.1 ml/min for 10 min); (B) lateral medullary "pressor" area (LMPA). Blockade of initial hypertension and tachycardia response of carbachol by chlorisondamine. Further complete blockade by combined pretreatment with chlorisondamine and ethybenztropine (2 mg/ml, 0.1 ml/min for 10 min) of both the hypertension with tachycardia and the delayed hypotension with bradycardia.

TABLE I

CARDIOVASCULAR EFFECTS OF CHOLINERGIC DRUGS SUPERFUSED INTO "PRESSOR" AREA IN THE LATERAL MEDULLARY RETICULAR FORMATION IN CATS

Drug	Drug concentration (μg/ml)	Pretreatment	No. of animals	Initial response		Delayed response	
				Mean change in blood pressure (mm Hg ± S.E.)	Mean change in heart rate (bpm ± S.E.)	Mean change in blood pressure (mm Hg ± S.E.)	Mean change in heart rate (bpm ± S.E.)
Carbachol	500	—	5	+22.6 ± 2.1	+12.1 ± 2.2	−25.3 ± 2.8	−40.8 ± 5.6
		Chlorisondamine*	3	−16.3 ± 1.8	−28.6 ± 3.2	−26.2 ± 3.4	−52.8 ± 9.3
		Chlorisondamine* + ethybenztropine*	3	No effect	No effect	—	—
Acetylcholine	500	Physostigmine**	4	+36.3 ± 5.4	+40.0 ± 4.1	−33.8 ± 4.8	−10.0 ± 3.0
		Ethybenztropine*	4	+26.7 ± 2.3	+20.2 ± 3.4	+15.2 ± 2.8	+10.3 ± 2.1
		Chlorisondamine*	3	−17.5 ± 2.5	−10.2 ± 2.2	−32.5 ± 7.6	−18.1 ± 4.2
Nicotine	250	—	4	+70.4 ± 9.8	+54.6 ± 5.3	−52.3 ± 4.8	−38.2 ± 4.3
		Ethybenztropine*	3	+80.2 ± 10.3	+50.4 ± 4.8	−49.7 ± 5.3	−40.6 ± 3.2
		Chlorisondamine*	4	−28.2 ± 4.2	−22.3 ± 3.2	−41.6 ± 7.7	−35.5 ± 4.9
Oxotremorine	200	—	5	−28.3 ± 2.8	−42.4 ± 7.8	−20.4 ± 3.7	−32.2 ± 4.9
		Ethybenztropine*	3	No effect	No effect	—	—

*2 mg/ml, 0.1 ml/min for 10 min.
**1 mg/ml, 0.1 ml/min for 10 min.

acetylcholine and nicotine was observed following local treatment with chlorisondamine superfusion in the LMPA. However, while ethyl benztropine pretreatment could block the depressor phase and the bradycardia induced by acetylcholine and oxotremorine, ethybenztropine failed to block the depressor response and bradycardia induced by nicotine superfusion (Table I).

Superfusion of cholinergic drugs in the posterior hypothalamus (PH)

The cardiovascular effects of superfusion of carbachol, nicotine and oxotremorine in the PH were investigated before and after pretreatment with local superfusion of cholinergic blocking agents and the results are shown in Table II. Carbachol superfusion (500 μg/ml) in PH evoked a pressor response associated with tachycardia in 3 cats. The peak effects were observed in 5—10 min (33 mm Hg and 17 bpm) and lasted for 25—30 min. Nicotine superfusion (250 μg/ml) also evoked an excitatory cardiovascular response (33 mm Hg and 40 bpm) in 3 cats. On the other hand, oxotremorine superfusion (200 μg/ml) in the PH failed to evoke any cardiovascular response in 2 cats. Furthermore, pretreatment with superfusion of chlorisondamine (2 mg/ml) in the PH blocked the excitatory cardiovascular response to both carbachol and nicotine superfusion.

TABLE II

CARDIOVASCULAR EFFECTS OF CHOLINERGIC DRUGS SUPERFUSED INTO THE POSTERIOR HYPOTHALAMUS OF CATS

Drug	Drug concentration (μg/ml)	Pretreatment	No. of animals	Mean change in blood pressure (mm Hg ± S.E.)	Mean change in heart rate (bpm ± S.E.)
Carbachol	500	—	3	+33.4 ± 4.5	+16.6 ± 3.4
		Chlorisondamine*	2	No effect	No effect
Nicotine	250	—	3	+33.3 ± 2.4	+40.0 ± 5.8
		Chlorisondamine*	2	No effect	No effect
Oxotremorine	200	—	2	No effect	No effect

*Concentration: 2 mg/ml, 0.1 ml/min for 10 min.

DISCUSSION

In the present study, superfusion of acetylcholine in the "pressor" area of the lateral medullary reticular formation (LMPA) of physostigmine-pretreated cats, evoked a biphasic cardiovascular response. This response consisted of an initial excitatory phase of hypertension and tachycardia followed by delayed hypotension and bradycardia. The initial excitatory cardiovascular response to acetylcholine was due to activation of nicotinic receptors in the LMPA since it was blocked by prior superfusion of the LMPA with a nicotinic blocking agent, chlorisondamine. Furthermore, the acetylcholine-induced delayed inhibitory responses, hypotension and bradycardia, were due to stimulation of muscarinic receptors as they could be blocked by pretreatment with ethybenztropine, a muscarinic blocking agent. Similarly, carbachol superfusion in the LMPA resulted in a biphasic cardiovascular response. The initial excitatory effect of carbachol was also blocked by local superfusion with chlorisondamine and the delayed inhibitory response with ethybenztropine. Thus these observations suggested the presence of both nicotinic excitatory and muscarinic inhibitory cholinoceptors in the LMPA which may be involved in cardiovascular regulation.

Brezenoff and Jenden (1970) also demonstrated the presence of both excitatory nicotinic and inhibitory muscarinic receptors in the brain stem of rats since intramedullary and 4th ventricular injections of carbachol and oxotremorine elicited a biphasic and a pure depressant cardiovascular response respectively. However, Guerstzenstein (1973) observed a depressor effect of carbachol when applied topically to the ventral surface of the medulla of cats. The latter is failure to demonstrate an excitatory cardiovascular effect of carbachol could be due to failure of the drug to reach active "nicotinic" sites in the medullary reticular "pressor" area. On the contrary, Sinha et al. (1967) demonstrated in dogs, a blockade by atropine of the pressor response to topical application of acetylcholine to the floor of the 4th ventricle by atropine; this suggested the presence of excitatory muscarinic receptors in the medulla. The blockade of the pressor effect of centrally administered acetylcholine by atropine could also have resulted from a non-specific procaine-like effect of atropine on brain stem neurons (Curtis and Phillis, 1960). That the muscarinic receptors in the LMPA were inhibitory was further confirmed by the observation that oxotremorine superfusion in the LMPA evoked a depressor and bradycardia response which was blocked by pretreatment with ethybenztropine. Similarly, the presence of excitatory nicotinic receptors for cardiovascular control in the LMPA was further demonstrated by the blockade of the initial pressor response and tachycardia induced by local superfusion of nicotine by chlorisondamine pretreatment. However, nicotine superfusion in the LMPA also evoked a delayed depressor response and bradycardia. This inhibition by nicotine was not due to an activation of the muscarinic receptors in the LMPA since it was not blocked by prior local superfusion of ethybenztropine. Moreover, nicotine is devoid of muscarinic receptor agonist activity. The depressor and bradycardia response to nicotine superfusion in the LMPA may, on the other hand, be due to a central release of catecholamines (Phillipu et al., 1971, 1974) as noradrenaline superfusion in the LMPA has been shown to cause hypotension and bradycardia (Bhargava, 1975).

The present study further demonstrated the presence of excitatory nicotinic receptors in the PH of cats since local superfusion of carbachol and nicotine elicited hypertension and bradycardia which were blocked by chlorisondamine pretreatment. On the contrary, the presence of muscarinic receptors in the PH seems unlikely since oxotremorine superfusion failed to evoke any cardiovascular response. Centrally administered ganglion blocking agents have been found to block pressor responses to intracerebroventricular injection of nicotine in cats (Armitage et al., 1967; Pradhan et al., 1967) and hypothalamic injection of carbachol in rats (Brezenoff, 1972).

Thus it may be concluded that cholinoceptors are present in the PH and in the LMPA which may be concerned in cardiovascular regulation. While excitatory nicotinic receptors are distributed in both the PH and the LMPA, inhibitory muscarinic receptors occur only in the LMPA.

SUMMARY

The role and nature of central cholinoceptors in the cardiovascular regulation were investigated in the present study by superfusing cholinoceptor agonists and antagonists into the posterior hypothalamus (PH) and "pressor" area in the lateral medullary reticular formation (LMPA) in pentobarbitone anaesthetized cats pretreated with atropine methylnitrate (1 mg/kg i.v.). Superfusion of acetylcholine, carbachol, nicotine and oxotremorine in the LMPA and the PH demonstrated the presence of excitatory nicotinic receptors in both these areas. On the other hand, inhibitory muscarinic cholinoceptors could only be found in the LMPA. The significance of these observations is discussed.

REFERENCES

Armitage, A.K. and Hall, G.H. (1967) Effect of nicotine on systemic blood pressure when injected into the cerebral ventricles of cat. *Int. J. Neuropharmacol.*, 6: 143—149.

Armitage, A.K., Hall, G.H., Milton, A.S. and Morrison, C.F. (1967) Effects of nicotine injected into and perfused through the cerebral ventricles of the cat. *Ann. N.Y. Acad. Sci.*, 142: 27—39.

Bhargava, K.P. (1975) Central α- and β-adrenoceptors in cardiovascular regulation. In *Recent Advances in Hypertension. Vol. 2*, P. Milliez and M. Safar (Eds), Boehringer, Ingelheim, pp. 109—127.

Brezenoff, H.E. (1972) Cardiovascular response to intrahypothalamic injections of carbachol and certain cholinesterase inhibitors. *Neuropharmacology*, 11: 637—644.

Brezenoff, H.E. and Jenden, D.J. (1970) Changes in arterial blood pressure after micro-injection of carbachol into the medulla and IV ventricle of rat brain. *Neuropharmacology*, 9: 341—348.

Curtis, D.R. and Phillis, J.W. (1960) The action of procain and atropine on spinal neurones. *J. Physiol. (Lond.)*, 153: 17—34.

De Robertis, E., De Iraldi, A.P., De Lores Arnaiz, R.G. and Salganicoff, L.(1962) Cholinergic and non-cholinergic nerve endings in rat brain. I. Isolation and subcellular distribution of acetylcholine and acetyl cholinesterase. *J. Neurochem.*, 9: 23—35.

Feldberg, W. and Vogt, M. (1948) Acetylcholine synthesis in different regions of the central nervous system. *J. Physiol. (Lond.)*, 107: 372—381.

Guerstzenstein, P.G. (1973) Blood pressure effects obtained by drugs applied to the ventral surfaces of brain stem. *J. Physiol. (Lond.)*, 229: 395—408.

Lang, W.J. and Rush, M.L. (1973) Cardiovascular response to injections of cholinomimetic drugs into cerebral ventricles of unanaesthetized dogs. *Brit. J. Pharmacol.*, 47: 196—205.

Merlis, J.K. (1940) The effect of changes in the calcium content of cerebrospinal fluid on spinal reflex activity in the dog. *Amer. J. Physiol.*, 13: 67—72.

Phillipu, A., Przuntek, H., Heyd, H. and Burger, A. (1971) Central effects of sympathomimetic amines on the blood pressure. *Europ. J. Pharmacol.*, 15: 200—208.

Phillipu, A., Przuntek, H. and Roesberg, W. (1973) Superfusion of the hypothalamus with gamma-aminobutyric acid. *Naunyn Schmiedeberg's Arch. exp. Path. Pharmak.*, 276: 103—118.

Phillipu, A., Demmeler, R. and Roensberg, G. (1974) Effects of centrally applied drugs on pressor responses to hypothalamic stimulation. *Naunyn Schmiedeberg's Arch. exp. Path. Pharmak.*, 282: 389—400.

Pradhan, S.N., Bhattacharya, I.C. and Atkins, K.S. (1967) Effects of intraventricular administration of nicotine on blood pressure and some somatic reflexes. *Ann. N.Y. Acad. Sci.*, 142: 50—66.

Shute, C.C.D. and Lewis, P.R. (1967) The ascending cholinergic reticular system: neocortical, olfactory and sub-cortical projections. *Brain*, 90: 497—520.

Sinha, J.N., Dhawan, K.N., Chandra, O. and Gupta, G.P. (1967) Role of acetylcholine in central vasomotor regulation. *Canad. J. Physiol. Pharmacol.*, 45: 503—507.

Central Action of some Cholinergic Drugs (Arecaidine Esters) and Nicotine on Blood Pressure and Heart Rate of Cats

A.J. PORSIUS and P.A. VAN ZWIETEN

Department of Pharmacy, Division of Pharmacotherapy, University of Amsterdam, Amsterdam (The Netherlands)

INTRODUCTION

Since it became known that antihypertensive drugs like clonidine and α-methyldopa exert their pharmacological activity by stimulating central α-adrenergic receptors, many investigations have been performed in order to test a possible central hypotensive action of drugs. However, little information is available concerning the central action of cholinergic drugs. Therefore, we investigated the influence of a number of structurally related cholinergic drugs on blood pressure and cardiac frequency after infusion into the left vertebral artery of the cat. Recently, the pharmacological actions of various synthetized arecaidine esters and related compounds on isolated atria (Christiansen, 1967), on the isolated ileum (Gloge et al., 1966) and on systemic blood pressure (Kummer et al., 1966) were quantified. Additionally, structure—activity relationships have been considered (Mutschler and Hultzsch, 1973). Therefore, it was of interest to investigate the possible central action of these esters on blood pressure and heart rate in order to compare their peripheral and central activities. Moreover, we studied the central effects of nicotine on the afore-mentioned cardiovascular parameters, since little information is available in this respect. The experimental results may yield evidence as to whether cholinergic mechanisms contribute to central regulation of blood pressure and heart rate.

MATERIALS AND METHODS

(a) Influence on blood pressure and heart rate

The experiments were carried out on cats of either sex (weight 2—4 kg), anaesthetized with 60 mg α-chloralose/kg. Blood pressure was recorded continuously from a femoral artery via a pressure transducer connected to a Hellige recorder. Heart rate was evaluated from the pulse waves in the femoral artery. A femoral vein was cannulated for intravenous administration of drugs. The technique of drug infusion into the vertebral artery of the cat has been described previously in detail (Van Zwieten, 1975).

132

(b) Distribution of nicotine in the brain

The distribution of [N-methyl-^{14}C]nicotine D-bitartrate was established after injection of 10 μg of the radioactive drug per kg into the left vertebral artery. The drug solution (0.1 ml/kg) was infused for 1 min. One minute after the injection, the circulation was arrested by occluding the aorta between the left ventricle and the brachiocephalic trunk. Various brain regions were isolated and weighed. Radioactivity was measured after dissolving the brain tissues in Soluene-100 and adding Insta-Gel (Packard).

RESULTS

The intravenous administration of the cholinergic drugs shown in Fig. 1 (arecaidine esters) caused a dose dependent reduction in mean arterial pressure of the cat. This hypotensive effect could be blocked by pretreatment with intravenously injected methylatropine (300 μg/kg). However, pretreatment with centrally administered atropine (30 μg/kg) or D-benzethimide (10 μg/kg) did not prevent the hypotensive action of these drugs. Dose-response curves of the peripherally induced blood-pressure lowering effect were established and the ED-25 was calculated (Table I). Injection of these cholinergic drugs into the vertebral artery also reduced arterial pressure in a dose dependent manner. This

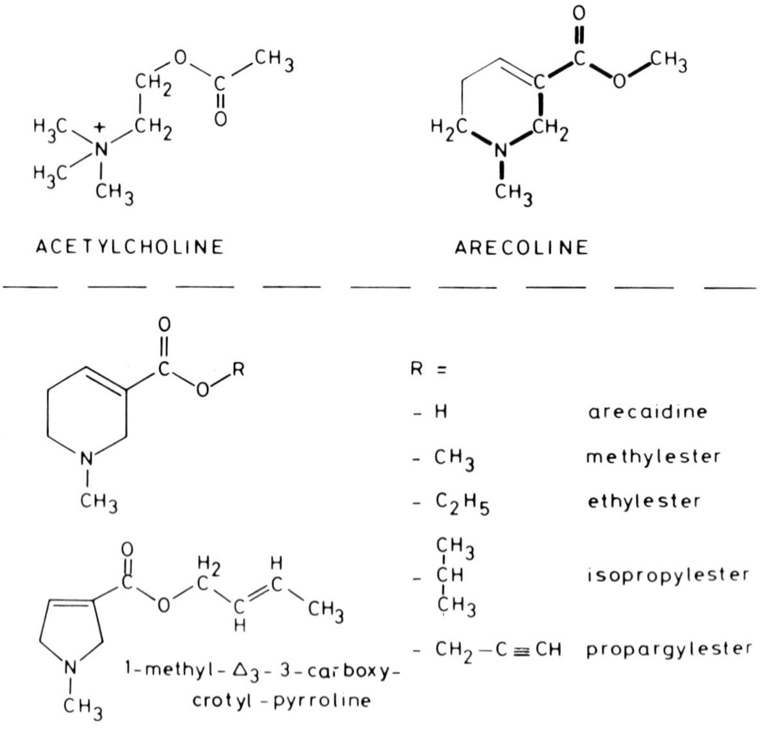

Fig. 1. Arecaidine esters.

TABLE I

CENTRAL AND PERIPHERAL HYPOTENSIVE ACTIVITIES
OF SOME CHOLINERGIC ESTERS

Ester	ED -25 moles/kg vertebral artery	ED -25 moles/kg femoral vein
Arecaidine-propargylester	1.0×10^{-9}	1.4×10^{-9}
Arecaidine-ethylester	2.0×10^{-9}	4.2×10^{-9}
Arecaidine-methylester (arecoline)	15.1×10^{-9}	18.6×10^{-9}
(chemical structure depicted)	631×10^{-9}	590×10^{-9}
Arecaidine-isopropylester	1040×10^{-9}	1200×10^{-9}

centrally induced hypotensive effect was not inhibited by pretreatment with intravenous methylatropine (300 μg/kg). However, pretreatment with atropine (50 μg/kg) and D-benzethimide (10 μg/kg), both administered via the vertebral artery, blocked the central hypotensive action of these derivatives. Bilateral vagotomy did not influence the centrally induced hypotensive effect. Pretreatment with the α-blocking agent yohimbine (300 μg/kg) did not affect the action of the centrally applied arecaidine esters. Dose-response curves of the central hypotensive effect were established and the ED-25 was calculated (Table I). Only in relatively high doses did intravenous injection of these drugs cause a decrease in cardiac frequency. Central application had no effect on heart rate, even in high doses.

After injection into the vertebral artery nicotine caused a dose dependent decrease of both blood pressure and heart rate. Central administration of 5 μg nicotine base/kg caused a reduction in mean arterial pressure by $40.3 \pm 6.0\%$, whereas the decrease in cardiac frequency amounted to $34.3 \pm 6.2\%$ (mean $\pm$ S.E.M., n = 8). Both effects were neither influenced by pretreatment with yohimbine nor by atropine. However, pretreatment with metoprolol (1 mg/kg) or mecamylamine (50 μg/kg) both administered via the vertebral artery blocked these centrally induced cardiovascular effects of nicotine completely. Bilateral vagotomy did not influence the hypotensive effect, but abolished the negative chronotropic action of nicotine. One minute after the injection of 10 μg [^{14}C]nicotine bitartrate/kg into the vertebral artery, the concentrations of nicotine (calculated as percentage of the administered dose/100 mg tissue) in various brain regions were as follows: medulla oblongata 0.58 ± 0.10, pons 0.33 ± 0.06, hypothalamus 0.039 ± 0.013, cortex

0.027 ± 0.015, pituitary gland 0.024 ± 0.006, cerebellum 0.26 ± 0.13 (mean ± S.E.M., n = 7).

DISCUSSION

The present study demonstrates the cardiovascular effects of some structurally related cholinergic drugs after central administration. Drugs injected into the left vertebral artery are distributed to the rhombencephalon, where the vasomotor centres are located (Van Zwieten, 1975). Because of their high lipophilicity, the arecaidine esters easily penetrate the blood—brain barrier. The resulting hypotensive effect can be attributed to stimulation of central muscarinic receptors in the brain stem, since peripherally administered methylatropine does not counteract the hypotensive action, whereas centrally applied anticholinergic drugs like atropine and D-benzethimide block the effect. Recently, dose-response curves of the negative inotropic action (Christiansen, 1967) and the stimulating action on the isolated ileum (Gloge et al., 1966) of these drugs were established. When the intrinsic activities and affinities of these esters towards peripheral muscarinic receptors are compared with those towards central muscarinic receptors, it can be concluded that a striking similarity exists between centrally and peripherally located muscarinic receptors. Drugs with a high affinity (intrinsic activity) towards the peripheral muscarinic receptor (heart, ileum) possess a high affinity (intrinsic activity) towards the central muscarinic receptor (compare Table I). Since bilateral vagotomy does not affect the central blood pressure lowering effect, the central hypotensive action may probably be attributed to a decrease in sympathetic outflow. The fact that cardiac frequency is not influenced suggests that stimulation of central muscarinic receptors in the brain stem does not increase vagal activity.

In contrast to the cardiovascular effects of peripherally administered nicotine, this alkaloid causes a significant decrease of both blood pressure and heart rate after central application. Severe hypotensive and cardiodepressive effects of nicotine occur from relatively low doses. The experiments with [^{14}C]nicotine demonstrate the distribution of this drug to the rhombencephalon after central administration. The hypothalamus for instance contains only an insignificant amount of nicotine at the moment of maximal pharmacological response. Since yohimbine or anticholinergic drugs do not influence these cardiovascular actions, it is concluded that neither central α-receptors nor central muscarinic receptors are involved. Mecamylamine blocks both biological actions, indicating that stimulation of central nicotine receptors is responsible for the afore-mentioned actions. Pretreatment with atropine or bilateral vagotomy abolishes the cardiodepressive action but not the hypotensive effect. Therefore, it is plausible, that the reduction in sympathetic outflow, which gives rise to hypotension, is accompanied by a stimulation of the vagus nerves, resulting in a bradycardia. The inhibition of the centrally induced cardiovascular effects by the specific β-sympatholytic agent metoprolol is not clear and is the subject of further investigation. Our experimental results demonstrate that interaction of both central muscarinic and nicotinic receptors with their respective agonists gives rise to potent cardiovascular effects. It is suggested that physiologically released acetylcholine in the brain stem may play an important part in regulating both blood pressure and heart rate by stimulating central nicotinic and muscarinic receptors.

SUMMARY

The influence of various structurally related cholinergic drugs (arecaidine esters) and of nicotine on arterial pressure and cardiac frequency was tested following central administration via the left vertebral artery of the cat. A comparison is made of the effects following intravenous injection. Arecaidine esters possess a central hypotensive action by stimulating central muscarinic receptors in the brain stem, but do not influence cardiac frequency. It is postulated that peripheral muscarinic receptors behave in the same way as central muscarinic receptors towards their agonists. After injection into the vertebral artery, nicotine accumulates mainly in the brain stem and causes potent hypotensive and cardiodepressive effects by stimulating central nicotinic receptors. The experimental results suggest that acetylcholine may play an important part in the central regulation of blood pressure and heart rate.

ACKNOWLEDGEMENT

The arecaidine esters and the related compound (Fig. 1) were kindly supplied by Prof. Dr. Dr.E. Mutschler, Frankfurt, G.F.R.

REFERENCES

Christiansen, A. (1967) *Untersuchungen über Struktur-Wirkungs-Beziehungen von Arecaidinderivaten an isolierten Vorhöfen von Meerschweinchen.* Dissertation, Kiel.

Gloge, H., Lüllmann, H. and Mutschler, E. (1966) The action of tertiary and quaternary arecaidine and dihydroarecaidine esters on the guinea pig isolated ileum. *Brit. J. Pharmacol.,* 27: 185—195.

Kummer, B., Lüllmann, H. und Mutschler, E. (1966) Über die Wirkung von Arecaidinestern auf den Blutdruck der Katze. *Naunyn-Schmiedeberg's Arch. exp. Path. Pharmak.,* 254: 159—169.

Mutschler, E. und Hultzsch, K. (1973) Über Struktur-Wirkungs-Beziehungen von ungesättigten Estern des Arecaidins und Dihydro-arecaidins. *Arzneim.-Forsch.,* 23: 732—737.

Van Zwieten, P.A. (1975) Antihypertensive drugs with a central action. *Progr. Pharmacol.,* 1: 1—63.

Central Angiotensin in the Control of Water Intake and Blood Pressure

J.L. ELGHOZI, J.T. FITZSIMONS, P. MEYER and S. NICOLAÏDIS

(J.T.F.) Physiological Laboratory, Cambridge (Great Britain) and (S.N.) Collège de France and (P.M. and J.L.E.) Hôpital Necker, INSERM U7, Paris (France)

INTRODUCTION

The action of angiotensin II on the central nervous system has at least 4 different effects. These are (1) thirst, (2) neurogenic pressor action, (3) antidiuretic hormone (ADH) release, and (4) sodium (Na) appetite. For the first three of these actions there is good evidence that sensitive structures in the brain are accessible to blood-borne hormone as well as to angiotensin injected directly into the brain. The case of Na appetite is a little different. Firstly, it is by no means clear that the slight increase in Na intake produced by intracranial angiotensin is physiologically significant. Secondly, activation of the renal renin—angiotensin system does not stimulate Na appetite. Thirdly, the amount of an aversive concentration of saline that is drunk in response to intracranial angiotensin increases with repeated injections of angiotensin suggesting that there is an addictive or learned component to the intake.

Though there are obvious uncertainties regarding different aspects of each of these 4 actions of angiotensin they can all be regarded as contributing to the control of extracellular fluid volume. The pressor response, for example, favours the shift of interstitial fluid into the plasma. All 4 actions would therefore be useful in situations where the blood volume is reduced and it is of course well established that hypovolaemia activates the renal renin—angiotensin system. But it has also been established that there is a cerebral isorenin—angiotensin system which is quite independent of the renal system. In view of the sensitivity of brain structures to angiotensin this raises the question of the possible role of the cerebral renin—angiotensin system in eliciting these 4 actions of angiotensin under physiological conditions. The remainder of this paper will be devoted to certain aspects of two of these actions of angiotensin on the central nervous system, namely thirst and the neurogenic pressor response, together with a consideration of what is known about involvement of the cerebral renin—angiotensin system in these responses.

ANGIOTENSIN IN THE CONTROL OF WATER INTAKE

Circulating angiotensin II, or angiotensin injected directly into the brain, causes drinking by water-replete animals in all species so far tested (Fitzsimons,

138

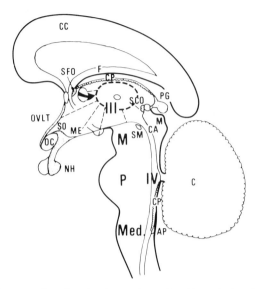

Fig. 1. Schematic diagram showing brain regions implicated in the central actions of angiotensin II (paramedian sagittal section, cerebral hemispheres omitted, dotted areas lie outside the blood—brain barrier). Arrow comes from lateral ventricle and represents the flow of CSF into the third ventricle. III, third ventricle; CA, cerebral aqueduct; IV, fourth ventricle; CP, choroid plexus; Dotted lines, thalamus and hypothalamus; CC, corpus callosum; F, fornix; OC, optic chiasm; M, mesencephalon; P, pons; Med, medulla; C, cerebellum; SFO, subfornical organ; OVLT, organum vasculosum of the lamina terminalis; SO, supraoptic nucleus; ME, median eminence; NH, neurohypophysis; SCO, subcommissural organ; PG, pineal gland; SM, subnucleus medialis; AP, area postrema.

1975). The parts of the brain that are most sensitive to the dipsogenic action of angiotensin are two highly vascular circumventricular structures that lie outside the blood—brain barrier, the subfornical organ (Simpson and Routtenberg, 1973) and the organum vasculosum of the lamina terminalis which lies in the wall of the anterior third ventricle (Nicolaïdis and Fitzsimons, 1975)(Fig. 1). The fact that the most sensitive structures appear to lie outside the blood—brain barrier could explain how blood-borne angiotensin causes drinking since it is clear that the octapeptide cannot cross the barrier (Osborne et al., 1971; Ganten et al., 1975).

It was suggested that activation of the renal renin—angiotensin system might contribute to drinking induced by extracellular dehydration (Fitzsimons, 1966, 1969). According to this view a deficit of extracellular fluid causes a change in sensory information from receptors in thoracic capacitance vessels. This results in stimulation of brain structures involved in thirst and also in increased renin secretion and generation of angiotensin II (Fig. 2). The increased circulating angiotensin acts directly on the brain to augment drinking induced by the extracellular deficit. However, the discovery of a cerebral isorenin—angiotensin system (Fischer-Ferraro et al., 1971; Ganten et al., 1971) allows other interpretations of the significance of intracranial sensitivity to angiotensin. It is possible that the cerebral isorenin system is a peptidergic neurotransmitter system activated by local changes in the brain and that this is the only way in

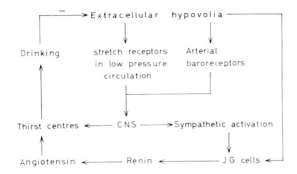

Fig. 2. Possible mechanisms for drinking caused by extracellular dehydration. In addition to increased drinking of water there is also a delayed increase in sodium appetite not indicated on the figure. (From Fitzsimons, 1970.)

which angiotensin normally causes drinking. Present evidence is that circulating angiotensin contributes to thirst induced by certain extracellular stimuli, whereas up to now it has not been possible to show whether the cerebral system ever affects water intake.

The cerebral isorenin—angiotensin system does, however, allow us to explain the rather surprising finding that renin, renin substrate and angiotensin I are at least as effective intracranial dipsogens as angiotensin II (Fitzsimons, 1971). The cerebral system would ensure the local generation of angiotensin II when components of the renin—angiotensin system other than angiotensin II itself are injected. By injecting the antibody to angiotensin II or peptide antagonists of the reactions that lead to the generation of angiotensin II, just before injecting one of the precursor components, it has been shown that this explanation is correct (Fitzsimons et al., 1976). As far as the shorter chain analogues of angiotensin are concerned, the requirements for dipsogenic activity are similar to those for other biological actions (Fitzsimons, 1971). The (2—8) heptapeptide retains much of the activity of the octapeptide but the absence of phenylalanine at the C-terminal end of the molecule in the (1—7) heptapeptide results in an inactive compound (Fig. 3). The (3—8) hexapeptide is relatively inactive, and the (4—8) pentapeptide and the (1—4) and (5—8) tetrapeptide fragments of angiotensin II are devoid of any activity. The D-arginine^2 substituted octapeptide is also ineffective. It is apparent that shortening the octapeptide chain, particularly removal of phenylalanine at the C-terminal end, results in a loss of dipsogenic activity.

The properties of the angiotensin-sensitive dipsogenic receptor therefore resemble those of the myotropic receptor. This and the fact that the subfornical organ and the organum vasculosum, the structures most sensitive to the dipsogenic action of angiotensin, are highly vascularised would support a hypothesis that drinking induced by angiotensin is mediated by an effect on the blood vessels in these structures. Though angiotensin far outstripped other vasoactive substances as a dipsogen in reliability and efficacy, it is also evident that a variety of agents affecting the smooth muscle of arterioles elsewhere in the body sometimes cause drinking when injected into the brain (Table I).

140

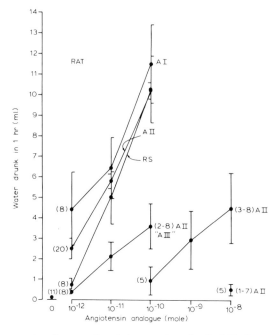

Fig. 3. The mean amounts of water drunk by rats in 1 hr (± S.E.M., number of observations in parentheses) in response to various doses of angiotensin II (AII) and its analogues. AI = angiotensin I; RS = renin substrate. (Fitzsimons, 1971 and unpublished observations.)

In order to test this hypothesis further, drinking in response to either angiotensin or to an equidipsogenic dose of carbachol (another potent intracranial dipsogen) was measured before and after the injection of various vasoactive agents including vasoplegics (Nicolaïdis and Fitzsimons, 1975). It was found that a variety of vasoactive substances, mainly vasodilator, antagonizes the dipsogenic action of angiotensin without affecting that of carbachol (Table II). The action of vasopressin was not fully explored because the combination of angiotensin and vasopressin seemed to induce a catatonic-like state which necessarily interfered with drinking and which made the interpretation of results difficult. The mean quantities drunk during control periods and after the injection of three vasoactive substances are illustrated in Fig. 4. A highly significant reduction in angiotensin-induced drinking occurred after pretreatment with papaverine, sodium nitrite or sodium nitroprusside injected into the anterior third ventricle or the subfornical organ but none of these agents affected carbachol-induced drinking of similar magnitude.

The most important findings revealed by vasoactive substances may be summarized as follows. (1) Many vasoconstrictors and vasodilators cause some drinking when injected into certain regions of the brain but none approach angiotensin in effectiveness. (2) The most sensitive regions are two vascular structures in the brain lying outside the blood—brain barrier, the subfornical organ and the organum vasculosum of the lamina terminalis. (3) Vasoplegics such as papaverine, sodium nitrite, sodium nitroprusside and prostaglandin E_2 interfere with angiotensin-induced drinking but not with carbachol-induced

TABLE I

INCIDENCE OF DRINKING 0.5 ML OR MORE WITH A LATENCY OF 6 MIN OR LESS FOLLOWING INTRACRANIAL
INJECTIONS OF VARIOUS SUBSTANCES

(From Nicolaïdis and Fitzsimons, 1975.)

	Dose	Number of injections	Number of drinking responses	% age of drinking responses	Maximum intake Dose in parentheses
0.9% NaCl	1–6 μl	47	0	0	—
Angiotensin II	1–100 × 10^{-12} mole	39	39	100	19 ml (50 × 10^{-12} mole)
Carbachol	821–3285 × 10^{-12} mole	8	8	100	17.5 ml (1642 × 10^{-12} mole)
Papaverine	53–318 × 10^{-3} mole	45	8	17.8	12.5 ml (106 × 10^{-3} mole)
NaNO$_2$	20–80 × 10^{-9} mole	16	1	6.25	9.1 ml (80 × 10^{-9} mole)
Nitroprusside	10–100 × 10^{-9} mole	14	2	14.3	7.6 ml (20 × 10^{-9} mole)
ADH	1–10 mU	16	7	43.7	10.3 ml (5 mU)
PGE$_2$	10–40 μg	11	3	27.3	4.6 ml (10 μg)

TABLE II

INCIDENCE OF COMPLETE BLOCK (intake of less than 0.5 ml in 30 min) OF
ANGIOTENSIN- OR CARBACHOL-INDUCED DRINKING BY VARIOUS AGENTS
GIVEN 6 MIN BEFORE THE DIPSOGEN THROUGH THE SAME INTRACRANIAL
CANNULA

(From Nicolaïdis and Fitzsimons, 1975.)

	Angiotensin II			Carbachol		
	Number of injections	Number blocked	% age blocked	Number of injections	Number blocked	% age blocked
0.9% NaCl	39	0	0	8	0	0
Papaverine	31	16	51.6	14	1	7.1
NaNO$_2$	13	7	53.8	3	0	0
Nitroprusside	8	7	87.5	6	0	0
ADH	5	2	40	0	—	—
PGE$_2$	9	4	44.4	3	0	0

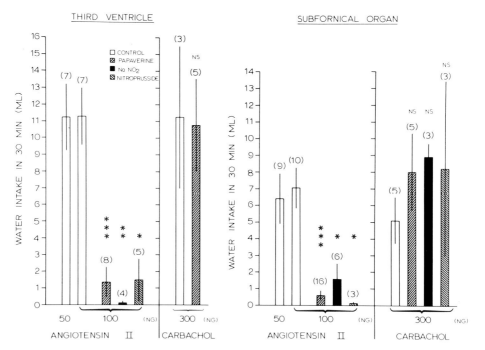

Fig. 4. The mean amounts of water drunk by rats with permanent cannulae either in the
anterior third ventricle or in the subfornical organ after injection of angiotensin II or
carbachol receded by 0.9% NaCl (1–4 μl), papaverine (53–318 x 10^{-3} mole), NaNO$_2$ (20–
40 x 10^{-9} mole) or sodium nitroprusside (10–100 x 10^{-9} mole) given through the same
intracranial cannula. The doses of dipsogen are given on the abscissa. The vertical bars are
twice the S.E.M. and the numbers of experiments are given in parentheses. The levels of
significance are, the comparison being made with the dose of 50 ng in the case of
angiotensin: * $P < 0.05$; ** $P < 0.01$; *** $P < 0.001$; NS, not significant. (From Nicolaïdis
and Fitzsimons, 1975.)

drinking. (4) With the exception of renin substrate there is extraordinarily good parallelism between the dipsogenic efficacy of the different analogues of angiotensin and their effect on blood pressure. Renin substrate is as good a dipsogen as angiotensin II but has only 10% of the pressor activity. The reason for this discrepancy could be that renin substrate injected into the brain is rapidly acted upon by the cerebral isorenin angiotensin system to yield angiotensin II which then exerts its dipsogenic effect.

If it can be accepted by this evidence that angiotensin-sensitive dipsogenic receptors are in fact myotropic receptors in the walls of blood vessels in circumventricular organs lying outside the blood—brain barrier, then it is attractive to speculate that these organs are extracellular volume receptors, though not necessarily the only ones in the body. According to this hypothesis any mechanical deformation of these cavernous structures causes thirst, and it is interesting in this regard that the removal of a small amount of cerebrospinal fluid induces drinking (Nicolaïdis, 1974). However, the adequate or physiological stimulus to the subfornical organ and the organum vasculosum is deformation produced by reduced filling as it occurs in hypovolaemic or as a consequence of angiotensin-induced vasoconstriction in the structure itself. Presumably stretch receptors in the walls of the blood vessels signal the changes, however, these may be induced.

ANGIOTENSIN IN THE CONTROL OF BLOOD PRESSURE

The increase in arterial blood observed after administration of angiotensin II results (1) mainly from its powerful vasoconstrictor action on vascular smooth muscle, (2) perhaps from its stimulating action on the peripheral sympathetic system, and (3) from an action on the central nervous system. The central pressor action of angiotensin was first demonstrated by Bickerton and Buckley (1961) who found that the injection of larger doses of angiotensin II into the carotid artery of the vascularly isolated dog's head with intact neural connections to the rest of the body caused an increase in systemic arterial pressure which was prevented by a systemic α-adrenergic blockade. Subsequently it was established that infusion of angiotensin into the vertebral artery in doses that are non-pressor when given intravenously causes a rise in blood pressure (Dickinson and Lawrence, 1963). This central hypertensive effect of angiotensin II was also obtained following injections of hormone into the cerebral ventricular system but not after injections into the subarachnoid space (Severs et al., 1966; Scroop and Lowe, 1969). The characteristics of the central pressor response depend on the route of administration. Intravertebral angiotensin causes an immediate rise in blood pressure which lasts as long as the infusion, whereas the rise produced by intraventricular infusion is slower in onset, is not sustained and shows tachyphylaxis after repeated infusions. The intravertebral pressor response is mediated by increased sympathetic discharge to the arterioles, but in the greyhound and perhaps in other animals in which resting vagal tone to the heart is high, diminution in parasympathetic discharge also plays a part. The mechanism of the intraventricular pressor response is less clear. Section of the spinal cord in the cervical region abolishes the response

(Smookler et al., 1966; Rosendorff et al., 1970), which suggests that the rise in blood pressure is caused by increased sympathetic tone. However, at least part of the intravertebral pressor response is mediated by release of vasopressin since the rise in blood pressure is less after hypophysectomy (Severs et al., 1970). Finally angiotensin also inhibits reflex vasodilatation by acting centrally. It prevents the baroreceptor inputs, which come via the sensory vagal centres, from compensating for the increased sympathetic tone caused by the direct action of angiotensin on the area postrema (Sweet and Brody, 1970).

Central sites of action for the pressor response to angiotensin II are in the medulla, the midbrain and possibly the hypothalamus. The sensitive site for the intravertebral pressor response is the area postrema, as evidenced by the following. (1) Thermocoagulation (Joy and Lowe, 1970) or selective cooling (Ferrario et al., 1972) of the area postrema abolishes the pressor response induced by intravertebral angiotensin II. (2) Intravertebral angiotensin causes increased electrical activity of neurones in the area postrema (Ueda et al., 1972). (3) Injection of angiotensin II directly into the area postrema causes a rise in blood pressure (Ueda et al., 1972). There is also good evidence that the area postrema responds to angiotensin generated as a result of the activation of the renal renin—angiotensin system. Thus, in the dog the regulation of blood pressure after haemorrhage is imperfect after ablation of the area postrema, but in the nephrectomized dog the regulation is imperfect both before and after ablation (Katic et al., 1971). Also, the increase in arterial pressure caused by clamping the renal artery in the dog is reduced to one-half after ablation of the area postrema, although the rise in plasma renin is the same (Scroop et al., 1975).

The sensitive site for the intraventricular pressor response appears to be in the midbrain. The pressor effect of the injection of angiotensin II into the lateral ventricle of the cat is abolished by anterior midbrain section, or by cannulation of the cerebral aqueduct (Severs et al., 1966). Injections of angiotensin into the anterior aqueduct are pressor whereas those into the posterior aqueduct are not (Deuben and Buckley, 1970). Electrolytic destruction of the subnucleus medialis in the midbrain abolishes the pressor response to intraventricular angiotensin II (Deuben and Buckley, 1970). This mesencephalic site and the area postrema appear to function independently in the cat since bilateral destruction of the area postrema does not abolish the pressor response to intraventricular angiotensin II, nor does mesencephalic section modify the pressor response to intravertebral injection of angiotensin II (Gildenberg et al., 1973).

The hypothalamus may also play a role in the central pressor response to angiotensin because of the connections it makes with the mesencephalon and because it controls the release of vasopressin. It is significant that rats with hereditary diabetes insipidus have been reported not to respond to the central action of angiotensin (Ganten et al., 1975).

As in the case of the control of drinking behaviour by angiotensin, the discovery of a cerebral isorenin—angiotensin system has posed new questions and changed our view of the possible significance of the rise in blood pressure produced by stimulation of regions in the central nervous system by angiotensin. It is now fairly clear that circulating angiotensin does not readily penetrate the blood—brain and blood—cerebrospinal fluid barriers (Ganten et al., 1975). All the radioactivity found in the cerebrospinal fluid 0—6 min after intravenous injection of tritiated angiotensin II represented angiotensin fragments. This of course presents no particular problems as far as the intravertebral response is concerned because the area postrema is a circumventricular organ that lies outside the blood—brain barrier and is accessible to blood-borne hormone. But the mesencephalic site is not accessible to blood-borne angiotensin; it can only be reached from the cerebrospinal fluid. This of course immediately implicates the cerebral isorenin system which is the sole source of angiotensin in the cerebrospinal fluid, and it is therefore extremely interesting that Ganten and his colleagues (1975) have found higher than normal concentrations of angiotensin II in the cerebrospinal fluid of spontaneously hypertensive rats. It is tempting to think that increased activation of the cerebral isorenin—angiotensin system may be the cause of some sorts of hypertension. Ganten and his colleagues also found that intraventricular perfusion of the angiotensin II (AII) antagonist Sar^1, Ala^8-AII (P 113) caused a fall in blood pressure in spontaneously hypertensive rats but not in normotensive animals.

The importance of this finding is evident and prompted the following experiments in conscious normotensive or spontaneously hypertensive rats of the Okamoto strain fitted with chronically implanted ventricular cannulae and femoral arterial cannulae for recording blood pressure (Elghozi et al., 1976). Intraventricular injections of the angiotensin antagonist, Sar^1, Thr^8-AII or Sar^1, Ile^8-AII, in doses from 1 to 5000 ng into normotensive or spontaneously hypertensive rats did not cause any drop in arterial blood pressure (Fig. 5). The stereotaxic coordinates and numbers of hypertensive animals used are given in Table III; 5 normotensive rats were also used. The mean arterial blood pressure ranged from 150 to 180 mm Hg in conscious spontaneously hypertensive rats at an age of 30 weeks. One experiment was performed in a 10-week-old rat with a blood pressure of 200 mm Hg. Mean blood pressure in conscious normotensive rats ranged from 100 to 120 mm Hg. Although the AII antagonists did not cause a drop in arterial pressure (or drinking), angiotensin II itself injected by the same route into these animals caused a rise in arterial pressure and increased drinking behaviour except when the angiotensin injections were repeated at close intervals. In Fig. 5A it may be seen that 14 min after the last injection of

TABLE III

NUMBERS OF SPONTANEOUSLY HYPERTENSIVE
RATS USED

Stereotaxic coordinates (Albe-Fessard et al., 1971):
VL, A 7 mm, L 1.5 mm, H—4 mm; VIII, A 8.5, L 0,
H—7 mm.

	Sar^1, Thr^8-AII	Sar^1, Ile^8-AII
VL	2	3
VIII	6	1

146

1000 ng Sar^1, Ile^8-AII in a normotensive rat, the injection of 100 ng of AII in the same lateral ventricle caused a 30 mm Hg rise in blood pressure and a drinking response. A second injection of AII did not produce any further rise in blood pressure but led to an arhythmia with extrasystoles probably the consequence of increased sympathetic activity. This is seen more clearly on the

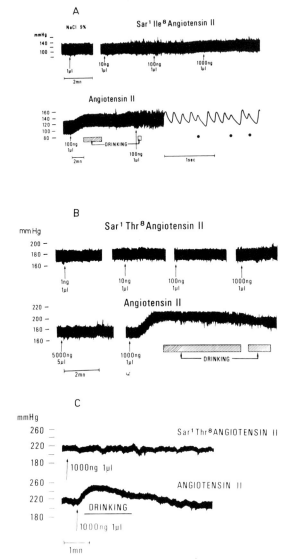

Fig. 5. A: the femoral arterial pressure in a normotensive rat after injection of Sar^1, Ile^8-AII (1—1000 ng) or angiotensin II (100 ng) into the lateral ventricle. The black dots on the faster record indicate extrasystoles. B: arterial pressure in a spontaneously hypertensive rat after injection of Sar^1, Thr^8-AII (1—5000 ng) or angiotensin II (1000 ng) into the lateral ventricle. C: arterial pressure in a spontaneously hypertensive rat after injection of Sar^1, Thr^8-AII (1000 ng) or angiotensin II (1000 ng) into the lateral ventricle. Note that the angiotensin antagonists did not produce any lowering in blood pressure though angiotensin II itself by the same route caused a rise in pressure and drinking. (From Elghozi et al., 1976.)

higher speed recording where the extrasystoles are indicated by black dots. The drinking response to the second injection was brief. Fig. 5B illustrates the rise in blood pressure and drinking in response to a very large dose (1000 ng) of angiotensin given into the lateral ventricle of a spontaneously hypertensive rat 20 min after injection of 5000 ng Sar^1, Thr^8-AII into the same lateral ventricle.

The failure of two antagonists of angiotensin to lower the blood pressure in hypertensive or in normotensive rats is in disagreement with the results of Ganten et al. (1975). The absence of effect of AII antagonists when given alone should be contrasted with their effectiveness in blocking the effect of exogenous AII when this is given within 10 min of the antagonist. Since exogenous AII can reach sensitive sites in the brain to cause drinking and a rise in blood pressure, AII antagonists given by the same route should also reach these sensitive regions and antagonize the effects of AII generated by the cerebral isorenin—angiotensin system. The fact that they do not argues against a role for the cerebral system in spontaneous hypertension of this type.

CONCLUSIONS

The actions of angiotensin II on structures in the brain which result in drinking and an increase in arteriolar tone contribute to the regulation of blood volume. Other actions of angiotensin not considered here also help regulate the blood volume. These include Na retention by the kidney, brought about by renin—angiotensin—aldosterone, ADH release, increased intestinal Na reabsorption and possibly increased Na appetite. Angiotensin II can therefore be regarded as the hormone of blood volume regulation (Fitzsimons, 1976). These actions, however, all refer to the renal system. The role of the cerebral renin—angiotensin system and its relationship with the renal system remain to be elucidated.

SUMMARY

The physiological significance of drinking and the rise in blood pressure produced by angiotensin II (AII) is uncertain. Also uncertain is the role of the cerebral isorenin—angiotensin system in these responses, and the relationship between the cerebral and renal systems.

It has been reported that intracranial injection of the angiotensin antagonist Sar^1, Ala^8-AII causes a fall in arterial blood pressure. In the present experiments neither Sar^1, Ile^8-AII nor Sar^1, Thr^8-AII injected into the brain caused a drop in femoral arterial pressure in conscious normotensive or spontaneously hypertensive rats of the Okamoto strain. On the other hand AII was dipsogenic and pressor in these rats. The lack of a hypotensive effect of intracranially applied blockers suggests that cerebral isorenin does not contribute to the maintenance of vascular tone nor to the development of spontaneous hypertension.

The regions of the brain most sensitive to the action of blood-borne and intracranial AII are vascularised periventricular structures lying outside the blood—brain barrier. Injection of vasoplegics such as papaverine, $NaNO_2$, sodium nitroprusside or prostaglandin E_2 into the subfornical organ or the organum vasculosum of the lamina terminalis blocked the dipsogenic action of AII injected through the same cannula. The effect of these substances on the AII pressor response is not known. Antagonism of AII by substances known to relax vascular smooth muscle supports the hypothesis that AII acts by altering stretch receptor discharge from these special cavernous structures.

REFERENCES

Albe-Fessard, D., Stutinsky, F. and Libouban, S. (1971) *Atlas Stéréotaxique du Diencéphale du Rat Blanc*, CNRS, Paris.

Bickerton, R.K. and Buckley, J.P. (1961) Evidence for a central mechanism in angiotensin-induced hypertension. *Proc. Soc. exp. Biol. (N.Y.)*, 106: 834—836.

Deuben, R.R. and Buckley, J.P. (1970) Identification of a central site of action of angiotensin II. *J. Pharmacol. exp. Ther.*, 175: 139—146.

Dickinson, C.J. and Lawrence, J.R. (1963) A slowly developing pressor response to small concentrations of angiotensin. Its bearing on the pathogenesis of chronic renal hypertension. *Lancet*, 1: 1354—1356.

Elghozi, J.L., Altman, J., Devynck, M.A., Liard, J.F., Grünfeld, J.P. and Meyer, P. (1976) Lack of hypotensive effect of central injection of angiotensin inhibitors in SH and normotensive rats. *Clin. Sci. molec. Med.*, in press.

Ferrario, C.M., Gildenberg, P.L. and McCubbin, J.W. (1972) Cardiovascular effects of angiotensin mediated by the central nervous system. *Circulat. Res.*, 30: 257—262.

Fischer-Ferraro, C., Nahmod, V.E., Goldstein, D.J. and Finkielman, S. (1971) Angiotensin and renin in rat and dog brain. *J. exp. Med.*, 133: 353—361.

Fitzsimons, J.T. (1966) Hypovolaemic drinking and renin. *J. Physiol. (Lond.)*, 186; 130—131P.

Fitzsimons, J.T. (1969) The role of a renal thirst factor in drinking induced by extracellular stimuli. *J. Physiol. (Lond.)*, 201: 349—368.

Fitzsimons, J.T. (1970) The renin-angiotensin system in the control of drinking. In *The Hypothalamus*, L. Martini, M. Motta and F. Fraschini (Eds.), Academic Press, New York, pp. 195—212.

Fitzsimons, J.T. (1971) The effect on drinking of peptide precursors and of shorter chain peptide fragments of angiotensin II injected into the rat's diencephalon. *J. Physiol. (Lond.)*, 214: 295—303.

Fitzsimons, J.T. (1975) The renin-angiotensin system and drinking behavior. In *Hormones, Homeostasis and the Brain, Progress in Brain Research, Vol. 42*, W.H. Gispen, Tj. B. van Wimersma Greidanus, B. Bohus and D. de Wied (Eds.), Elsevier, Amsterdam, pp. 215—233.

Fitzsimons, J.T. (1976) The physiological basis of thirst. *Kidney Int.*, 10:3—11.

Fitzsimons, J.T., Epstein, A.N. and Johnson, A.K. (1977) The peptide specificity of receptors for angiotensin-induced thirst. In *International Symposium on the Central Actions of Angiotensin and Related Hormones*, J.P. Buckley and C. Ferrario (Eds.), Pergamon, Oxford, in press.

Ganten, D., Marquez-Julio, A., Granger, P., Hayduk, K., Karsunky, K.P., Boucher, R. and Genest, J. (1971) Renin in dog brain. *Amer. J. Physiol.*, 221: 1733—1737.

Ganten, D., Hutchinson, J.S. and Schelling, P. (1975) The intrinsic brain iso-renin-angiotensin system in the rat. *Clin. Sci. molec. Med.*, 48: 265S—268S.

Gildenberg, P.L., Ferrario, C.M. and McCubbin, J.W. (1973) Two sites of cardiovascular action of angiotensin II in the brain of the dog. *Clin. Sci.*, 44: 417—420.

Joy, M.D., and Lowe, R.D. (1970) Evidence that the area postrema mediates the central cardiovascular response to angiotensin II. *Nature (Lond.)*, 228: 1303—1304.

Katic, F., Joy, M.D., Lavery, H., Lowe, R.D. and Scroope, G.C. (1971) Role of central effects of angiotensin in response to haemorrhage in the dog. *Lancet* 2: 1354–1356.

Nicolaïdis, S. (1974) Y a-t-il une régulation et des récepteurs distincts d'un espace hydrique extracellulaire non vasculaire (ECNV). *J. Physiol. (Paris)*, 69: 166A.

Nicolaïdis, S. et Fitzsimons, J.T. (1975) La dépendance de la prise d'eau induite par l'angiotensine II envers la fonction vasomotrice cérébrale locale chez le rat. *C. R. Acad. Sci. (Paris)*, 281D: 1417–1420.

Osborne, M.J., Pooters, N., Anglès d'Auriac, G., Epstein, A.M., Worcel, M. and Meyer, P. (1971) Metabolism of tritiated angiotensin II in anaesthetized rats. *Pflügers Arch. ges. Physiol.*, 326: 101–114.

Rosendorff, C., Lowe, R.D., Lavery, H. and Cranston, I. (1970) Cardiovascular effects of angiotensin mediated by the central nervous system of the rabbit. *Cardiovasc. Res.*, 4: 36–43.

Scroop, G.C. and Lowe, R.D. (1969) Efferent pathways of the cardiovascular response to vertebral artery infusions of angiotensin in the dog. *Clin. Sci.*, 37: 605–619.

Scroop, G.C., Katic, F.P., Brown, M.J., Cain, M.D. and Zeegers, P.J. (1975) Evidence for a significant contribution from central effects of angiotensin in the development of acute renal hypertension in the greyhound. *Clin. Sci. molec. Med.*, 48: 115–119.

Severs, W.B., Daniels, A.E., Smookler, H.H., Kinnard, W.J. and Buckley, J.P. (1966) Interrelationship between angiotensin II and the sympathetic nervous system. *J. Pharmacol. exp. Ther.*, 153: 530–537.

Severs, W.B., Summy-Long, J., Taylor, J.S. and Connor, J.D. (1970) A central effect of angiotensin: release of pituitary pressor material. *J. Pharmacol. exp. Ther.*, 174: 27–34.

Simpson, J.B. and Routtenberg, A. (1973) Subfornical organ: site of drinking elicitation by angiotensin II. *Science*, 181: 1172–1175.

Smookler, H.H., Severs, W.B., Kinnard, W.J. and Buckley, J.P. (1966) Centrally mediated cardiovascular effects of angiotensin II. *J. Pharmacol. exp. Ther.*, 153: 485–494.

Sweet, C.S. and Brody, M.J. (1970) Central inhibition of reflex vasodilation by angiotensin and reduced renal pressure. *Amer. J. Physiol.*, 219: 1751–1758.

Ueda, H., Katayama, S. and Kato, R. (1972) Area postrema, angiotensin sensitive site in brain. *Advanc. exp. Med. Biol.*, 17: 109–116.

Effect of Saralasin and Atropine on Thirst induced by Water Deprivation

WILLIAM HOFFMAN, PIERRE SCHELLING and DETLEV GANTEN

Department of Pharmacology, University of Heidelberg, 6900 Heidelberg (G.F.R.)

In the rat, two compounds have been reported to produce a short-latency drinking response when injected into the brain. These two drugs are angiotensin II (AII) (Epstein et al., 1970; Severs et al., 1970) and carbachol, a muscarinic agonist (Grossman, 1960; Hoffman and Phillips, 1976). The dipsogenic responsiveness of the rat to low doses of these drugs suggests that there may be a physiological basis for the responses. However, there is no evidence to date that blockade of central AII or muscarinic receptors will inhibit physiological thirst. We have investigated the role of central muscarinic and AII receptors in the mediation of thirst produced by water deprivation.

Twenty-six 250 g male Sprague—Dawley rats were implanted with chronic brain cannulae which passed through the ventricles and ended in the hypothalamus. Thirst was produced by 48 hr of water deprivation, with food available. Intracranial infusions of saralasin (Sar^1-Ala^8-AII analogue) and atropine sulfate were used to block angiotensin and muscarinic receptors. The drugs were infused at a rate of 1.4 μg/min and 0.7 μg/min respectively. The volume of the infusions for both drugs was 1.4 μl/min and the experimental conditions were compared to artificial cerebrospinal fluid (CSF) infusions alone. Intracranial infusions of the drugs or cerebrospinal fluid were started 10 min before access to water and were continued for 30 min.

The infusion of either saralasin or atropine alone had no significant effect on the water intake of the animals during the infusion period (Fig. 1). However, when the two blocking agents were combined into the same intracranial infusion, a significant 70% decrease in water intake was observed. The reduction in the drinking response with the infusion of both drugs together is apparently a specific effect since no change in milk intake of food deprived rats was found with saralasin plus atropine infusions. The results suggest that there are central physiological mechanisms involving both, AII and muscarinic receptors in the thirst response produced by water deprivation. An interrelationship of these two is indicated by the fact that both systems must be blocked in order to show a significant reduction in thirst drive. This is consistent with previous findings that the central AII or muscarinic receptors can be blocked independently (Fitzsimons and Settler, 1975). It would appear likely that the cholinergic thirst system blocked is of central origin. This is probably also true for angiotensin since AII does not readily cross the blood—brain barrier (Ganten et al., 1975), and an isorenin—angiotensin system

152

has been reported to be endogenous to the brain (Ganten et al., 1975). Recent findings in this laboratory indicate that the brain isorenin—angiotensin system is stimulated by water deprivation and support the idea of local brain angiotensin being involved in thirst mechanisms.

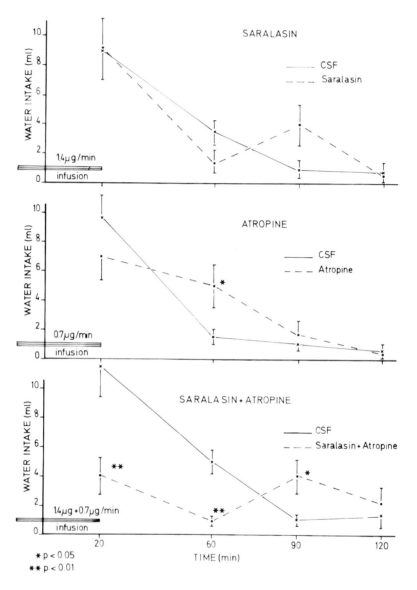

Fig. 1. Effect of saralasin and atropine on water intake. Water intake following 48 hr of water deprivation. Drug infusions were started 10 min before water was given and continued for 30 min. All groups are compared to CSF test infusions in the same animal. Comparisons were made by Student's t-test. Top: saralasin infused at a rate of 1.4 μg/min (n = 8). Middle: atropine sulfate infused at a rate of 0.7 μg/min (n = 10). Bottom: saralasin (1.4 μg/min) plus atropine (0.7 μg/min) infused together (n = 8).

SUMMARY

The role of central muscarinic and angiotensin II receptors in a physiological thirst response was investigated. The thirst challenge was 48 hr of water deprivation. Intracranial infusions of 1.4 μg/min of saralasin, a specific angiotensin II antagonist, had no effect on water intake. Atropine sulfate infused intracranially at a rate of 0.7 μg/min for 30 min also had no significant effect on drinking. Both drugs infused together, however, produced a 70% decrease in water intake. An interaction of central cholinergic and angiotensin II thirst mechanisms in the rat is suggested by these results.

ACKNOWLEDGEMENTS

This work has been supported by grants from the German Research Foundation (SFB 90) and an Individual Cardiovascular Research Fellowship No. H 107007 to W.E.H.

REFERENCES

Epstein, A.N., Fitzsimons, J.T. and Rolls, B. (1970) Drinking induced by injection of angiotensin into the brain of the rat. *J. Physiol. (Lond.)*, 210: 457—474.

Fitzsimons, J.T. and Settler, P.E. (1975) The relative importance of central nervous catecholaminergic and cholinergic mechanisms in drinking in response to angiotensin and other thirst stimuli. *J. Physiol. (Lond.)*, 250: 613—631.

Ganten, D., Hutchinson, J.S., Schelling, P., Ganten, U. and Fischer, H. (1976) The iso-renin angiotensin systems in extrarenal tissue. *Clin. exp. Pharmacol. Physiol.*, 3: 103—126.

Grossman, S.P. (1960) Eating or drinking elicited by direct adrenergic or cholinergic stimulation of the hypothalamus. *Science*, 132: 301—302.

Hoffman, W.E. and Phillips, M.I. (1976) A pressor response to intraventricular injections of carbachol. *Brain Res.*, 105: 157—162.

Severs, W.B., Summy-Long, J., Taylor, J.S. and Connor, J.P. (1970) A central effect of angiotensin: release of pituitary pressor material. *J. Pharmacol. exp. Ther.*, 174: 27—34.

The Brain Isorenin–Angiotensin System: Localization and Biological Function

DETLEV GANTEN, KJELL FUXE, URSULA GANTEN, THOMAS HÖKFELT and PER BOLME

(D.G. and U.G.) Department of Pharmacology, University of Heidelberg, 6900 Heidelberg (G.F.R.) and (K.F., T.H. and P.B.) Department of Histology, Karolinska Institutet, Stockholm 60 (Sweden)

The kidney renin—angiotensin system exerts its effects on arterial blood pressure in the periphery and the brain. In addition, the isorenin—angiotensin system probably has a local function in the brain (for review see Ganten et al., 1976). Catecholamines, including dopamine, noradrenaline and adrenaline also participate in the regulation of arterial blood pressure by acting at peripheral and central sites (Davies and Reid, 1975). In view of the multiple interactions between catecholamines and the renin-angiotensin system (Palaic and Khairallah, 1968; Boadle et al., 1969; Zimmermann et al., 1972; for review see Severs and Daniels-Severs, 1973), we have investigated whether the localization of components of the isorenin—angiotensin system, especially angiotensin II, in the brain permits interaction with various known neurotransmitter systems.

Ultracentrifugation studies for subcellular localization of renin and isorenin were carried out in parallel with kidney and brain tissue following the techniques of Whittaker (1969) and Koenig et al. (1964). Briefly, fresh kidney tissue, frontal cortex and caudate nucleus of dog brains were obtained. Tissue was homogenized with teflon pestles, 0.64 and 0.28 clearance. Centrifugation at (a) $900 \times g$, 10 min, (b) $11,500 \times g$, 20 min; (c) $74,500 \times g$, 80 min, yielded the following primary cell fractions: nuclei, mitochondria and microsomes, respectively. The primary mitochondrial fraction was submitted to a discontinuous sucrose density gradient centrifugation with densities of 0.29, 0.8, 1.2 and 1.4 M sucrose (Whittaker, 1969). The synaptosomes obtained by this technique represent isolated nerve terminals. Isorenin concentrations in the subfractions are given in terms of relative specific activity (RSA), the primary mitochondrial fraction being taken as 1; thus, RSA greater than unity shows relative enrichment of enzyme activity.

Angiotensin II was localized in the brain tissue of rats, using immunohistofluorescence techniques. Antibodies were obtained by coupling ileu[5]—angiotensin II to bovine serum albumin and this complex was injected into rabbits. Cross-reactivity of the antibody, as tested by radioimmunoassay, with somatostatin, bradykinin, substance P, thyrotropin-releasing factor and luteinizing hormone-releasing factor was less than 0.01%, with angiotensin I 1%, with 2—8, 3—8, 4—8 angiotensin II fragments 100% and with desasp—ala[8]—angiotensin II 0.01%. For control of specificity the antibodies were adsorbed with bovine serum albumin and with angiotensin II before the

TABLE I

RELATIVE SPECIFIC ACTIVITY (RSA, % of enzyme activity/% of protein; **primary** mitochondrial fraction = 1) IN SUBFRACTIONS OF THE PRIMARY MITOCHONDRIAL OF FRONTAL CORTEX AND CAUDATE NUCLEUS OF DOG BRAIN AND KIDNEY CORTEX

Main constituents of subfractions of primary mitochondrial fraction	Sucrose molarity	Frontal cortex (RSA)	Frontal cortex (osmotic shock) (RSA)	Caudate nucleus (RSA)	Renal cortex (RSA)
(A) Myelin	0.3—0.8	0.62	1.37	0.50	0.2
(B) Synaptosomes	0.8—1.2	1.14	0.69	1.08	0.2
(C) Synaptosomes + mitochondria	1.2—1.4	0.62	0.66	1.17	0.27
(D) Dense granules "lysosomes"	1.4	2.55	1.11	2.30	2.59

immunohistochemical procedure. Specific immunofluorescence disappeared using this treatment and this is therefore probably due to the presence of angiotensin II or angiotensin II related peptides. Histochemical procedure involved the indirect technique with fluoresceine isothiocyanate conjugated sheep anti-rabbit immunoglobulins (for details see Fuxe et al., 1976).

The distribution of enzyme concentrations in primary cell fractions showed a similar pattern in the brain and kidney: the highest concentrations were found in the mitochondrial fractions, followed by nuclear and microsomal fractions in the frontal cortex and in the caudate nucleus of the brain and in the kidney cortex. The results were obtained by subfractionation of the primary mitochondrial fraction on a discontinuous sucrose density gradient and are described in Table I. Renin from the kidney cortex and isorenin from the brain were enriched in the dense granule fraction. There was, however, additional enzyme activity localized in less dense fractions of the gradient, representing nerve terminal-rich subfractions of the primary mitochondrial fraction and purified synaptosomes (Whittaker, 1969). Resuspension of these fractions in water ("osmotic shock"), rather than isotonic sucrose, liberated the particle-bound enzyme from osmotically sensitive synaptosomes and from

Fig. 1. Angiotensin II-like immunofluorescence in untreated male Sprague—Dawley rats. 1: strong angiotensin II-like immunofluorescence in nerve terminals of sympathetic lateral column of spinal cord, sagittal section, high density. × 120. 2: strong angiotensin II-like immunofluorescence in nerve terminals of substantia gelatinosa of the dorsal horn (DG); transverse section, high density. × 300. 3: strong angiotensin II-like immunofluorescence in descending axons of the lateral funiculus of the spinal cord, innervating sympathetic lateral column. Accumulation of specific fluorescence (between arrowheads) is seen cranial to a spinal cord transection one week earlier. × 120. 4: weak angiotensin II-like immunoreactivity in nerve terminals of nucleus dorsomedialis hypothalami, moderate density. × 300.

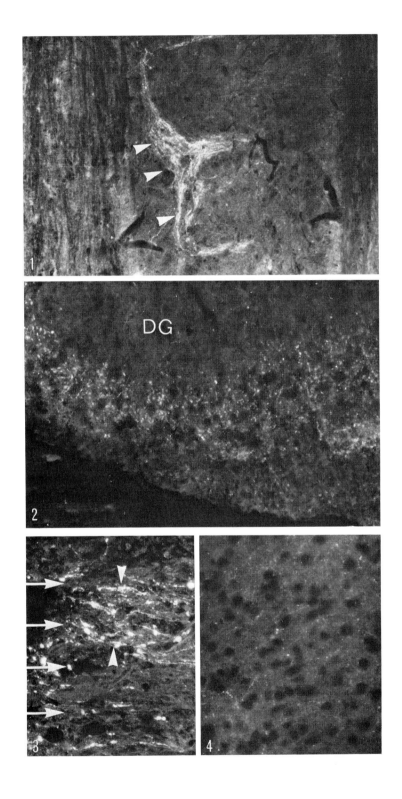

the dense granule fraction. The enzyme released by this hypoosmotic treatment then appeared in the supernatant. The question of whether the cellular enzyme distribution could be due to non-specific binding to cell organelles has also been tested by the addition of exogenous renin to the tissue homogenate. No selective surface binding to any of the subfractions could be detected. The results indicate that isorenin is not confined to vasculature but occurs in neural elements of the brain and is enriched in nerve terminals.

Since angiotensinogen has been found in brain tissue and angiotensin-like peptides have been extracted from whole brain homogenate by several authors (for review see Severs and Daniels-Severs, 1973 and Ganten et al., 1976), the occurrence of isorenin in synaptosomes would indicate that nerve terminals possess the capacity to synthetize angiotensin enzymatically. Indeed, angiotensin II positive immunofluorescence was found in several brain regions.

High density: substantia gelatinosa of the spinal cord, and of the nucleus tractus spinalis nervi trigemini, median eminence (medial external layer), nucleus amygdaloideus centralis, sympathetic lateral column.

Moderate density: locus coeruleus.

Scattered terminals: periventricular mesencephalic grey, hypothalamus, preoptic area, subcortical limbic structures (amygdaloid cortex, septal area), limbic cortex, thalamus (midline area), ventral midbrain, substantia nigra, reticular formation, raphe region, the nucleus tractus solitarius, nucleus dorsalis motorius nervi vagi, periventricular area of pons and medulla oblongata.

No immunofluorescence: parts of the neocortex, cortex cerebelli.

The results show that isorenin and angiotensin II are located intracellularly in nerve endings. The question of angiotensin's mechanism(s) of action within the brain now assumes more importance. Specific angiotensin II receptive neurons have been described in the brain (Sakai et al., 1974; Phillips and Felix, 1976). A stimulating effect of brain angiotensin II on cardiovascular centers has been made probable by the finding that blood pressure decreases following central angiotensin II receptor blockade in spontaneously hypertensive rats (Ganten et al., 1975). The presence of angiotensin II positive neurons in the locus coeruleus, which is built up of noradrenaline cell bodies, may indicate the participation of angiotensin II in the control of norepinephrine pathways, controlling blood pressure, wakefulness and positive reinforcement, functions ascribed to this noradrenaline system (see Fuxe et al., 1976). The high density of angiotensin II terminals in the substantia gelatinosa would suggest a role of angiotensin II in the control of sensory information. The discovery of rich networks of angiotensin II positive nerve terminals in the external layer of the median eminence may suggest a neuroendocrine function for this peptide (Fuxe et al., 1976).

The localization of angiotensin II in synaptosomes, points to its possible role as a neurotransmitter itself or a modulator of the action of other neurotransmitters (Minnich et al., 1972). The effect of angiotensin on catecholamine release and synthesis, as well as on the metabolism of other transmitters, and the effect of angiotensin on membrane permeability (calcium, sodium, potassium) (Severs and Daniels-Severs, 1973) indicate a regulatory potential of the peptide in the function of the central nervous system.

SUMMARY

All components of an isorenin—angiotensin system, including angiotensinogen, isorenin, angiotensin I, angiotensin I converting enzyme, angiotensin II, angiotensin receptors and angiotensinases are present in brain tissue. Highly purified synaptosomes were obtained from primary mitochondrial cell fractions of the dog brain and were found to contain high isorenin concentrations. Angiotensin II positive immunofluorescence was found in varicose nerve terminals of several regions in rat brain. Thus, enzyme analysis and effector peptide localization yield compatible results and indicate intracellular localization of the isorenin angiotensin system in neural elements of the brain.

ACKNOWLEDGEMENTS

This work has been supported by grants from the German Research Foundation (SFB 90) and from the Swedish Medical Research Council (04X-4246).

REFERENCES

Boadle, M.C., Hughes, J. and Roth, R.H. (1969) Angiotensin accelerates catecholamine biosynthesis in sympathetically innervated tissues. *Nature (Lond.)*, 222: 987—988.

Davies, D.S. and Reid, J.S. (Eds.), (1975) *Central Action of Drugs in Blood Pressure Regulation*, Pitman Medical, London.

Fuxe, K., Ganten, D., Hökfelt, T. and Bolme, P. (1976) Immunohistochemical evidence for the existence of angiotensin II-containing nerve terminals in the brain and spinal cord of the rat. *Neurosci. Lett.*, 2: 229—234.

Ganten, D., Hutchinson, J.S. and Schelling, P. (1975). The intrinsic brain iso-renin angiotensin system: its possible role in central mechanisms of blood pressure regulation. *Clin. Sci. molec. Med.*, 48: 265S—268S.

Ganten, D., Hutchinson, J.S., Schelling, P., Ganten, U. and Fischer, H. (1976) The iso-renin angiotensin system in extrarenal tissue. *Clin exp. Pharmacol. Physiol.*, 2: 103—126.

Koenig, H., Gaines, D., McDonald, T., Gray, R. and Scott, J. (1964) Studies of brain lysosomes. I. Subcellular distribution of five acid hydrolases, succinate dehydrogenase and gangliosides in rat brain. *J. Neurochem.*, 11: 729—735.

Minnich, J.L., Ganten, D., Barbeau, A. and Genest, J. (1972) Subcellular localization of cerebral renin-like activity. In *Hypertension '72*, J. Genest and E. Koiw (Eds.), Springer, Heidelberg, pp. 432—435.

Palaic, D. and Khairallah, P.A. (1968) Inhibition of norepinephrine re-uptake by angiotensin in brain. *J. Neurochem.*, 15: 1195—1202.

Phillips, M.I. and Felix, D. (1976) Specific angiotensin II receptive neurons in the cat subfornical organ. *Brain Res.*, 109: 531—540.

Sakai, K.K., Marks, B.H. George, J. and Koestner, A. (1974) Specific angiotensin II receptors in organ-cultured canine supra-optic nucleus cells. *Life Sci.*, 14: 1337—1344.

Severs, W.B. and Daniels-Severs, A.E. (1973) Effects of angiotensin on the central nervous system. *Pharmacol. Rev.*, 25: 415—449.

Whittaker, V.P. (1969) The synaptosome. In *Handbook of Neurochemistry, Vol. 2*, A. Lajtha (Ed.), Plenum Press, New York, pp. 327—353.

Zimmermann, B.G., Gomer, S.K. and Ji Chia Liao (1972) Action of angiotensin on vascular adrenergic nerve endings: facilitation of norepinephrine release. *Fed. Proc.*, 31: 1344—1350.

Endogenous Angiotensin in the Brain

JOHN S. HORVATH, CLAIRE BAXTER, FIONA FURBY and
DAVID J. TILLER

Renal and Hypertension Units, Royal Prince Alfred Hospital, Camperdown, N.S.W. 2050
(Australia)

INTRODUCTION

A renin—angiotensin system in the brain was first reported by Fischer-Ferraro et al. (1971) and Ganten et al. (1971) who reported the presence of renin and renin substrate in dog and rat brain extracts and angiotensin in concentrations of 2.7—11.2 ng/g of brain tissue. Levels of renin, angiotensin and renin substrate in these reports were determined using the rat pressor bioassay. Following these reports the presence of a renin—angiotensin system in the brain was generally accepted (Severs and Daniels-Severs, 1973; Dickenson and Ferraro, 1974), however, there has been no evidence to indicate that the components of the renin—angiotensin system interact to produce angiotensin II (AII) in the brain. Although there is conflicting evidence to support the hypothesis that AII is produced in the brain, pharmacological doses of AII administered via the cerebral ventricles cause a marked pressor response (Severs and Daniels-Severs, 1973) and this response can be abolished by the simultaneous infusion of the AII competitive inhibitor saralasin acetate (P113). The effect of in vivo administration of P113 and other peptide inhibitors have yielded conflicting results. Ganten et al. (1975) have reported that intraventricular injections of AII inhibitors will cause a fall in blood pressure in spontaneously hypertensive rats whereas Elghozi et al. (1976) failed to demonstrate this effect. Malayan and Reid (1975) also failed to demonstrate a fall in blood pressure when intraventricular P113 was given to normal dogs.

Whilst attempting to clarify the role of endogenous AII in the brain we have compared measurements of angiotensin I (AI) and AII in brain tissue of 3 species by radioimmunoassay (RIA) and rat pressor bioassay.

PREPARATION AND ASSAY OF BRAIN TISSUE FOR ANGIOTENSIN

Normal rats and rats that had been nephrectomized 48 hr previously were decapitated and their heads immediately frozen in liquid nitrogen. After freezing, the brains were removed and pools of two or more brains were homogenized with cold 80% ethanol (5 ml 80% ethanol/g of brain tissue). The supernatants were collected and dried and reconstituted in Tris—acetate buffer (pH 7.0) for RIA. Rabbit and dog brains were prepared in a similar fashion but were not collected into liquid nitrogen but homogenized immediately on collection.

Those samples that were to be both bioassayed and measured by RIA were further purified by chromatography of Dowex 50W as described by Ganten et al. (1971) and on a Sephadex G25 column standardised with AII. The eluates were lyophilized and reconstituted for RIA in Tris buffer, pH 7.0.

AI was measured in the brain extracts by the method of Haber et al. (1969) and AII by a modified method of Ruiz-Maza et al. (1974). The limits of sensitivity of these assays were 0.1 ng of AI/g of brain and 0.02 ng of AII/g of brain.

RECOVERY OF EXOGENOUS ANGIOTENSIN AFTER EXTRACTING PROCEDURE

^{125}I-angiotensin I and ^{125}I-angiotensin II were injected into whole rat brains before homogenization and there was 78% ± 4% recovery of counts in the ethanol extracts. Similarly ^{125}I-angiotensin I or ^{125}I-angiotensin II was added to the homogenates and recovery in the ethanol extracts was 82 ± 2%. Further studies were carried out by injecting cold AI and AII into rat brains. There was a 107 ± 16% recovery by RIA after allowing for recovery of radioactive angiotensin, and there was no loss of immunoreactivity of the angiotensin. Recovery of internal standards of angiotensin added to the extracts before RIA was 104 ± 16%. The recovery data indicate that angiotensin was not lost or altered during the extraction process.

ANGIOTENSIN LEVELS IN BRAIN EXTRACTS

Neither AI nor AII was detected by RIA in brain extracts prepared from normal or nephrectomized rats or rabbits, indicating that the total

TABLE I

AI AND AII MEASURED BY RIA, AND BY BIOASSAY PRESSOR ACTIVITY IN BRAIN EXTRACTS FROM RATS, RABBITS AND DOGS

No difference was found between normal and nephrectomised rats and rabbits and results for these are pooled. Bioassay pressor activity is expressed in AII equivalents.

| Species | Radioimmunoassay (ng/g brain) | | Bioassay pressor activity AII (ng/g brain ± S.D.) |
	AI	AII	
Rat N = 14	< 0.1	< 0.02	21.6 ± 7.1
Rabbit N = 6	< 0.1	< 0.02	20.2 ± 7.2
Dog N = 3	< 0.1	0.03 ± 0.016	6.8 ± 7.5

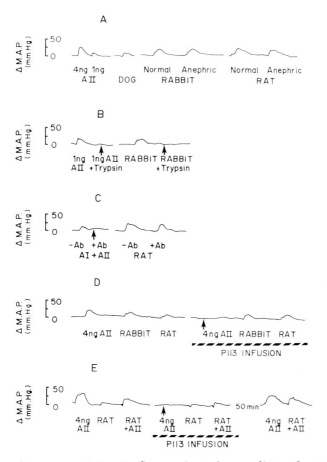

Fig. 1. Bioassay of pressor activity. A: Grass polygraph recordings of responses in mean arterial pressure of rats to injections of AII and brain extracts. B: the effect of trypsin on pressor activity. C: effect of AI and AII antibodies on pressor activity of brain extract. D: effect of infusion of P113 on responses to AII and brain samples. E: effect of P113 infusion on pressor responses to brain extracts from bisected brains.

concentration of these peptides was less than 0.12 ng/g of brain. Small amounts of AII (< 0.05 ng/g of brain) were detected in the dog brain (see Table I), however, as the removal of dog brains was technically difficult, contamination of the brain tissue with blood was a possible cause for the low levels of AII detected.

Bioassay of these brain extracts demonstrated potent pressor activity equivalent to 6.8 ± 7.5 ng of AII/g of brain in dogs, 21.6 ± 7.1 ng of AII/g of brain in rats with similar levels in rabbits (see Fig. 1 and Table I).

ANGIOTENSIN BLOCKADE IN THE BIOASSAY

In order to further characterize the pressor substance in the brain extracts, saralasin acetate (P113) was infused at the rate of 10 μg/kg/min into the rat preparation during bioassay. This dose of P113 was sufficient to block a 4 ng

AII standard pressor response. There was no decrease of pressor response to the brain extract during P113 infusion (pressor response before infusion 13 ± 8 mm Hg and during P113 infusion 13 ± 3 mm Hg). The preparation demonstrated normal responsiveness to AII both before and after P113 infusion (Fig. 1). Similarly treatment of brain extracts prior to injection into the bioassay with specific antibodies to AI and AII failed to block the pressor response of brain extracts (see Fig. 1).

In further studies brains were bisected and half of each brain was injected with AII 14 ng/g of brain, then brain extracts were bioassayed both before and during P113 infusion. There was no decrease in pressor response in the brains without exogenous AII, however, there was a reduction in pressor response during P113 infusion in those brain extracts with AII added. The extent of the reduction in pressor response observed is accounted for by the injected AII (see Fig. 1).

The pressor effect of brain extracts could be abolished by pretreatment of the extracts with trypsin in a concentration of 0.25 mg/ml for 60 min at $20°C$ before bioassay (see Fig. 1). The effect of trypsin on the pressor substance suggests that its structure is that of a peptide.

DISCUSSION

Although the brain isorenin system has been described and individual components of this system isolated, it has not been demonstrated that they can interact in vivo to produce AII. The studies reported to date have required the addition of components of the system (Fischer-Ferraro et al., 1971; Ganten et al., 1971; Malayan and Reid, 1976). Furthermore, although pharmacological responses to the central administration of AII have been described the physiological significance of the brain renin—angiotensin system remains unclear.

Our results indicate that the total concentration of brain AI and AII is below 0.15 ng/g of brain which conflicts with the results of Ganten et al. (1971) and Fischer-Ferraro et al. (1971), however, these studies were carried out using bioassay pressor techniques and not the more specific measurements that can be obtained using RIA. We have demonstrated similar levels of pressor substance in brain tissue, however, in our bioassay system the pressor response could not be abolished by the specific AII inhibitor P113 or specific antibodies to AI and AII. These results combined with the low values for AI and AII measured by RIA lead us to conclude that the pressor substances we have described is not AI or AII. We have found a pressor substance in brain tissues of a similar molecular weight to angiotensin that is inactivated by trypsin. It is possible that this peptide is vasopressin, however, it is present in brains which do not have hypothalamic or pituitary tissue present. Work is currently in progress to identify this peptide.

SUMMARY

We have examined the concentration of AI and AII in brain using RIA. Normal and nephrectomised rats were decapitated and their heads frozen immediately in liquid N_2. Brains were extracted with 80% ethanol and extracts chromatographed on Dowex 50W and Sephadex G25. Brains from dogs and normal and anephric rabbits were treated similarly. In all species the total concentration of AI and AII as measured in the extracts by RIA was < 0.15 ng/g of brain. When the extracts were examined for pressor activity by bioassay, the brain levels were, in AII equivalents, 21.6 ± 7.1 ng/g, 20.2 ± 7.2 ng/g and 6.8 ± 7.5 ng/g in the rat, rabbit and dog with no difference between normal and anephric animals. The pressor activity was unaffected by P113 or AI and AII antibodies but was destroyed by trypsin. Our results suggest that the pressor activity in brain extracts cannot be attributed to angiotensin but to another peptide with a similar molecular weight.

ACKNOWLEDGEMENT

Eaton Laboratories for kindly supplying the saralasin-acetate used in these studies.

REFERENCES

Dickinson, C.J. and Ferraro, C.M. (1974) Central neurogenic effects of angiotensin. In *Angiotensin, Handbook of Experimental Pharmacology, XXXVII*, Springer, Berlin, pp. 408—416.

Elghozi, J.L., Altman, J., Devynck, M.A., Laird, J.F., Grunfeld, J.P. and Meyer, P. (1976) Lack of hypotensive effect of central injection of angiotensin inhibitors in S.H. and normotensive rats. *IVth Meeting of the Int. Soc. and Hypertension, Sydney*, Abstr. 52.

Fischer-Ferraro, C., Nahmod, V., Goldstein, D. and Finkielman, S. (1971) Angiotensin and renin in rat and dog brain. *J. exp. Med.*, 133: 353—361.

Ganten, D., Marquez-Julio, A., Granger, P., Hayduk, K., Korsushy, K.P., Boucher, R. and Genest, J. (1971) Renin in dog brain. *Amer. J. Physiol.*, 221: 1733—1737.

Ganten, D., Hutchinson, J.S. and Schelling, P. (1975) The intrinsic brain iso-renin-angiotensin system in the rat: its possible role in central mechanisms of blood pressure regulation. *Clin. Sci. molec. Med.*, 48: 265S—268S.

Haber, E., Koener, T., Page, L.B., Kliman, B. and Pernode, A. (1969) Application of a radioimmunoassay for AI to the physiological measurement of plasma renin activity in normal human subjects. *J. Clin. Endocr.*, 28: 1349—1358.

Malayan, S.A. and Reid, I.A. (1976) Antidiuresis produced by injection of renin into the third cerebral ventricle of dog. *Endocrinology*, 98: 329—335.

Riuz-Maza, F., Tiller, D.J. and Walker, W.G. (1974) Measurement of angiotensin II in ultrafiltrate of plasma. *Johns Hopk. Med. J.*, 135: 211—228.

Severs, W. and Daniels-Severs, A. (1973) Effects of angiotensin on the central nervous system. *Pharmacol. Rev.*, 25: 415—449.

SESSION III

BRAIN DAMAGE AND HYPERTENSION: EXPERIMENTAL AND CLINICAL

Chairmen: O. Magnus (Wassenaar)
D.J. Reis (New York, N.Y.)

Brain Lesions and Hypertension: Chronic Lability and Elevation of Arterial Pressure Produced by Electrolytic Lesions and 6-Hydroxydopamine Treatment of Nucleus Tractus Solitarii (NTS) in Rat and Cat

DONALD J. REIS, NOBUTAKA DOBA, DAVID W. SNYDER and MARC A. NATHAN

Laboratory of Neurobiology, Department of Neurology, Cornell University Medical College, New York, N.Y. 10021 (U.S.A.)

INTRODUCTION

Over the past several years, our laboratory has been pursuing a new strategy in developing models of sustained neurogenic hypertension in experimental animals. This has been achieved through impairing CNS centers critical in circulatory control. Our objectives have been two-fold. First, we have sought to establish the *fact* that imbalances within cardiovascular centers of the brain produced by destructive lesions, and which would lead to a preponderance of pressor systems, can result in chronic neurogenic hypertension. Secondly, we have been seeking to ascertain whether discrete biochemical defects of the brain also can result in a sustained elevation of arterial pressure. Such demonstrations, we believe, are necessary to establish the validity of the hypothesis that dysfunction of the CNS, structural or chemical, can be a possible causal mechanism in essential hypertension in man. To date no models exist of sustained hypertension produced by neural dysfunction (see Reis and Doba, 1974).

Our investigations primarily have focused on one particular area of the brain stem, the nucleus of the tractus solitarii (NTS). Attention has been directed to this nucleus because of the fact that it serves as a primary site of termination of baroreceptors (Cottle, 1964; Humphrey, 1967; Crill and Reis, 1968; Miura and Reis, 1969; Seller and Illert, 1969). Thereby it plays an important role in integrating inhibitory regulation of the sympathetic nervous system. Furthermore, since the NTS receives an important input from catecholamine neurons (e.g., Dahlström and Fuxe, 1965; Chiba and Doba, 1975, 1976), it also is a useful place wherein to start an examination of the effects of a disordered balance of neurotransmitters on blood pressure.

In the following paper we shall review our efforts to produce experimental neurogenic hypertension in laboratory animals by electrolytic and chemical lesions of the brain. We shall demonstrate that it is indeed possible to produce chronic hypertension by lesions of NTS, thereby validating the hypothesis that central neural imbalances can result in hypertension. We shall also report recent studies demonstrating that selective destruction of the noradrenergic innervation of NTS by the drug 6-hydroxydopamine (6-OHDA), which will selectively destroy noradrenergic terminals (Thoenen and Tranzer, 1968;

Ungerstedt, 1968; Bloom et al., 1969; Uretsky and Iversen, 1970) can result in the development of marked lability of the arterial pressure. This would suggest that defects of chemical neurotransmission within the CNS could possibly contribute to conditions favoring development of hypertension.

FULMINATING ARTERIAL HYPERTENSION PRODUCED BY ELECTROLYTIC LESIONS OF NTS IN RAT

The observation by Miura and Reis (1972) that small bilateral lesions of NTS at the level of the obex in anesthetized cat will abolish all baroreceptor reflexes led Doba and Reis (1973) to attempt to determine whether neurogenic hypertension could be produced in the rat by central deafferentation of baroreceptors. In their initial investigation experiments were performed on rats in whom intravascular cannulae were inserted while the animals were briefly anesthetized with halothane. Cardiovascular activity was determined following discontinuation of the anesthesia and then, after a brief reanesthetization, lesions were placed in the NTS, the anesthesia again was discontinued, and the ensuing cardiovascular changes followed.

(1) Cardiovascular effects

Lesions restricted to the NTS bilaterally (Fig. 1) and abolishing baroreceptor reflexes (Fig. 2) invariably resulted in the development of arterial hypertension.

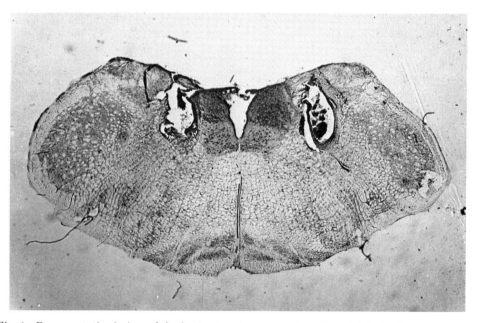

Fig. 1. Representative lesion of the brain stem in a rat that produced fulminating neurogenic hypertension. This section was taken just rostral to the obex. Note destruction of NTS bilaterally.

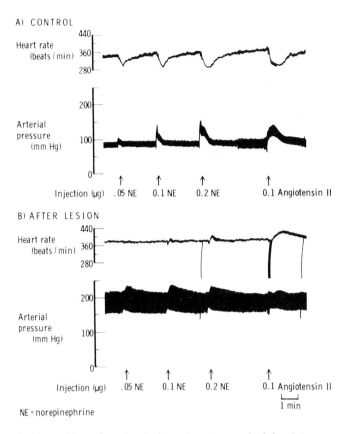

Fig. 2. Reflex bradycardia and systemic hypertension evoked by intravenous injection of different doses of norepinephrine (NE) and angiotensin II before (A) and after (B) production of bilateral lesions of the NTS in the anesthetized rat (alpha-chloralose 30 mg/kg, i.v.). Before lesions, both agents produced a graded bradycardia associated with hypertension. After lesions, the reflex bradycardia was no longer elicited, and tachycardia and arrhythmias were observed with injections of norepinephrine and angiotensin II. (From Doba and Reis, 1973.)

The elevation of arterial pressure appeared within 5 min after discontinuation of the anesthesia and achieved maximal levels of systolic pressure, over 200 mm Hg, within 30 min. The hypertension produced by NTS lesions was entirely attributable to a 2—3-fold increase in peripheral resistance. The elevated peripheral resistance produced an overload of the left ventricle, a consequent reduction of stroke volume, an increase in left ventricular end-diastolic pressure, and as a result a fall of the cardiac output to approximately 60% of normal values. Central venous pressure was also elevated. These events occurred within 30 min after the placement of the lesion. The elevated peripheral resistance and the incipient congestive heart failure ultimately evolved. By 4—6 hr the animals rapidly developed acute pulmonary edema and died. The evolution of the hypertension in a typical animal is shown in Fig. 3.

The hypertension produced by NTS lesions in rat is neurogenic and primarily

172

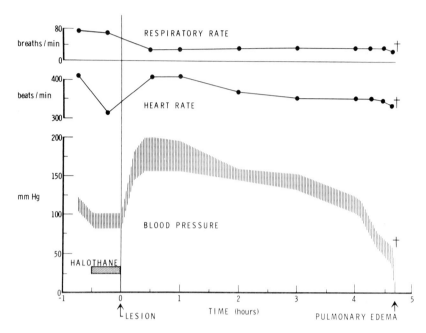

Fig. 3. Time course of changes in systemic arterial blood pressure, heart rate, and respiratory rate in a representative unanesthetized rat after production of bilateral lesions in the NTS. Just prior to death the rat developed pulmonary edema. (From Doba and Reis, 1973.)

due to increased sympathetic discharge. It is neither attributable to changes in blood gases nor to release of pressor substances from the kidneys nor the adrenal glands since prior removal of these organs does not reduce the magnitude of the hypertension. On the other hand, the hypertension can be entirely blocked by prior treatment with ganglionic blocking agents, α-adrenergic blockade with phentolamine, or the destruction of peripheral sympathetic neurons by 6-OHDA in association with adrenalectomy (Doba and Reis, 1974).

The activation of the sympathetic nervous system after NTS lesions appears to be largely differentiated. It results primarily from increased activity of sympathetic neurons innervating blood vessels. Thus, there is no evidence of widespread sympathetic activation, as for example mydriasis, proptosis or piloerection, nor is there tachycardia. Recent studies (Snyder, Doba and Reis, unpublished) in which the distribution of regional blood flow has been measured by the use of an isotope dilution method have demonstrated that the vasoconstriction is maximal within skin, skeletal muscles and some abdominal viscera particularly the lower bowel.

(2) Central neural mechanisms

(a) Suprasegmental mechanisms

All evidence suggests that NTS lesions produce the release of sympathetic neural activity by damage to the central projections of baroreceptors within the

NTS and/or conceivably to relays from NTS neurons to tonic sympathetic areas elsewhere. One of the characteristic features of NTS hypertension in rat is its dependence on the integrity of structures lying above the midbrain: midcollicular decerebration will abort the development of hypertension before NTS lesions are placed or abolish the hypertension once the lesions are established (Doba and Reis, 1973). The importance of rostral regions of the brain in mediating the hypertension parallels the observation that the reflex hypertension elicited by sino-aortic denervation or carotid occlusion is reduced or abolished by decerebration (Manning, 1965; Reis and Cuénod, 1965). The findings support the contention (Miura and Reis, 1969; Spyer, 1972) that baroreceptors, after terminating in the medulla, engage in long-loop cardiovascular reflexes within higher brain areas. The precise localization of the rostrally situated regions necessary for the expression of the hypertension remains to be established.

(b) Central catecholamine mechanisms

While the precise pathways mediating hypertension produced by NTS lesions in rat remain to be elucidated, there is evidence that its expression depends upon the integrity of at least one of the central neural systems that synthesize,

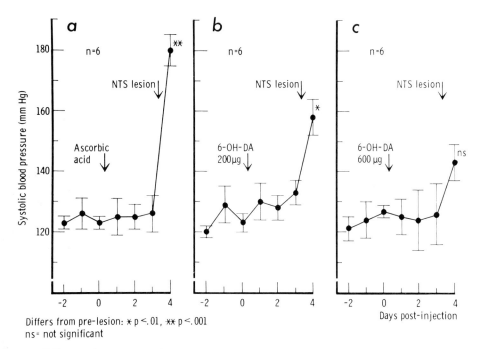

Fig. 4. Effects of 6-OHDA administered intracisternally on systolic blood pressure before and after NTS lesions. Blood pressure was measured by a tail cuff method for 3 consecutive days before the intracisternal injection of 6-OHDA. Control rats (a) were treated with ascorbic acid vehicle alone. Other rats received 200 μg (b) and 600 μg (c) of 6-OHDA in 10 μl of ascorbic acid vehicle. Blood pressure was measured for 4 days and then bilateral lesions of the NTS were placed. Note that 6-OHDA in the higher dose blocked and in the lower dose attenuated the NTS hypertension. (From Doba and Reis, 1974.)

store and release a catecholamine neurotransmitter, probably norepinephrine (NE) (Doba and Reis, 1974). Intracisternal injection of 6-OHDA will block the development of NTS hypertension even when the adrenal glands are intact (Fig. 4). This finding is consistent with the observations of others that intracisternal 6-OHDA will abort the hypertension produced by sino-aortic denervation (Chalmers and Reid, 1972), the evolution of the genetic form of hypertension (SHR rats) (Finch et al., 1972; Haeusler et al., 1972), and even some renal forms of hypertension (Lewis et al., 1973).

While it is not absolutely certain which central catecholamine system is necessary for maintaining the elevated arterial pressure, the evidence strongly suggests that it is a descending noradrenergic pathway. Bilateral intra-hypothalamic injections of 6-OHDA which interrupt dopaminergic as well as noradrenergic projections locally as well as those ascending through the hypothalamus to innervate the forebrain (Ungerstedt, 1971) will not alter the arterial pressure and fail to influence NTS hypertension (Doba and Reis, 1974). On the other hand, low doses of intracisternal 6-OHDA capable of lowering the content of norepinephrine only in the spinal cord (Doba and Reis, 1974) are successful in aborting the syndrome.

CHRONIC LABILE HYPERTENSION PRODUCED BY NTS LESIONS IN CATS

While our experiments in rats demonstrated that lesions of CNS could elevate the blood pressure, the inability of the animals to survive more than a few hours obviously limits their utility as an animal model. However, the rapid death of rats appears to be a consequence of the sudden load imposed upon the heart by the intense peripheral vasoconstriction and not to the lesion *per se*. Reasoning that a larger animal might have the myocardial reserve capable of weathering the initial autonomic storm, we examined the circulatory effects of bilateral lesions in NTS in cats (Nathan and Reis, 1976).

In these studies, cats were anesthetized with halothane and under aseptic conditions cannulas were placed in the carotid artery and jugular vein and electrodes occasionally implanted for measurements of EEG, the neck muscle EMG, and extraocular movements. The animals were permitted to recover from surgery and, over the next several weeks, arterial pressure, heart rate and bioelectric activity were recorded during spontaneously occurring behavior or in response to presentation of environmental stimuli. The animals were then reanesthetized and, in the experimental group, electrical lesions were placed bilaterally in NTS. In other animals that served as controls, the brain stem was exposed but no lesions were made. The animals were permitted to recover and observations of cardiovascular activity were made. At present, animals with bilateral NTS lesions have been observed up to 3 months.

Arterial pressure and heart rate were also analyzed by the generation of frequency histograms similar to those developed by Cowley et al. (1973). By this method it was possible to obtain information as to the mean of the arterial pressure and heart rate over a selected time period and to assess lability in two ways: graphically, by inspection of the histograms; numerically, by calculation of the standard deviation of the arterial pressure, and also the correlation coefficient.

(1) Acute phase

Within minutes after termination of anesthesia the arterial pressure of cats with NTS lesions began to rise, reaching on the average a level of 144 mm Hg mean arterial pressure and gradually declining thereafter (Fig. 5). It gradually returned to normal by 24—48 hr. Lesioned cats also developed a tachycardia

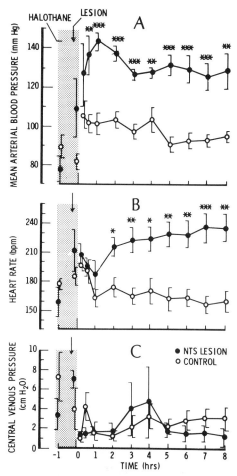

Fig. 5. Acute effects of NTS lesions on the mean arterial blood pressure (A), heart rate (B) and central venous pressure (C) in cats. All cats were anesthetized for the period of time indicated by the shaded area. The data points on the left edge of the shaded area represent the responses recorded 1 hr before placement of the lesions. The data points on the right edge of the shaded area represent the responses in the experimental group (●, n = 6) after placement of NTS lesions or in the control group (○, n = 7) after sham lesions. At time 0, the anesthesia was stopped and the time course of cardiovascular activity for the next 8 hr was followed. Each data point signifies a mean value and the bars indicate ± S.E. The significance of differences from the control at each time point is represented by asterisks: * = $P < 0.05$; ** = $P < 0.01$; *** = $P < 0.001$. (From Nathan and Reis, 1976.)

TABLE I

EFFECTS OF NTS LESIONS IN CAT ON MEANS AND STANDARD DEVIATIONS OF
ARTERIAL PRESSURE AND HEART RATE DURING DAY AND NIGHT

All values expressed as ±S.E. Figures in parentheses = number of animals. NS = not significant.

	Day	Night	% Difference (night/day)	P
Mean arterial pressure (mm Hg)				
Control	80 ± 1.5 (6)	77 ± 3.3 (5)	96	NS
Lesion	114 ± 2.4 (5)	96 ± 4.7 (4)	84	<0.02
% Difference (lesion/control)	143	125	—	—
P	<0.001	<0.02	—	—
Standard deviation of arterial pressure (mm Hg)				
Control	4 ± 0.4 (6)	5 ± 0.4 (5)	125	NS
Lesion	18 ± 2.3 (5)	6 ± 0.5 (4)	33	<0.05
% Difference (lesion/control)	450	120	—	—
P	<0.001	NS	—	—
Heart rate (bpm)				
Control	154 ± 8.1 (6)	149 ± 6.4 (5)	97	NS
Lesion	191 ± 5.6 (5)	181 ± 1.4 (4)	95	NS
% Difference (lesion/control)	124	121	—	—
P	<0.01	<0.05	—	—
Standard deviation of heart rate (bpm)				
Control	10 ± 1.3 (6)	7 ± 1.2 (5)	70	NS
Lesion	7 ± 1.7 (5)	7 ± 1.2 (4)	100	NS
% Difference (lesion/control)	70	100	—	—
P	NS	NS	—	—

(Fig. 5, Table I) which persisted unabated. In cat, in contrast to rat, venous
pressure was almost never elevated. Thus cats, in contrast to rats, were able to
survive the initial phase of acutely elevated arterial pressure and could enter a
chronic state totally compatible with life.

(2) Chronic phase

Cats with bilateral lesions of the NTS, after recovery from the acute effects
of surgery, appeared to be behaviorally normal. However, they developed
several marked changes in cardiovascular performance which may be
summarized.

(a) Lability

The most striking feature of the chronic NTS cat is the lability of arterial
pressure. Lability appears by 8—16 hr following placement of the lesion and

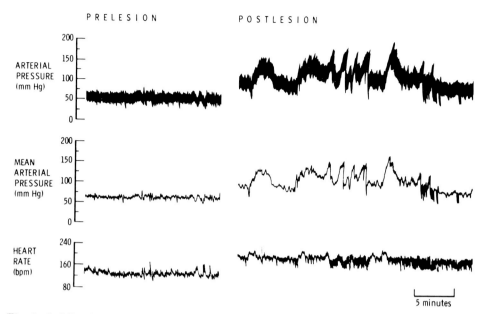

Fig. 6. Labile changes in arterial pressure following NTS lesions in cat. The prelesion tracing was taken 2 days before placement of the lesions when the cat was in quiet wakefulness and lying down. The postlesion result is taken 1 week after the lesion with the cat in the same behavioral state. Note the extreme lability of the arterial pressure.

continues unabated for the rest of the animal's life. Marked spontaneous fluctuations of systolic, diastolic and mean arterial pressures, both elevations and depressions, and sometimes as great as 100 mm Hg (Fig. 6), were common. The lability was also present over longer periods of time as seen in the histogram of Fig. 7, where the distribution of values of arterial pressure in an individual animal and in groups of lesioned cats (recorded during the daytime) was spread over a much larger range of values than those in controls. One striking feature of the lability is that it was seen primarily during daytime hours, but not at night (Table I). Whether this daily variation represents a true biorhythm or is merely related to the fact that the animals were housed in a busy laboratory and were therefore exposed to greater levels of environmental stimulation during the daytime remains to be established.

(b) Sustained hypertension

In addition to increased daytime lability of the arterial pressure, NTS lesioned cats maintained an elevation in their average arterial pressure both during the day (averaging 114 mm Hg) and at night (averaging 96 mm Hg) (Table I). The presence of elevated pressures during the nighttime, when lability had disappeared (Table I), indicates that lability *per se* is not necessary for the maintenance of the elevation in arterial pressure.

(c) Exaggerated cardiovascular responses in behavior

Lesions of the NTS in the cat not only altered the stability of arterial pressures during quiet repose but they also profoundly altered the reactive

178

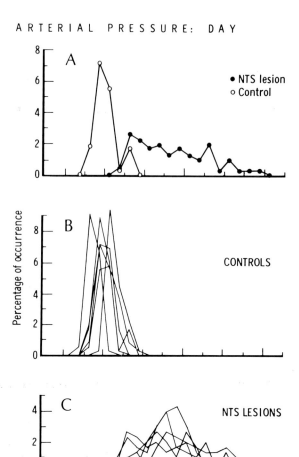

Fig. 7. Daytime frequency histogram of mean arterial pressure in normal and NTS-lesioned cats. A: individual cat before (○) and 1 week after (●) placement of the lesions. B: overlay of 6 normal cats 1 week after the sham operation. C: overlay of 5 cats 1 week after placement of NTS lesions. Note the increased lability of the mean arterial pressure in the NTS-lesioned cats. (From Nathan and Reis, 1976.)

changes of pressure associated with the expression of other spontaneously occurring or elicited behaviors. While the direction of the arterial pressure associated with specific behaviors was comparable in lesioned animals and controls the magnitude of the responses and their duration were greatly exaggerated in the lesioned group. For example, during grooming (Fig. 8), in response to petting or in orienting to a novel stimulus the normal and modest elevation of arterial pressure could be markedly exaggerated, elevations of over 100 mm Hg systolic were often observed. Likewise the fall of pressure seen in the rapid eye movement (REM) phases of sleep (Guazzi and Zanchetti, 1965) was also enhanced (Fig. 9).

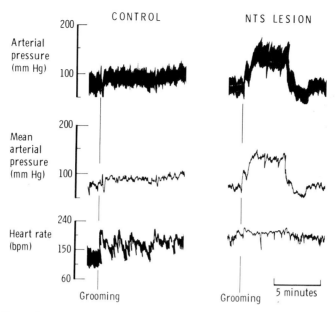

Fig. 8. Facilitation of pressor response to grooming after NTS lesion. (From Nathan and Reis, 1976.)

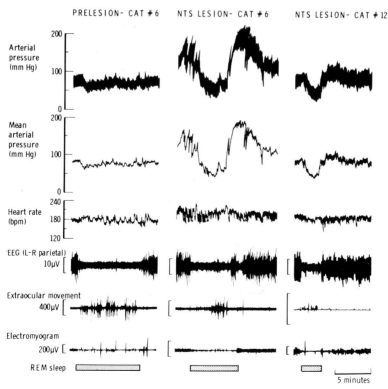

Fig. 9. Facilitation of depressor response during REM sleep. (From Nathan and Reis, 1976.)

(d) Fixed tachycardia

The heart rate of lesioned animals remains elevated both in day and night throughout the period under which they have been observed. There was no change in lability (Table I).

This study therefore indicates that NTS lesions in cats can lead to a sustained elevation of arterial pressure associated with lability, exaggerated responsivity and tachycardia. Since the NTS lesions abolished baroreceptor reflexes in cat it would be reasonable to assume that the syndrome was a consequence of disruption of central baroreceptor mechanisms. If so it would be of interest to compare the effects of NTS lesions with those resulting from sino-aortic denervation. Theoretically the brain lesion could differ from the peripheral one in that the central lesion would destroy not only inputs from baroreceptors of the carotid sinus and aortic depressor nerves, but those in the vagus, in NTS and also possibly suprasegmental inputs into the area of the NTS. At present such comparisons are not possible since no study has been undertaken in the same laboratory comparing the effects of the two procedures in the same species observed under controlled environmental conditions and using identical modes of graphic and numerical analysis. It is of interest, however, that lability and exaggerated reactivity appear to be results of sino-aortic denervation in dog (Cowley et al., 1973) but sustained hypertension is probably not.

LABILE ARTERIAL PRESSURE PRODUCED IN RATS BY CHEMICAL LESIONS OF NORADRENERGIC PROJECTIONS INTO NTS

Since destructive lesions of NTS can, in cat, result in chronic labile hypertension we have recently sought to determine if imbalances in neurotransmitters within the nucleus can also result in abnormalities of arterial pressure. It is well established that the NTS is richly innervated by the terminals of catecholamine-containing neurons (Dahlström and Fuxe, 1965; Chiba and Doba, 1975, 1976). The nucleus and adjacent areas of the dorsal medulla contain a rich plexus of catecholamine-containing fibers. In rat, cells containing catecholamines are also located within the area of NTS but the majority of fibers arise from cell groups located elsewhere, particularly the A2 and possibly A1 groups (Dahlström and Fuxe, 1965). It has been presumed on the basis of histofluorescence that most of the fibers innervating NTS are noradrenergic. However, recent immunocytochemical (Hökfelt et al., 1974) and biochemical evidence (Saavedra et al., 1974, 1976) have suggested that some of the cells in the area of NTS and some of the terminals within the nucleus contain the enzyme phenylethanolamine N-methyl transferase (PNMT) raising the possibility that the NTS is innervated by adrenergic (i.e. epinephrine containing) fibers.

In view of the role of the NTS in the regulation of arterial pressure and the fact that many centrally acting hypertensive agents such as clonidine and L-DOPA act through central adrenergic mechanisms (Haeusler, 1973; Phillipu et al., 1973; Day and Roach, 1974) possibly even within NTS (Haeusler, 1973; Phillipu et al., 1973). Doba and Reis (1974) sought to examine the effects of the microinjection of 6-OHDA directly into the NTS of rats. Twelve μg of

6-OHDA was injected into the NTS in anesthetized animals and on subsequent days systolic arterial pressure was recorded from the tail artery by an indirect cuff method.

The effect of the injection resulted in elevation of systolic arterial pressure seen by the third day which persisted for about a week with recovery. The study therefore suggested that the noradrenergic innervation of NTS served to facilitate baroreceptor mechanisms and hence was inhibitory to the arterial pressure. The findings were also consistent with the demonstration that the microinjection of norepinephrine directly into the NTS in rat resulted in a dose-dependent fall of the arterial pressure (De Jong, 1974; De Jong et al., 1975). Our findings also suggested that within the NTS the effect of norepinephrine was opposite in direction with respect to the arterial pressure as was the same transmitter acting within the spinal cord.

Since NTS lesions in the cat result in profound alterations in the lability and reactivity as well as modest elevations of the average pressure it was possible that some of these changes in cardiovascular function could not be detected by indirect means. Thus it is essential to chronically record arterial pressure intravascularly.

We have therefore undertaken a much more detailed examination of the effects of selective destruction of the noradrenergic innervation of the NTS by 6-OHDA in the unanesthetized freely moving rat. In these studies rats were chronically instrumented with indwelling carotid arterial and jugular cannulas. Some animals were observed prior to microinjection of 6-OHDA into NTS. Others either received 6-OHDA at the time of instrumentation, received vehicle alone, or were uninjected controls. Frequency distribution histograms of arterial pressure and heart rate were plotted over 1 hr during daytime hours. The average standard deviations were calculated as an index of lability. The sensitivity of the baroreceptor reflex was also assessed by determination of the reflex fall of heart rate produced by the graded injections of a pressor dose of phenylephrine (Smyth et al., 1969).

The introduction of 4 μg of 6-OHDA in 1 μl of vehicle into the NTS bilaterally in rats resulted in persistent changes in cardiovascular activity. During the first 24 hr treated animals demonstrated a modest increase in the mean arterial pressure (Fig. 10) but not of heart rate (Fig. 11). However, by 48 hr and up to 16 days, the longest period of observation, the arterial pressure (Fig. 10) as well as the heart rate (Fig. 11) of treated rats did not differ from controls.

The treated animals, however, developed within 24 hr an exaggerated lability of the arterial pressure (Fig. 10) but not of the heart rate (Fig. 11). An example of lability is seen in Fig. 12. Lability was evident graphically, in the frequency histograms (Fig. 13), as an increase in the range of arterial pressure, and numerically by an elevation of the standard deviation of arterial pressure around the mean (Fig. 10). The increased lability appeared relatively permanent and persistent. Treated rats also demonstrated an exaggerated reactivity of the arterial pressure during spontaneous and elicited behaviors.

The effect of 6-OHDA on the arterial pressure could not be attributed to the destruction of arterial baroreceptor reflexes. When tested in unanesthetized freely moving animals by measurement of the reflex fall of heart rate in

182

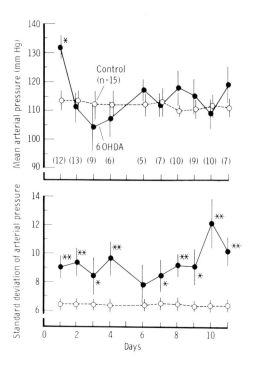

Fig. 10. Time course of changes in the mean (upper panel) and variability (S.D.) (lower panel) of arterial pressure in awake, freely moving rats following microinjection of 6-OHDA into NTS on day 0. Means (±S.E.) and standard deviations (±S.D.) were computed from frequency distribution curves recorded daily over a 1 hr period during the day. Note that the arterial pressure is elevated only during the first 24 hr but that variability (lability) persists. Controls: n = 15. Number of treated animals examined on any day indicated in parentheses in upper panel. * = $P < 0.05$; ** = $P < 0.01$.

response to increasing pressor doses of phenylephrine, the baroreceptor reflex in treated animals was present, although the gain of the system was somewhat depressed (Fig. 14). Thus unlike electrolytic lesion of NTS the 6-OHDA treatment did not appear to impair the baroreceptor reflex arc.

The 4 μg of 6-OHDA appeared relatively selective in its effects on catecholamine neurons. There was no evidence on histological examination of the NTS from treated animals observed 1—2 weeks after treatment of any neuronal damage. Moreover, biochemical examination of the NTS demonstrated a reduction in the activity of dopamine-β-hydroxylase (DBH) to 40% of control without significant changes in the activity of cholineacetyltransferase, a marker of cholinergic neurons (Fig. 15). Since 6-OHDA is believed not to affect the adrenergic innervation of NTS the results would suggest that most of the DBH which was abolished by the 6-OHDA must lie within central noradrenergic neurons.

This study therefore provides evidence that the noradrenergic innervation of NTS serves to modulate rather than to mediate baroreceptor reflexes. The fact that its interruption results in lability of the arterial pressure and does not affect the heart rate suggests that one of the principal functions of this system

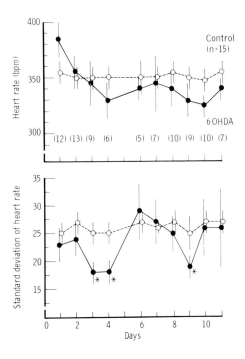

Fig. 11. Time course of changes in the mean (upper panel) and variability (S.D.) (lower panel) of heart rate in awake, freely moving rats following microinjection of 6-OHDA into NTS on day 0. Means (±S.E.) and standard deviations (±S.D.) were computed from frequency distribution curves recorded daily over a 1 hr period during the day. Note that the mean heart rate is unchanged. There is a tendency on several days for the heart rate to stabilize. Number is same as Fig. 10. * = $P < 0.05$.

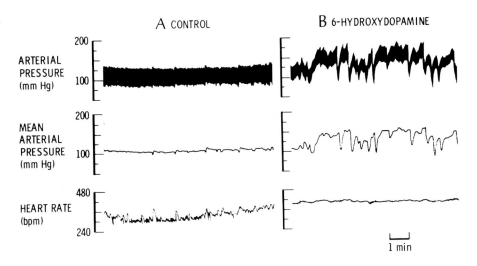

Fig. 12. Labile changes in arterial pressure in awake quiet rat before and 1 week following bilateral microinjection of 6-OHDA into NTS in rat.

184

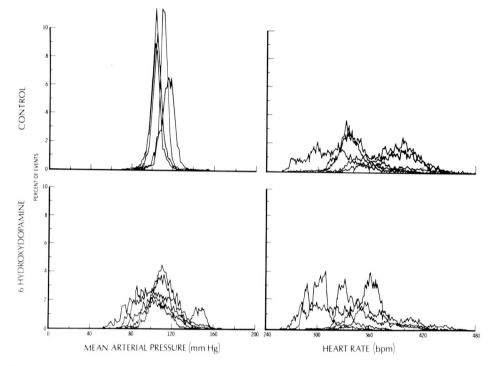

Fig. 13. Frequency distribution curves of mean arterial pressure and heart rate in control and 6-OHDA treated rats. Upper panels: overlay of 5 control rats 4 days after vehicle (0.8 mg/ml ascorbic acid) was microinjected into NTS. Lower panels: overlay of 5 rats 4 days after 6-OHDA (4 µg in 1 µl) was microinjected into NTS. Note the increased lability of the mean arterial pressure after 6-OHDA treatment.

	Control (N = 5)		6-OHDA (N = 5)	
	Mean ± S.D.	S.D. ± S.E.	Mean ± S.D.	S.D. ± S.E.
Arterial pressure (mm Hg)	108 ± 5	6 ± 0.8	107 ± 8	15 ± 4**
Heart rate (bpm)	342 ± 31	25 ± 5	330 ±27	18 ± 3*

*Significantly different from control $P < 0.05$.
**Significantly different from control $P < 0.01$.

is to tonically facilitate the function of baroreceptor reflexes in stabilizing arterial pressure.

At present we have not found that persistent hypertension can be produced by chemical lesions of NTS. Thus the effect of selective denervation in rat does not reproduce the effects of destructive lesion in the same species nor, if such comparisons can be made, in cat. However, two facts should be borne in mind. First, at present, we have only observed our animals during the daytime and thus, during periods in which the psychomotor activity of this nocturnal species is reduced. In view of the finding of exaggerated reactivity of the arterial pressure after 6-OHDA treatment it is possible that arterial pressure

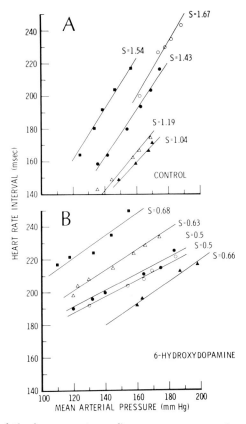

Fig. 14. Comparison of the baroreceptor reflex response curves in unanesthetized 6-OHDA treated and control rats. The increased mean arterial blood pressure produced by graded injections of phenylephrine is plotted against the heart rate interval. Each line represents a different animal. Note that the gain of the reflex indicated by the slopes (S) is reduced following 6-OHDA treatment.

might be elevated during periods of enhanced motor activity and behaviors. Second, it is also possible that lability, if persistent over prolonged periods of time, could lead to the development of fixed hypertension. Thus at this stage, our experiments, while not demonstrating persistent hypertension, do show that regional defects of central noradrenergic transmission can lead to disturbances of the arterial pressure which might be considered as predisposing to hypertension.

SUMMARY AND CONCLUSIONS

Neurogenic hypertension can be produced in rat and cat by bilateral electrolytic lesions of the NTS. Such lesions abolish arterial baroreceptor reflexes. In rat NTS lesions result in a profound, immediate, and partially differentiated excitation of sympathetic neurons, leading to increased peripheral resistance, elevated arterial pressure, cardiac overload, congestive

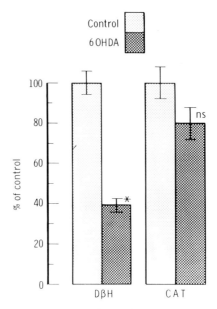

Fig. 15. Changes in enzyme activities 14 days after microinjection of 4 μg of 6-OHDA into NTS of rats. The area of NTS of one animal was removed bilaterally by microdissection and probed. Dopamine-β-hydroxylase (DBH) was assayed by a modification of the method of Reis and Molinoff (1972). Choline acetyltransferase (CAT) was assayed by a modification of the method of Schrier and Shaster (1967). Enzyme activities are expressed as percent of control (N = 6). Control DBH = 388.1 ± 25.6 nmoles octopamine/g/hr. Control CAT = 6.6 ± 0.5 μmoles ACh/g/hr. Note that DBH activity is significantly (* = P < 0.001) reduced without change in CAT activity indicating the specificity of the action of this dose of 6-OHDA on only catecholamine neurons.

failure and death within 4—6 hr. In cat the lesions produce similar acute changes in arterial pressure which are not lethal. After the first 24 hr cats enter a chronic and persistent state characterized by: (a) marked lability of the arterial pressure; (b) fixed elevations of the average arterial pressure; (c) exaggerated cardiovascular responses to naturally occurring and evoked behaviors; (d) tachycardia.

The syndrome of NTS hypertension cannot be accounted for as a consequence of selective destruction of the noradrenergic innervation of the NTS. Selective destruction of major portions of the noradrenergic input of NTS in rat by 6-OHDA results in the development of persistent lability and exaggerated reactivity of the arterial pressure, without changes in its average level. Baroreceptor reflexes remain intact and heart rate is unchanged. Thus the catecholamine innervation of NTS, probably noradrenergic, seems to modulate rather than mediate, baroreceptor reflexes by facilitating the role of baroreceptors in stabilizing the arterial pressure.

We conclude that chronic neurogenic hypertension can result from imbalances in the CNS which result in disinhibition of sympathetic vasomotor outflow. Specific biochemical defects of neurotransmitter systems particularly of the noradrenergic innervation of the NTS could possibly lead over time to the development of hypertension.

ACKNOWLEDGEMENTS

Dr. Tong Joh provided help in the biochemical assays. Mr. Lewis Tucker provided excellent technical assistance.

The research was supported by grants from the National Institutes of Health (HL 18974, HL 18195, and NS 06911). David Snyder is a recipient of "The John R. Raben" Fellowship of the New York Heart Association. Marc A. Nathan is a recipient of a Research Career Development Award from the National Heart and Lung Institute.

REFERENCES

Bloom, F.E., Algeri, S., Groppetti, A., Revuelta, A. and Costa, E. (1969) Lesions of central norepinephrine terminals with 6 OH-dopamine: biochemistry and fine structure. *Science*, 166: 1284—1286.

Chalmers, J.P. and Reid, J.L. (1972) Participation of central noradrenergic neurons in arterial baroreceptor reflexes in the rabbit: a study with intracisternally administered 6-hydroxy-dopamine. *Circulat. Res.*, 31: 789—804.

Chiba, T. and Doba, N. (1975) Catecholaminergic axon varicosities and their synaptic structure in the nucleus tractus solitarii: possible roles in the regulation of cardiovascular reflexes. *Brain Res.*, 84: 31—46.

Chiba, T. and Doba, N. (1976) Catecholaminergic axo-axonic synapses in the nucleus of the tractus solitarii (pars commissuralis) of the cat: possible relation to presynaptic regulation of baroreceptor reflexes. *Brain Res.*, 102: 255—265.

Cottle, M.A. (1964) Degeneration studies of the primary afferents of IXth and Xth cranial nerves in cat. *J. comp. Neurol.*,122: 329—343.

Cowley, A.W., Jr., Liard, J.F. and Guyton, A.C. (1973) Role of the baroreceptor reflex in daily control of arterial blood pressure and other variables in dogs. *Circulat. Res.*, 32: 564—576.

Crill, W.E. and Reis, D.J. (1968) Distribution of carotid sinus and depressor nerves in the cat brainstem. *Amer. J. Physiol.*, 214: 269—276.

Dahlström, A. and Fuxe, K. (1965) Evidence for the existence of monoamine neurons in the central nervous system. II. Experimentally induced changes in the intraneuronal amine levels of bulbo-spinal neuron systems. III. Distribution of monoamine nerve terminals in the central nervous system. *Acta physiol. scand.*, 247: 1—87.

Day, M.D. and Roach, A.G. (1974) Central adrenoreceptors and the control of arterial blood pressure. *Clin. exp. Pharmacol. Physiol.*, 1: 347—360.

De Jong, W. (1974) Noradrenaline, central inhibitory control of blood pressure and heart rate. *Europ. J. Pharmacol.*, 29: 179—181.

De Jong, W., Zandberg, P. and Bohus, B. (1975) Central inhibitory noradrenergic cardiovascular control. In *Hormones, Homeostasis and the Brain, Progr. in Brain Res., Vol. 42*, W.H. Gispen, Tj.B. van Wimersma Greidanus, B. Bohus and D. De Wied (Eds.), Elsevier, Amsterdam, pp. 285—298.

Doba, N. and Reis, D.J. (1973) Acute fulminating neurogenic hypertension produced by brainstem lesions in the rat. *Circulat. Res.*, 32: 584—593.

Doba, N. and Reis, D.J. (1974) Role of central and peripheral adrenergic mechanisms in neurogenic hypertension produced by brainstem lesions in rat. *Circulat. Res.*, 34: 293—301.

Finch, L., Haeusler, G. and Thoenen, H. (1972) Failure to induce experimental hypertension in rats after intraventricular injection of 6-hydroxy-dopamine. *Brit. J. Pharmacol.*, 44: 356—357.

Fuxe, K., Hökfelt, T. and Nilsson, O. (1965) A fluorescence microscopical and electron microscopic study on certain brain areas rich in monoamine terminals. *Amer. J. Anat.*, 117: 33—46.

Guazzi, M. and Zanchetti, A. (1965) Blood pressure and heart rate during natural sleep of the cat and their regulation by carotid sinus and aortic reflexes. *Arch. ital. Biol.*, 103: 789—817.

Haeusler, G. (1973) Activation of the central pathway of the baroreceptor reflex, a possible mechanism of the hypotensive action of clonidine. *Naunyn-Schmiedeberg's Arch. exp. Path. Pharmak.*, 278: 231—246.

Haeusler, G., Finch, L. and Thoenen, H. (1972) Central adrenergic neurons and the initiation and development of experimental hypertension. *Experientia (Basel)*, 28: 1200—1203.

Hökfelt, T., Fuxe, K., Goldstein, M. and Johansson, O. (1974) Immunohistochemical evidence for the existence of adrenaline neurons in the rat brain. *Brain Res.*, 66: 235—251.

Humphrey, D.R. (1967) Neuronal activity in the medulla oblongata of cat evoked by stimulation of the carotid sinus nerve. In *Baroreceptors and Hypertension*, P. Kezdi (Ed.), Pergamon, Oxford, pp. 131—167.

Lewis, P.J., Reid, J.L., Chalmers, J.P. and Dollery, C.T. (1973) Importance of central catecholaminergic neurons in the development of renal hypertension. *Clin. Sci.*, 45: 111S—118S.

Manning, J.W. (1965) Cardiovascular reflexes following lesions in medullary reticular formation. *Amer. J. Physiol.*, 208: 283—288.

Miura, M. and Reis, D.J. (1969) Termination of secondary projections of carotid sinus nerve in the cat brainstem. *Amer. J. Physiol.*, 217: 142—153.

Miura, M. and Reis, D.J. (1972) Role of the solitary and paramedian reticular nuclei in mediating cardiovascular reflex responses from carotid baro- and chemoreceptors. *J. Physiol. (Lond.)*, 223: 525—548.

Nathan, M.A. and Reis, D.J. (1976) Chronic labile hypertension produced in cat by lesion of nucleus tractus solitarii. *Circulat. Res.*, in press.

Philippu, A., Rosenberg, W. and Przuntek, H. (1973) Effects of adrenergic drugs on pressor responses to hypothalamic stimulation. *Naunyn-Schmiedeberg's Arch. exp. Path. Pharmak.*, 278: 373—386.

Reis, D.J. and Cuénod, M. (1965) Central neural regulation of carotid baroreceptor reflexes in the cat. *Amer. J. Physiol.*, 209: 1267—1277.

Reis, D.J. and Doba, N. (1974) The central nervous system and neurogenic hypertension. *Progr. Cardiovasc. Dis.*, 17: 51—71.

Reis, D.J. and Molinoff, P.B. (1972) Brain dopamine-β-hydroxylase: regional distribution and effects of lesions and 6-hydroxy-dopamine on activity. *J. Neurochem.*, 19: 195—204.

Saavedra, J.M., Palkovits, M., Brownstein, M.J. and Axelrod, J. (1974) Localisation of phenylethanolamine N-methyl transferase in rat brain nuclei. *Nature (Lond.)*, 248: 695—696.

Saavedra, J.M., Grobecker, H. and Axelrod, J. (1976) Adrenaline-forming enzyme in brainstem: elevation in genetic and experimental hypertension. *Science*, 191: 483—484.

Schrier, B.K. and Shuster, L. (1967) A simplified radiochemical assay for choline acetyltransferase. *J. Neurochem.*, 14: 977—985.

Seller, H. and Illert, M. (1969) The localization of the first synapse in the carotid sinus baroreceptor reflex pathway and its alteration of the afferent input. *Pflügers Arch. ges. Physiol.*, 306: 1—19.

Smyth, H. S., Sleight, P. and Pickering, G. W. (1969) Reflex regulation of arterial pressure during sleep in man: a quantitative method of assessing baroreflex sensitivity. *Circulat. Res.*, 24: 109—121.

Spyer, K. M. (1972) Baroreceptor sensitive neurones in the anterior hypothalamus of the cat. *J. Physiol. (Lond.)*, 224: 245—257.

Thoenen, H. and Tranzer, J. P. (1968) Chemical sympathectomy by selective destruction of adrenergic nerve endings with 6-hydroxydopamine. *Naunyn-Schmiedeberg's Arch. exp. Path. Pharmak.*, 261: 271—288.

Ungerstedt, U. (1971) Stereotaxic mapping of the monoamine pathway in the rat brain. *Acta physiol. scand.*, 82, Suppl. 367: 1—48.

Uretsky, N. J. and Iversen, L. L. (1970) Effects of 6-hydroxydopamine on catecholamine neurones in the rat brain. *J. Neurochem.*, 17: 269—278.

Acute and Chronic Hypertension after Lesions and Transections of the Rat Brain Stem

WYBREN DE JONG, PIETER ZANDBERG, MIKLÓS PALKOVITS* and
BÉLA BOHUS

*Rudolf Magnus Institute for Pharmacology, Medical Faculty, University of Utrecht, Utrecht
(The Netherlands)*

The control of arterial blood pressure by the brain has been a subject of interest for a period of more than 100 years. The importance of the central nervous system in hypertension often was neglected despite substantial experimental and clinical evidence (De Jong et al., 1975b; Julius, 1976). Recent findings as reported in this volume give new and substantial support to the role of the brain in hypertension.

Cyon and Ludwig (1866) first described the role of a depressor nerve in the rabbit. They already postulated that afferent neuronal information from the cardiovascular system exerts an inhibitory influence on blood pressure, and that this effect is mediated via the brain. Depressor responses can also be obtained by electrical stimulation of different sites in the brain stem. In the rat, a relatively small depressor area occupies caudal structures in the medulla oblongata, corresponding with the mediocaudal part of the nucleus tractus solitarii (NTS). The depressor response obtained by stimulation of the NTS was associated with a marked bradycardia (De Jong et al., 1975a, b). Stimulation of structures immediately below the depressor area resulted in distinct pressor responses, while the heart rate usually showed no major changes. The frequency dependence of the hypotensive response is shown in Fig. 1. A depressor response already occurred with a stimulation frequency of 1 Hz, while a maximal response was obtained with 10—20 Hz. The frequency characteristic for the pressor response following electrical stimulation of the reticular formation below the NTS is also shown. Pressor responses started to occur with 10—20 Hz and reached a maximum with 150 Hz. Current intensity which was needed to evoke a well-defined response was in general slightly higher for the pressor response (Fig. 1). These data may indicate that two different fiber systems were stimulated.

The depressor area of the NTS may well mediate a tonic inhibition of sympathetic tone and of reflex activity and thereby decrease blood pressure. We studied the cardiovascular effects of bilateral electrolytic lesions of the rat brain stem at the level of the obex (De Jong et al., 1975a, b). Blood pressure

*First Department of Anatomy, Semmelweis University Medical School, Tüzoltó u-58, 1450-Budapest-II (Hungary).

190

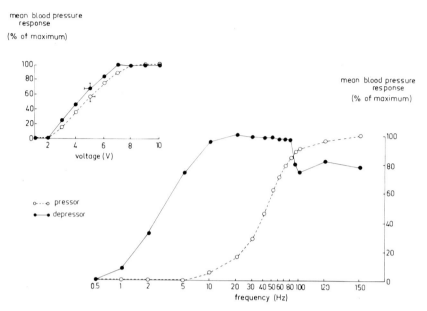

Fig. 1. Frequency dependence of depressor and pressor responses obtained by electrical stimulation of the medulla oblongata in the area of the nucleus tractus solitarii of rats anesthetized with urethane. The range of current intensities (V) and of frequencies (Hz) used is indicated on the abscissa. Data are means of 3—5 animals. Bars indicate S.E.M. (De Jong et al., 1975a).

was recorded from a permanent indwelling iliac cannula. The size of the lesions was approximately 1.0—1.2 mm. The lesions destroyed the most dorsal region of the medulla including the nucleus and tractus solitarius. Hypertension reached a maximum within a few minutes after the recovery from anesthesia and remained stable at a mean blood pressure level of 160—170 mm Hg during a period of 1 hr (Fig. 2). The increase in heart rate was not statistically

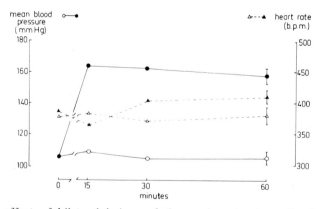

Fig. 2. Acute effect of bilateral lesions of the nucleus tractus solitarii on mean blood pressure and heart rate of 7 rats. Lesions were made under ether anesthesia, which was stopped directly after the operation. Closed symbols represent lesioned rats. Bars indicate S.E.M. (De Jong et al., 1975a).

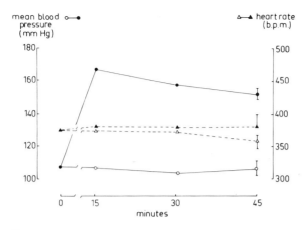

Fig. 3. Acute effect of bilateral transections of the medulla oblongata just lateral to the nucleus tractus solitarii on mean blood pressure and heart rate of 5 rats. Transections were made under ether anesthesia, which was stopped directly after the operation. Closed symbols represent rats with surgical cuts. Bars indicate S.E.M.

significant. Since the lesion destroyed the cells of the NTS as well as the tractus, the effect of frontal plane transections through the NTS was also investigated. The cuts were located at the level of the obex, 1—2 mm more rostral or 1—2 mm caudal of the obex. These transections failed to cause hypertension (De Jong et al., 1975b, De Jong and Palkovits, 1976). Thus, a mere interruption of the tractus at one of these levels is not sufficient to cause hypertension. Frontal plane transection rostral to the obex did not prevent the acute hypertension caused by a bilateral lesion of the NTS at the level of the obex. Thus, these transections are unlikely to have a non-specific inhibitory action preventing development of hypertension after damage to the NTS.

In order to see if fibers entering the NTS from laterally were more important in this respect we also performed a bilateral transection with cuts located just lateral to the NTS (De Jong and Palkovits, 1976). Following these bilateral surgical cuts hypertension developed the same way as after the bilateral lesion (Fig. 3). This may indicate that deafferentation of the NTS from lateral fibers was the cause of the hypertension. The location of the transection (tx_1) is depicted in Fig. 4. A more caudal transection (tx_2) did not elevate blood pressure.

The effect of several bilateral lesions of different parts of the NTS was investigated. The size of the lesions was approximately 0.8 mm. The location of the lesions is shown in Fig 4. Only the lesions at obex level (lesions number 3 and 5) were effective in causing hypertension. The caudal one of these two effective lesions, which was located at the level of the area postrema, also caused an increase in heart rate (Fig. 5). The more caudal and rostral lesions were ineffective. The lesion located more laterally apparently was too small to destroy a sufficient amount of incoming fibers.

The region destroyed by the effective lesions comprises the common projection site for the IXth and Xth cranial nerves. It may well be that both the effective lesions and transections caused hypertension by removal of an

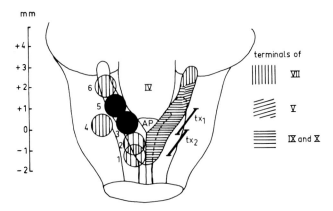

Fig. 4. Dorsal view of the medulla oblongata with schematic representation of the location of the different bilateral lesions (left side) and transections (right side). Projection sites of the cranial nerves are given according to Torvik (1956). AP = area postrema; IV = fourth ventricle.

inhibitory input via these nerves upon the cells of the NTS at the level of the obex. This possibility is also suggested by the observation that transection of these cranial nerves outside the medulla but within the skull caused a similar type of acute hypertension (De Jong, unpublished data). The region destroyed by the effective lesions is medial to the location of the effective transection (Fig. 4). The area postrema and this region are interconnected and it was often destroyed by the caudal effective lesion. For these reasons we also studied the effect of removal of the area postrema in rats. As can be seen in Fig. 6 removal of the area postrema did not affect blood pressure and heart rate. We also failed

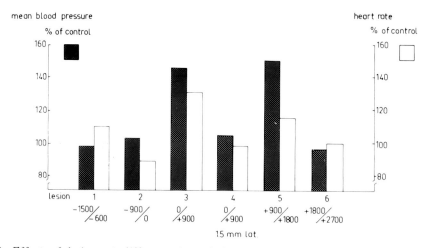

Fig. 5. Effect of lesions at different sites of the nucleus tractus solitarii on mean blood pressure and heart rate 30 min after the operation. The location of the lesions is shown in Fig. 4. Data of at least 4 rats are expressed as percentage of the value of sham-operated controls. The figures at the bottom indicate the caudal/rostral extension of the bilateral lesions. The level of the posterior tip of the area postrema was used as zero reference point.

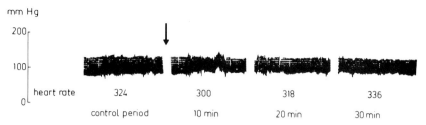

Fig. 6. Effect of removal of the area postrema (arrow) on blood pressure and heart rate of a rat. The ether anesthesia was stopped immediately after completion of the operation.

to show changes of baroreceptor function and of the heart rate response to diving after removal of the area postrema. The data summarized above clearly show that a part of the NTS serves to tonically inhibit blood pressure and that fibers entering the NTS laterally carry essential information in this respect. Neuroanatomical observations supporting the afferent nature of these fibers are reported elsewhere in this volume (Palkovits and Záborszky, 1977).

In order to see if the effective lesion (nr. 3, as shown in Fig. 4) also caused hypertension chronically, reserpine (i.p., 5 mg/kg) was administered before the operation in order to prevent the acute lethal rise of blood pressure. A moderate hypertension with a slight tachycardia did develop. Hypertension was still present after 6 weeks (Fig. 7) and was measured in conscious rats with a tail sphygmographic method as described earlier (Leenen and De Jong, 1971). There was no significant increase in heart weight. In a second chronic experiment, systolic blood pressure values obtained by the sphygmographic method were compared to direct measurements from an iliac cannula. For comparison, a group of renal hypertensive rats with a similar degree of hypertension was used. Hypertension was present in both groups of animals and the same blood pressure level was found with both methods.

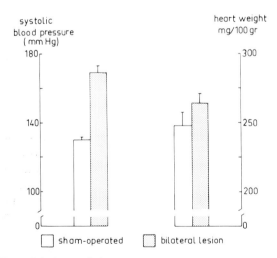

Fig. 7. Effect of bilateral lesions of the nucleus tractus solitarii on systolic blood pressure and relative heart weight 6 weeks after the operation. Data of 8 rats are given as means ± S.E.M.

DIVING REFLEX BRADYCARDIA

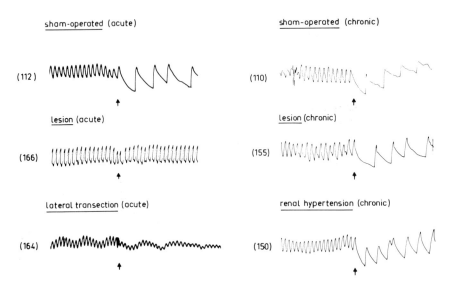

sham-operated (acute)   sham-operated (chronic)

(112)   (110)

lesion (acute)   lesion (chronic)

(166)   (155)

lateral transection (acute)   renal hypertension (chronic)

(164)   (150)

Fig. 8. Examples of diving reflex bradycardia of rats with acute or chronic bilateral lesions of the nucleus tractus solitarii or with bilateral transections of the medulla oblongata. A recording of a rat with chronic renal hypertension is shown for comparison. The arrow indicates the start of the diving procedure. The numbers in parentheses indicate the mean blood pressure. Blood pressure was recorded from a permanent iliac cannula.

In order to determine whether the lesion located at the level of the area postrema interfered with cardiovascular reflex regulation, the diving reflex-induced bradycardia was investigated. This reflex was obtained by keeping the nose of the rat immersed in water at $30°C$ for 5—10 sec (Lin, 1974). As shown in Fig. 8, an extreme bradycardia occurred in rats sham-operated 30 min before. The lesion acutely resulted in a complete absence of the diving reflex bradycardia. The acute bilateral transection at the level of the obex and the area postrema caused hypertension and also blocked the reflex bradycardia. Data obtained 6 weeks after operation are also shown in Fig. 8. Surprisingly, the diving reflex bradycardia reappears in rats with hypertension caused by the lesion and did not differ from the control response. A similar diving response was obtained in rats with renal hypertension.

Heart rate reflex responses were also studied 6 weeks after operation using bradykinin and angiotensin to induce a decrease and an increase of blood pressure respectively. The bradycardia after i.v. administration of angiotensin II and the tachycardia caused by i.v. administration of bradykinin are shown in Fig. 9. A sham-operated group as well as rats with renal hypertension were used for comparison. Bradykinin caused a similar decrease of blood pressure in all these groups. An increase in heart rate was observed in the sham-operated rats as well as in the renal hypertensive rats. In contrast, a decrease in heart rate was observed in the hypertensive rats with the lesion. The bradycardia induced by the angiotensin pressor response showed no significant difference in both groups of hypertensive rats as compared to the controls (Fig. 9).

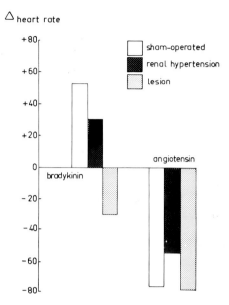

Fig. 9. Changes of heart rate in rats with a chronic bilateral lesion of the nucleus tractus solitarii and of rats with chronic renal hypertension. Heart rate changes were induced by hypotension following intravenous administration of 1.0 μg bradykinin or by abrupt blood pressure elevation following intravenous administration of 500 ng angiotensin II. Blood pressure and heart rate were recorded from a permanent iliac cannula. Data are means of at least 4 rats.

In summary, destruction of the cells of the NTS bilaterally at the level of the obex results in acute hypertension. Under chronic conditions hypertension is also observed in rats bearing a lesion. Acutely, reflex regulation appears to be almost completely disrupted. Chronically the diving reflex- and angiotensin-induced bradycardia are seen again. The transection studies indicate that a lateral deafferentation of the cells of the NTS is the cause of the hypertension. It appears that removal of an inhibitory input via part of the fibers of the IX and Xth cranial nerves is essential in this respect.

Although the acute phase of the hypertension after bilateral destruction of the NTS in several species appears not to be labile (Fallert and Bucher, 1966; Doba and Reis, 1973, 1974; De Jong et al., 1975a, b), a chronic labile hypertension may apparently result. The absence of an increase in heart weight may also reflect a labile hypertension. Labile hypertension after damage to the NTS has also been reported in man and in cats under chronic conditions (Magnus et al., 1977; Reis et al., 1977). A possible involvement of the area postrema (Ylitalo et al., 1974) could not be substantiated, either acutely after the operation or under chronic conditions.

SUMMARY

The effect of damage to the nucleus tractus solitarii (NTS) on blood pressure and heart rate and baroreceptor reflex responses was studied under acute and chronic conditions. When located at the level of the area postrema or just rostral from it, bilateral electrolytic lesions of the NTS of normotensive Wistar rats acutely caused hypertension. A slight tachycardia was observed in the first group. More extensive lesions also caused hypertension but no change of heart rate was found. Lesions located more caudally in the NTS and in the nucleus commissuralis were ineffective. A similar type of acute hypertension occurred after bilateral transections just lateral to the NTS at the level of the area postrema. Effective transections were found to extend into the reticular formation between the NTS and the nucleus tractus spinalis n. trigemini. Bilateral transection of the tractus failed to cause hypertension. Removal of the area postrema did not affect blood pressure and heart rate either. Electrical stimulation of the NTS caused frequency-dependent hypotension and bradycardia. These data may indicate that the cells of the NTS mediate a tonic inhibitory influence on blood pressure.

The effect of the lesions located at the level of the area postrema was also studied under chronic conditions. In these rats, moderate hypertension was found 6 weeks after operation without increase in heart weight. Although baroreceptor reflex responses and the diving reflex bradycardia were inhibited acutely, there was only slight alteration of these reflexes at 6 weeks following operation. The extreme, acute elevation of blood pressure observed after bilateral deafferentation or lesioning of the NTS indicates a major role of this nucleus in cardiovascular regulation. The area postrema does not seem to be directly involved in the observed hypertension.

REFERENCES

Cyon, E. und Ludwig, C. (1866) Die Reflexe eines der sensiblen Nerven des Herzens auf die Motorischen der Blutgefässe. *Ber. Verh. Konigl. Sachs. ges. Wiss. (Lpz.)*, 18: 307—328.

De Jong W., Nijkamp, F.P. and Bohus, B. (1975a) Role of noradrenaline and serotonin in the central control of blood pressure in normotensive and spontaneously hypertensive rats. *Arch. int. Pharmacodyn.*, 213: 272—284.

De Jong, W., Zandberg, P. and Bohus, B. (1975b) Central inhibitory noradrenergic cardiovascular control. In *Hormones, Homeostasis and the Brain, Progr. Brain Res.*, Vol. 42, W.H. Gispen, Tj.B. van Wimersma Greidanus, B. Bohus and D. De Wied (Eds.), Elsevier, Amsterdam, pp. 285—298.

De Jong, W. and Palkovits, M. (1976) Hypertension after localized transection of brainstem fibers. *Life Sci.*, 18: 61—64.

Doba, N. and Reis, D.J. (1973) Acute fulminating hypertension produced by brainstem lesions in the rat. *Circulat. Res.*, 32: 584—593.

Doba, N. and Reis, D.J. (1974) Role of central and peripheral adrenergic mechanisms in neurogenic hypertension produced by brainstem lesions in rat. *Circulat. Res.*, 34: 293—301.

Fallert, M. und Bucher, V.M. (1966) Lokalisation eines Blutdruck aktiven Substrats in der Medulla oblongata des Kaninchens. *Helv. physiol. Acta*, 24: 139—163.

Julius, S. (1976) Introduction. In *The Nervous System in Arterial Hypertension*, S. Julius and M.D. Esler (Eds.), Thomas, Springfield, Ill., pp. xii—xvi.

Leenen, F.H.H. and De Jong, W. (1971) A solid silver clip for induction of predictable levels of renal hypertension in the rat. *J. appl. Physiol.*, 31: 142—145.

Lin, Y.C. (1974) Autonomic nervous control of cardiovascular response during diving in the rat. *Amer. J. Physiol.*, 227: 601—605.

Magnus, O., Koster, M. and Van der Drift, J.H.A. (1977) Cerebral mechanisms and neurogenic hypertension in man: with special reference to baroreceptor control. In *Hypertension and Brain Mechanisms, Progr. Brain Res., Vol. 47,* W. De Jong, A.P. Provoost and A.P. Shapiro (Eds.), Elsevier, Amsterdam, pp. 199—218.

Palkovits, M. and Záborsky, L. (1977) Neuroanatomy of central cardiovascular control: nucleus tractus solitarii: afferent and efferent neuronal connections in relation to the baroreceptor reflex arc. In *Hypertension and Brain Mechanisms, Progr. Brain Res., Vol. 47,* W. De Jong, A.P. Provoost and A.P. Shapiro (Eds.), Elsevier, Amsterdam, pp. 9—34.

Reis, D.J., Doba, N., Snyder, B.W. and Nathan, M.A. (1977) Brain lesions and hypertension: chronic lability and elevation of arterial pressure produced by electrolytic lesions and 6-hydroxydopamine treatment of nucleus tractus solitarii (NTS) in rat and cat. In *Hypertension and Brain Mechanisms, Progr. Brain Res., Vol. 47,* W. De Jong, A.P. Provoost and A.P. Shapiro (Eds.), Elsevier, Amsterdam, pp. 169—188.

Torvik, A. (1956) Afferent connections to the sensory trigeminal nuclei; the nucleus of the solitary tracts and adjacent structures. *J. comp. Neurol.,* 106: 51—139.

Ylitalo, P., Karppanen, H. and Paasonen, M.K. (1974) Is the area postrema a control centre of blood pressure? *Nature (Lond.),* 247: 58—59.

Cerebral Mechanisms and Neurogenic Hypertension in Man, with Special Reference to Baroreceptor Control

O. MAGNUS, M. KOSTER and J.H.A. VAN DER DRIFT

Research Unit TNO for Clinical Neurophysiology, Ursula Kliniek, Wassenaar, and Department of Internal Medicine, University Hospital, Wilhelmina Gasthuis, Amsterdam (The Netherlands)

INTRODUCTION

The literature concerning clinical neurological disorders associated with hypertension will be reviewed and a comparison made with neurophysiological and neuropathological data. Previous reviews of the subject (i.a. Koster, 1952; Tyler and Dawson, 1961; Dickinson, 1965; Reis and Doba, 1974; De Jong et al., 1975) have served as valuable guides, however, we do not pretend to be able to cover the vast subject adequately.

In view of the fact that arterial hypertension and loss of baroreceptor control caused by lesions of the nucleus tractus solitarii (N.T.S.) have received particular emphasis during this Symposium, a few previously published case histories of patients with a comparable syndrome together with the neuropathological findings in one of these cases (Koster, 1952; Koster and Bethlem, 1961) will be presented in more detail.

Finally the role of cerebral disorders as a cause of transient arterial hypertension will be discussed.

HYPERTENSION ASSOCIATED WITH DISORDERS OF MEDULLA OBLONGATA AND PONS

The Cushing response

One of the earliest known types of arterial hypertension, due to intracranial processes, was studied in detail by Cushing (1901, 1902a, b, 1903). It had already been known for a long time that an acute increase of intracranial pressure (ICP) is associated with a rise of blood pressure (Duret, 1878; Naunyn and Schreiber, 1881; Spencer and Horsley, 1892; Kocher, 1901). In fact, according to Cushing (1902a and b) it was Kocher who encouraged him to make an experimental study of the subject; this was done in the Physiological Institute of Kronecker in Bern. Cushing was able to demonstrate the quantitative nature of the response, showing that it occurred with step-wise increases of the ICP as soon as this pressure exceeded the mean arterial blood pressure. Together with the increase of blood pressure, there occurred bradycardia and slowing and irregularities of respiration. In subsequent papers, Cushing (1902b, 1903) also reported clinical cases in which he had observed these phenomena. The triad of the Cushing phenomenon was at first generally accepted as a clinical danger signal of a critical increase of intracranial pressure. However, several authors observed that, in patients, the cerebral spinal fluid (CSF) pressure was rarely increased to a level even approaching the diastolic blood pressure. And on increasing the CSF pressure to levels close to the diastolic blood pressure (i.e. over 100 cm H_2O), blood pressure, pulse rate and respiration did not change significantly (Browder and Meyers, 1936, 1938; Evans et al., 1951). In 1959 Thompson and Malina demonstrated in dogs that the Cushing response could occur at levels considerably below the level of mean arterial pressure when there was no free passage of CSF between the supra- and the infratentorial space and when the increase of pressure in either compartment led to axial displacement of the lower brain stem. They concluded that when cardiorespiratory symptoms developed in the presence of increased intracranial pressure there was an acute dynamic axial distortion of the lower brain stem. This was confirmed by Weinstein et al. (1964) who showed in rhesus monkeys that with supratentorial expanding lesions, obstruction of communication of pressure from the supratentorial space to the posterior fossa by tentorial herniation consistently lowered the threshold of the vasopressor response (cf. also Weinstein et al., 1968).

This response has recently been studied more in detail. Hoff and Reis (1970) showed that carefully calibrated local shortlasting pressure applied with a fine metal probe within a clearly defined area of the floor of the fourth ventricle of anesthetized cats evoked the same graded increase of blood pressure and bradycardia with the same latency, < 10 sec, as did a subdural injection of saline, raising the ICP to 100—175 mm Hg. The threshold was also of the same order as that which was found for local pressure with a steel probe (165—200 mm Hg). The pressure-stretch sensitive area extends paramedially along the floor of the fourth ventricle from the obex to the facial colliculus. In this connection it is of interest that Spencer and Horsley (1892) obtained already an increase of the blood pressure by application of pressure on the floor of the IV ventricle in dogs. In an extension of this study, Doba and Reis (1972) found that an identical response could be produced by the rapid delivery of 1—3 μl of artificial CSF in a restricted area within the rostral medulla and caudal pons, lying deep to the probe-sensitive area on the surface of the fourth ventricle. The adequate stimulus appeared to be a transient distortion of tissue within the critical area. A similar response could also be evoked by punctate electrical stimulation restricted to the same area of the brain stem. The 'pressure' stimulus required for marked elevation of blood pressure was within the range of capillary pressure, indicating that such a response does not need large distorting pressures on the neuron. These findings appear to provide the physiological basis for the investigations of Thompson and Malina (1959) and of Weinstein et al. (1964); they also allow the sensitive area in the medulla to be located and to be limited to the pressure sensitive region under the floor of the fourth ventricle first outlined by Hoff and Reis (1970). In this context, cases of a tumor lying in the region of the floor of the fourth ventricle, and showing paroxysmal or reversible hypertension are of interest (Grimson, 1950). Evans et al. (1972) reported on such a case with paroxysmal hypertension and increased excretion of catecholamines. A pheochromocytoma could be excluded. There are several reports in the literature of an increased incidence of arterial hypertension in cases of posterior fossa tumors, sometimes leading to a wrong diagnosis of primary hypertension (Meyer, 1941) or pheochromocytoma (Cameron and Doig, 1970). Later Doba and Reis (1974) found that small lesions placed at the caudal end of the Cushing-sensitive region resulted in a fall of systemic blood pressure to the same levels to which the blood pressure falls with cervical transection. This suggests that the Cushing-sensitive region may coincide with the so-called vasomotor area of the lower brain stem, whose integrity is required for the maintenance of normal levels of blood pressure. Rowan and Johnston (1975) found that the substantial increase of blood pressure induced in baboons by cisterna magna infusion of mock CSF could not be attributed to a reduction of cerebral blood flow (CBF) or cerebral perfusion pressure (CPP). However, using cats, Hoff et al. (1975) showed that under various experimental conditions Cushing response only occurred when the CPP was reduced below 50mm Hg. They concluded that this response was due to reduction of medullary perfusion, approximating capillary closing pressure. McGillicuddy et al. (1975) obtained the same increases of blood pressure in rhesus monkeys with rapid increase of CSF pressure as with sudden ischemia and hypoxia. However, they remark that their findings do not necessarily contradict the findings that direct pressure or distortion of the brain stem can cause the Cushing response.

Though certainly not all problems concerning the 'Cushing response' have been solved the above experimental findings appear to explain to a considerable extent the discrepancies between clinical observations. It appears that neurologists and neurosurgeons are still justified in considering cardio-respiratory disturbances of the Cushing response type as a danger signal. The available data suggest that this indicates a combination of increased intracranial pressure with distortion (and/or ischemia) of the lower brain stem rather than elevation of the intracranial pressure to the level of the diastolic or mean arterial pressure.

Disturbances of baroreceptor control

It has been known since the investigations of Hering (1927) and of Heymans et al. (1933) that baroreceptors, particularly in the carotid sinus and also in the aortic arch, have an important influence on blood pressure regulation. The baroreceptor afferents enter the brain stem through the roots of the glosso-pharyngeal and vagus nerves and descend along the tractus solitarius to synapse within the nucleus tractus solitarii (NTS). In addition, there is, at least in the cat, a direct projection of carotid sinus afferents into the bulbar reticular formation, primarily to the large cells of the paramedian reticular nucleus (Miura and Reis, 1969). The baroreceptor reflexes are under a considerable degree of supra-segmental control, including the hypothalamus and the limbic system.

Though it is difficult to produce complete sino-aortic denervation in experimental animals, it has been possible to produce systemic hypertension with this procedure. Such a hypertension is characteristically labile.

In 1966 Fallert and Bucher showed that bilateral lesions of the NTS cause a rise of blood pressure in rabbits and in 1973 Doba and Reis showed that similar lesions in the rat at the level of the obex result in fulminating hypertension, not associated with any change in heart rate. Systolic pressure rose from 125 to 200 mm Hg. This was confirmed by De Jong et al (1975). They also showed that electrical stimulation of the NTS induces hypotension and bradycardia. Bilateral microinjections of noradrenaline into the NTS produced a dose-related decrease of the blood pressure and of the heart rate. The lowest dose of 1.2 nmoles caused a significant decrease of blood pressure without clear bradycardia. This effect could be prevented by a preceding injection of the alpha-receptor blocking agent, phentolamine. More recently, Reis et al. (1977) have shown that labile hypertension with loss of baroreceptor control can be produced by bilateral lesions of the NTS in chronic experiments in cats. Hypertension evoked by NTS lesions is dependent on the integrity of structures lying above the mid-brain. Mid-collicular decerebration before NTS lesions are placed, aborts the development of hypertension or once the lesions are established, abolishes the hypertension.

To our knowledge no cases have been described of loss of baroreceptor control due to medullary lesions. We should therefore like to discuss a few cases which have previously been reported by one of us (Koster, 1952), but for which the above findings provide a better interpretation.

The first patient, a woman of 50, was known to have a slowly progressing syringomyelia since the age of 33. Six months prior to admission to the hospital she developed nocturnal attacks of dyspnea which appeared to be very similar to cardiac asthma. On examination there were signs of mild cardiac decompensation. The blood pressure was 205/145 mm Hg. Moreover she had neurological signs of syringomyelia and syringobulbia, including analgesia and hypothermaesthesia of the right hand. Two days after admission she had an attack when she was lifted into her bed. She started to cry, became cyanotic, had a few facial jerks and became unconscious. She stopped breathing and there was no pulse on palpation and auscultation. After one minute she began

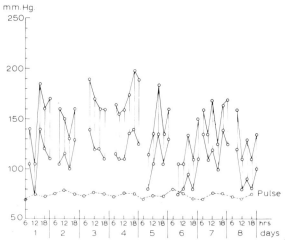

Fig. 1. Daily fluctuations in blood pressure during 8 successive days without significant variations of pulse rate.

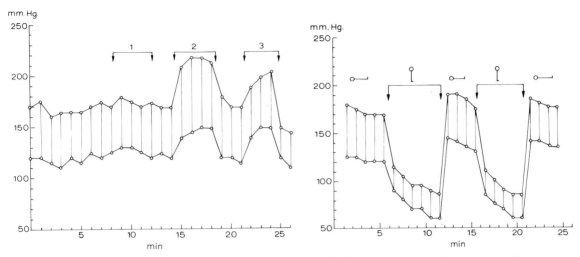

Fig. 2. Cold pressor test. At 1, the right hand, with hypothermaesthesia, is immersed in ice-water and no change in blood pressure is seen. At 2, the left, normal, hand is immersed in ice-water and a marked rise in blood pressure occurs. At 3, both hands are immersed in ice-water.

Fig. 3. In the upright position, a very marked fall in blood pressure occurred (orthostatic hypotension).

to recover gradually and the pulse rate increased from 12/min to 160/min. At that time she had a galop rhythm. Blood pressure increased to 290 mm Hg. The ECG, made shortly afterwards, was normal. Detailed investigations did not provide any evidence for the presence of a pheochromocytoma. Further observation showed that there were marked 'spontaneous' daily fluctuations of blood pressure. It varied between 105/75 and 200/140 mm Hg. (Fig. 1). These

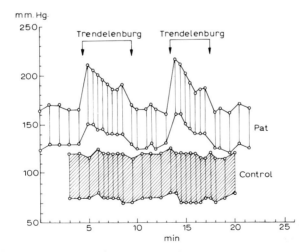

Fig. 4. When the patient is placed in the Trendelenburg position, an initial rise in blood pressure is followed by a gradual fall in blood pressure. There is hardly any change in blood pressure in a normal control.

variations were not accompanied by significant changes of the pulse rate. During the 'cold pressor test', immersion into ice-water of the left hand (in which thermaesthesia was unimpaired) showed an increase of the systolic pressure from 170 to 225 mm Hg (Fig. 2). Immersion of the right hand, in which there was no perception of temperature, had no effect. Emotion proved to be the most frequent cause of rises of blood pressure. Filling of the bladder also caused a strong rise of the blood pressure. There was a considerable orthostatic fall in blood pressure (Fig. 3) and a transient rise of blood pressure occurred when she was brought into the Trendelenburg position (Fig. 4). In order to check the possible causes of this phenomenon, the influence of CSF pressure changes was investigated. The Queckenstedt test caused a marked increase of blood pressure. This was neither seen in normals nor in patients with essential hypertension (Fig. 5). Intravenous injection of 40 ml of a hypertonic glucose solution, which is known to reduce CSF pressure, induced a gradual decrease of blood pressure (Fig. 6). Compression of the carotid sinus had no effect on the blood pressure.

The patient died 3 years later from pneumonia and congestive heart failure. At autopsy (Koster and Bethlem, 1961) no abnormalities were found in the brain. In the medulla oblongata, however, there was a slit on the right side, running in the ventrolateral direction from the caudal part of the floor of the fourth ventricle. The descending tract of the trigeminal nerve was interrupted. The greater part of the slit-like cavity was replaced by a neuroglial scar. The ganglion cells of the nuclei gracilis and cuneatus were degenerated. The slit descended into the first cervical segment. A smaller slit was present on the left side. In the cervical spinal cord there was a large cavity involving the dorsal parts of the ventral horn.

In view of the recent physiological findings, the original histological sections have been reexamined. It appeared that on the right side, the NTS was severely damaged by the neuroglial scar like formation (Fig. 7). The NTS was somewhat less affected on the left side.

A very similar case of syringomyelia and syringobulbia with spontaneously fluctuating hypertension and blood pressure varying with postural changes from 240/170 to 115/60 mm Hg has been studied. Filling of the bladder and CSF pressure changes had the same influence as in the previous patient. In this case no autopsy findings were obtained.

A third patient with syringomyelia served as control for these cases. At autopsy this patient, similarly to the first, proved to have a large cyst in the cervical region. The patient had had a normal blood pressure and no abnormal reaction to the tests for blood pressure regulation. There was no lesion in the lower brain stem and the NTS was intact on both sides.

When considering the data from the first patient and the available physiological data, it seems highly probable that the practically complete absence of baroreceptor control was due to the bilateral lesions of the NTS. The same explanation is assumed for the second patient, though no autopsy was available in this case. This view is supported by the extensive neuropathological studies of Ionesco-Sisesti (1932) and Greenfield (1963), that the type and location of the abnormalities found by Koster and Bethlem is fairly typical for

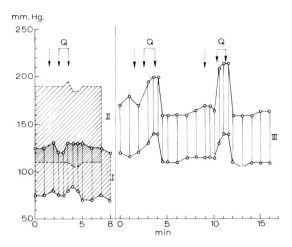

Fig. 5. Reaction of blood pressure to the Queckenstedt test. At ↓ the hands are put in position without compression of the jugular vein. At ↓↓ both jugular veins are compressed. No reaction of the blood pressure is seen in a normal control (I) or a patient with essential hypertension (II). A marked rise in blood pressure is seen in our patient (III).

syringobulbia. In their cases the fasciculus tr. solitarii was usually at least partially affected.

Bulbar vascular disturbances and arterial hypertension

Several authors have considered the possibility that ischemic lesions of the medulla oblongata could lead to arterial hypertension in man. In particular Dickinson (1965) has put forward the hypothesis of neurogenic arterial hypertension being caused by ischemia of the medullary vasomotor centers in cases of vertebral basilar atherosclerosis. This hypothesis was tested by Marshall (1966). He studied 679 cases with known brain lesions by comparing the casual blood pressure of patients with brain stem ischemia with that of patients with

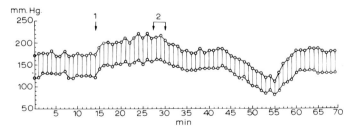

Fig. 6. Reaction of blood pressure to an intravenous injection of 40 ml hypertonic glucose solution (2). At 1, the patient sees the needle, with resulting rise in blood pressure.

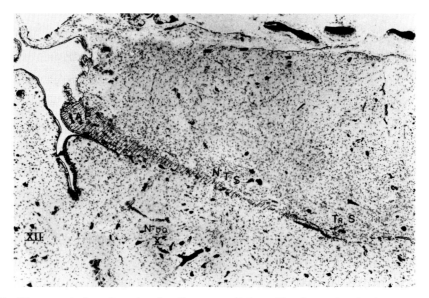

Fig. 7. Microscopical section showing the neuroglial scarlike formation in the region of the nucleus tractus solitarii (NTS). Tr.S. tractus solitarius; AP, area postrema; N do X, nucleus dorsalis nervi vagi; XII, nucleus nervi hypoglossi.

ischemia of a cerebral hemisphere. There was no consistent tendency for patients with brain stem ischemia to have a higher blood pressure than for those with ischemia of a cerebral hemisphere. When we now consider neuropathological studies of ischemic lesions caused by vertebro-basilar insufficiency we can perhaps understand why this should be the case.

In a very detailed recent anatomical study of 33 patients with bulbar infarctions Hauw et al. (1976) found bilateral lesions in only one patient and in this case the NTS was only slightly involved on one side. In 13 out of 31 cases unilateral involvement of the tractus solitarius and its nucleus was mentioned but only in one case was the nucleus specifically mentioned. It must therefore be extremely rare for the NTS to be affected bilaterally by vascular lesions. The NTS and the nucleus dorsalis nervi vagi are apparently relatively rarely destroyed by ischemic lesions, because these nuclei are supplied by dorsal as well as lateral arteries (i.e. short as well as long circumferential arteries). Fischer et al. (1961) described autopsy findings in 16 cases of unilateral lateral medullary infarct. Only in one case of unilateral dorsal infarct due to occlusion of the posterior inferior cerebellar artery was there a lesion in the area of the NTS, the tractus solitarius and the nucleus dorsalis nervi vagi. Clinically, this case was mainly characterized by hiccup. No abnormal findings were mentioned regarding blood pressure. Montgomery (1961) described 3 cases of vertebral basilar insufficiency with paroxysmal hypertension. Only in one case was autopsy performed: the basilar artery was markedly sclerotic and several miliary infarcts were seen microscopically among the nuclei of the medulla oblongata. Unfortunately, no further data were given concerning location of these infarcts.

Ito et al. (1973) investigated the relation between the location of cerebral vascular hemorrhages or infarcts and the difference between the blood pressure measured before and after the cerebral vascular accident. A marked increase was found, particularly in cases with a hemorrhage or infarct in the tegmentum pontis. In view of the findings of Hoff and Reis (1970) and of Doba and Reis (1972) it would seem possible that such vascular lesions affect the paramedial area under the floor of the fourth ventricle thus giving rise to arterial hypertension on stretch and distortion.

Tabes dorsalis

A neurological disease, tabes dorsalis, has not infrequently been observed to give rise to paroxysmal hypertension. Paroxysmal hypertension in association with tabetic crises, was first described by Pal in 1903 and reports on 18 cases are presented in his monograph of 1905. A number of other case histories were published soon afterwards by other authors. In most cases the acute hypertension occurred in association with the gastric crises. There were exceptions, however, and three such cases were described by Bennett and Heyman (1948). Only one of their patients also had gastric crises and in that instance the attack consisted only of nausea and vomiting, unaccompanied by pain. They were not able to find any consistent way of precipitating hypertension.

This was different in the case of the following patient: A man aged 54 on which Koster reported in 1952, had been known to suffer from tabes for 24 years and had complained of attacks of severe abdominal pain since the beginning of his illness. In recent weeks he had syncopal attacks characterized by unconsciousness, sweating and urinary incontinence. On admission the blood pressure was 160/120 mm Hg. There were no signs of pheochromocytoma. The blood pressure varied with postural changes between 70/55 mm Hg in the orthostatic position to 155/115 mm Hg in the Trendelenburg position. With the cold pressor test blood pressure changed from 150/120 to 190/165 mm Hg. The influence of the Queckenstedt test in this case was not convincing.

In this case of tabes dorsalis it is difficult to explain the disturbance of baroreceptor control. In the cases of tabes dorsalis with paroxysmal hypertension described in the literature, there was usually no postural hypotension and no abnormal reaction to the cold pressor test when this was done. However Bennett and Heyman (1940) mention one patient who had both paroxysmal hypertension and postural hypotension. It might be worthwhile to investigate cases of tabes dorsalis with paroxysmal hypertension in more detail using the tests mentioned above and to examine carefully the roots of the ninth and tenth cranial nerves and the region of the NTS when there is an opportunity for autopsy in such cases.

Porphyria

Baker and Watson (1945) described a case of porphyria with diffuse involvement of the nervous system. This patient had severe abdominal cramps, dysarthria, dysphagia, flaccid quadriplegia. His blood pressure was 180/120. In the subsequent remission it returned to normal. He died two years later of a recurrence. At autopsy, abnormalities were most marked in the medulla oblongata. The dorsal nucleus of the vagus revealed the most extensive changes. The NTS is not mentioned in this report. The spinal cord was free from changes but some of the most extensive alterations were observed in the peripheral nerves of the lower limbs. Kezdi (1954) suggested that the afferent pathway from the baroreceptors to the bulbar vasomotor center may have been affected in a case of porphyria with several periods of transient hypertension which were associated with involvement of the glosso-pharyngeal and vagus nerves.

Poliomyelitis

Periods of arterial hypertension in cases of poliomyelitis have been described by various authors (McDowell and Plum, 1951; Weinstein, 1957). Löblich (1950) carried out anatomical studies in 6 fatal cases of poliomyelitis whose case histories had been described by Lachmund (1950). Three of these cases had arterial hypertension and three were normotensive. Only the cases with arterial hypertension had bilateral lesions in the paramedian reticular formation. Lachmund mentioned 11 fatal cases of poliomyelitis with hypertension of varying duration, all of which had bilateral lesions in the reticular formation. Baker et al. (1950) examined the complete medulla oblongata in 80 cases of bulbar poliomyelitis. On the basis of the predominant injury to cell groups of the medulla it was possible to divide bulbar poliomyelitis into three types: (1) involvement of the nucleus ambiguus, resulting in dysphagia and dysarthria; (2) involvement of the small cells of the reticular formation, leading to disturbances of respiration and finally apnea; (3) involvement of the large cells in the ventromedial reticular formation which produced vasomotor disturbances.

All 7 patients, in whom severe bilateral damage of the large cells of the ventromedial formation was found, had shown vasomotor disturbances such as rapid irregular pulse, low pulse pressure and a labile blood pressure, varying from high to low levels and terminal shock. In bulbar poliomyelitis, when death was rapid both the small and large cells were always severely damaged.

Damage to the large cell portion of the reticular formation was also found in all 34 fatal cases of bulbar poliomyelitis described by Kemp (1957), in which high blood pressure had been documented. This area of the reticular formation corresponds with the paramedian areas in the cat, in which the large cells particularly receive a heavy input from baroreceptors (Miura and Reis, 1969).

DIENCEPHALON

Karplus and Kreidl showed as early as 1909 that electrical stimulation of the hypothalamus can cause an increase of blood pressure, an effect which disappeared after transection of the splanchnic nerves. In the period between 1930 and 1938 W.R. Hess showed that there is an area close to the caudal part of the third ventricle from which pressor responses could be obtained on electrical stimulation, whereas an area of depressor effects was situated rostro-laterally from the pressor regions (vide Hess, 1969). Ranson and Magoun (1939) also mapped the areas in the hypothalamus influencing blood pressure. Usually electrical stimulation of the brain at sites from which specific patterns of behavior can be evoked in chronically prepared anesthetized animals, will also elicit the appropriate pattern of circulation changes (Reis and Doba, 1974). Elevation of blood pressure of similar magnitude produced by stimulation at different sites may be associated with very different patterns of blood flow distribution. Folkow and Rubinstein (1965) performed electrical stimulation at sites from which the defense reaction or feeding behavior could be elicited when the animal was chronically prepared and unanesthetized. Under anesthesia, stimulation at each site produced an elevation of blood pressure. However, the stimulation from which the defense response was evoked, had as result an increase in muscle blood flow and a decrease in splanchnic blood flow, whereas stimulation at the feeding site produced opposite effects.

Folkow and Rubinstein (1966) also investigated the effect of chronic stimulation at sites from which the cardiovascular components of the defense reaction could be evoked. Six animals were stimulated repeatedly with 10 sec trains, once a minute for 12 hr a day over 17 weeks. The animals gradually developed arterial hypertension which was reversible when stimulation was stopped. The stimulation did not produce any obvious changes in behavior. No pathological changes were observed in the heart or kidneys. Endocrine factors cannot be ruled out, in these experiments.

Lesions principally involving the antero-medial hypothalamus can produce both chronic and acute fulminating forms of hypertension in the rat (Okamoto et al., 1964; Nozuka, 1966; Yamori, 1967). The hypertension develops over several weeks, is associated with increased adrenal weight and elevation of cortisol levels and may be abolished by adrenalectomy. Acute fulminating hypertension has been produced by Nathan and Reis (1975) by the placement of small bilateral lesions in the anterior hypothalamus of rats. When the animals awoke from anesthesia, the hypertension reached a peak within 90 min and was maintained for several hours until cardiac output failed. The hypertension was associated with a marked increase in motor activity, but persisted after the animal was paralyzed with curare. Hypertension but not local motor activity was abolished by adrenalectomy, adrenal demedullation or selective denervation of the adrenal glands. Hypertension of adrenomedullary origin in otherwise normal subjects is not a recognized human disease and appears to be a new type of neurogenic hypertension in animals.

Clinical observations

To our knowledge arterial hypertension due to a lesion of the hypothalamus has not been described. Efferent pathways from hypothalamus run not only to the medullary centers, but also to the hypophysis: the best known neurological cause of arterial hypertension is probably Cushing's syndrome, occurring in cases of basophilic and possibly also of chromophobe adenoma of the pituitary gland. This is, however, primarily a hormonal and not a nervous disease.

One of the best known examples of paroxysmal hypertension of diencephalic origin appeared to be a patient described by Penfield in 1929. It concerned a woman of 41, who had attacks characterized by restlessness, vasodilatation in an area supplied by the cervical sympathetic nerves, a sudden rise in blood pressure (from a systolic pressure of 100—210 mm Hg), lacrimation, sweating, salivation, mydriasis, tachycardia, occasional unconsciousness, hiccupping, transient shivering, Cheyne-Stokes breathing. There was never any movement of the body to suggest convulsions. Ventriculography showed an enormous symmetrical dilatation of both lateral ventricles. During one of the attacks ventricular puncture was performed which showed an extremely high pressure, following reduction of the pressure the patient regained consciousness. She died a few days later during an attack. At autopsy a small round cholesteatoma was found in the third ventricle, just between the two foramina of Monro. It apparently acted as a ball valve which intermittently occluded the foramina. Pressure appeared to have been exerted in the area of the dorsal nucleus of the thalamus but not on the hypothalamus. There were marked herniations in the temporal fossa and the cisterna magna. The brain and cerebellum were congested but the medulla and pons were strikingly white. The third and fourth ventricles were not dilated.

In view of these findings it would seem that there is not sufficient evidence to assume that these attacks were of an epileptic nature, as originally assumed by Penfield (1929). A more likely explanation seems to be that they were mainly due to CSF fluid obstruction in the lateral ventricles and that at least part of the symptoms including the arterial hypertension were due to a Cushing response. In this connection the ischemia of the medulla oblongata and pons in contrast with the marked congestion of the cerebral hemispheres and cerebellum are of particular interest.

CEREBRAL HEMISPHERES

Effects on blood pressure have been obtained in animals on stimulation of various regions of the cerebral hemispheres, notably from prefrontal and orbital frontal cortex, from the anterior cingular gyrus and the amygdala. Chapman (1960) has described an increase of blood pressure on stimulation of the region of the amygdala in conscious man. This occurred in association with other autonomic symptoms and with emotional symptoms. Van Buren (1961) studied effects of electrical stimulation with electrodes implanted in the amygdala in 11 patients with temporal lobe epilepsy. Surprisingly few autonomic responses appeared without evidence of central spread of epileptiform activity*. With most of the responses which appeared the patient also reported a visceral or somatic sensation from the same area. During

---

*The results are in accordance with similar findings of Andy et al. (1959) on electrical stimulation in unanesthetized cats.

post-stimulation ictal automatisms, the autonomic effects although varying in their time sequence nearly invariably resulted in autonomic changes moving in a similar direction. Thus hypertension, tachycardia, narrowing of the plethysmogram, swallowing and inhibition of respiration occurred if any changes appeared in these respective functions.

Van Buren (1958) also carried out careful polygraphic examinations, including automatic measuring of the blood pressure once per minute and ECG, during 20 temporal lobe seizures in 13 patients. Seven attacks occurred spontaneously, 3 were elicited by hyperventilation, 7 by Metrazol and 3 by electrical stimulation of implanted electrodes. A short-lasting increase of blood pressure usually associated with tachycardia was found in 11 out of 20 of these temporal lobe seizures. Though there was no fixed pattern, the general time sequence was usually as follows: a fall of skin resistance and/or swallowing tended to appear as the earliest features. Respiratory changes, usually expiratory apnea, were commonest of all, tachycardia with or without rise in blood pressure usually appeared somewhat later. Coincident with cardiovascular changes or even later came the patient's aura or unconsciousness. To our knowledge chronic or transient hypertension has not been described in cases of lesions of the cerebral hemispheres unless they were of a space-occupying character.

From the above experimental and clinical observations it must be concluded that chronic arterial hypertension is not a symptom of lesions of a cerebral hemisphere. A short-lasting moderate increase of the blood pressure, usually associated with tachycardia, apparently occurs not infrequently as one feature of partial seizures with complex symptomatology of temporal lobe origin. Such a transient hypertension will not be recorded in the large majority of cases. It appears to be more of theoretical than of practical interest to the neurologist.

DISCUSSION

Though there is so far no clear evidence that chronic arterial hypertension can be caused by a brain disease, there appear to be certain clinical neurological disorders associated with transient increased blood pressure. Clinical observations on such disorders have led to intensive neurophysiological and neuropathological investigations which have revealed several neuronal systems involved in the regulation of blood pressure at various levels. In the medulla oblongata at least 3 systems can be distinguished, which appear to have specific functions with regard to the regulation of blood pressure. Disturbance of each of these systems is associated with a different clinical condition.

The Cushing response, i.e., increased blood pressure, bradycardia and slowing and irregularity of the respiration occurring when the intracranial pressure reaches the level of the diastolic or mean arterial blood pressure, was already known when Cushing published the results of his detailed experimental studies in dogs and case histories which seemed to confirm the clinical importance of this triad. However, after some time it was pointed out by several investigators than even with intracranial hemorrhage or cerebral concussion, the intracranial pressure in man hardly ever reaches such high values and that when the CSF pressure was rapidly increased to values approaching to diastolic blood pressure, no significant change of the systemic blood pressure was found. However, clinical experience still showed regularly that the Cushing response occurred in cases of supra- or infratentorial lesions, usually when there was a rapid increase in intracranial pressure. Further research in animals showed that in such cases the important factor was axial displacement of the lower brain stem, occurring with blocking of free CSF communication between supra- and infratentorial space (Thompson and Malina, 1959). Weinstein et al. (1964, 1968) then demonstrated that in this situation the threshold for the Cushing response is markedly decreased. In a search for the structure responsible for this effect, Hoff and Reis (1970) found a pressor- or stretch-sensitive region, situated in a paramedian area below the floor of the fourth ventricle between the obex and the facial colliculus. Finally Reis and Doba (1972) demonstrated the precise location of the stretch-sensitive area in the cat by means of microinjections. This area also appears to be stimulated by interference with the capillary flow. That this region is important for the maintenance of blood pressure is shown by the fact that a bilateral lesion at its caudal end produces a condition of spinal shock.

Immediately caudal to the stretch-sensitive area lies another structure which is highly important for the regulation of blood pressure: the nucleus tractus solitarii (NTS). It appears to be the key-center for the baroreceptor reflexes.

Since Hering (1927) and Heymans et al. (1933) described the carotid sinus reflexes their importance for the regulation of blood pressure has been recognized. These reflexes have also received considerable attention from specialists in internal medicine and neurology, but mainly because increased sensitivity due to atherosclerotic changes in the wall of the carotid bifurcation leads to a sudden fall of blood pressure after physiologically occurring intravascular or extravascular stimulation of the carotid sinus. This not infrequently leads to syncopal attacks.

There are no clear descriptions in the literature of cases of loss of baroreceptor control due to intramedullary disorders in patients. To our knowledge the first well-documented cases of loss of baroreceptor control associated with a labile hypertension in patients with lesions in the medulla oblongata were described by Koster in 1952. This was found in two patients with syringobulbia and in a patient with tabes dorsalis. In one of the patients with syringobulbia autopsy could be carried out after death several years later (Koster and Bethlem, 1961). This revealed, apart from a cyst in the cervical medulla (which could not be the cause of the baroreceptor disturbances) a cavity and glial scarlike formation extending from the distal part of the floor of the fourth ventricle ventro-caudally on both sides.

At that time nothing was yet known about the function of the nucleus tractus solitarii (NTS) for baroreceptor control. Following the initial observation of Fallert and Bucher (1966), investigations by Reis and collaborators and by De Jong clarified the function of this extremely important structure (Reis et al., 1977; De Jong et al., 1977). It is specially interesting that the NTS is richly innervated with noradrenergic terminals and contains cell bodies of noradrenergic neurons. Bilateral microinjections of noradrenaline into the NTS cause a marked dose-related decrease of blood pressure. This is prevented by a preceding injection of the alpha-receptor blocking agent phentolamine (De Jong et al., 1975). Further details, particularly concerning the biochemical aspects of neurogenic hypertension, can be found in reviews by Reis and Doba (1974), Doba and Reis (1973), De Jong et al. (1975) and in the relevant chapters of this volume. Of particular significance are the experiments by Reis and collaborators in chronic cats in which the NTS had been destroyed bilaterally producing a syndrome of labile hypertension without changes of heart rate, a result identical to the symptomatology observed by Koster (1952) in the patients with syringobulbia. Reexamination of the microscopic slides of the first of these patients showed that there was severe bilateral damage to the NTS. It does not seem far fetched to assume that a similar lesion was the cause of the same symptomatology in the second patient with syringobulbia.

At this time it is not possible to explain the mechanism of the loss of baroreceptor control in the patient with tabes dorsalis and gastric crises. Though paroxysmal hypertension, usually associated with gastric crises, has been described repeatedly since the original observation of Pal (1903), loss of baroreceptor control is apparently usually not part of this syndrome. Several authors mention that no orthostatic hypotension was observed, with, as exception, a single case reported by Bennett and Heyman (1948).

Transient hypertension in porphyric crises has been observed in one case (Kezdi, 1954) which was associated with recurrent disturbances of function of the ninth and tenth cranial nerves. In this case it would seem that recurrent disturbance of the baroreceptor afferents had to be implicated. In a case with porphyria and transient hypertension reported by Baker and Watson (1945) destruction of nuclei in the medulla oblongata including the dorsal nucleus of the N. vagus was found, but the NTS was not mentioned.

A third type of transient arterial hypertension which is associated with tachycardia and, in fatal cases, leads to terminal shock, has repeatedly been described in cases of bulbar poliomyelitis. Though it frequently occurred in cases with respiratory disturbances and artificial ventilation the same type of hypertension was seen in other patients who were well ventilated and/or did not need artificial respiration. Neuropathological studies by several investigators led to the consistent finding that in these cases, the magnocellular nucleus in the medial part of the bulbar reticular formation was severely damaged (Lachmund and Löblich, 1950; Baker et al., 1950; Kemp, 1957). Though the exact function of this structure is apparently not known it appears to have mainly a vasodilatator effect on the peripheral circulation. It is of particular interest that at least in the cat this nucleus receives a substantial baroreceptor input.

The possible role of ischemia of the vertebro-basilar system in causing arterial hypertension in man has been particularly defended by Dickinson (1965). It has been meanwhile shown by several investigators that a Cushing type of response can be induced by anoxia or ischemia of the lower brain stem. The threshold for the ischemic response appears to be reached when perfusion pressure falls below the level to maintain adequate capillary flow. It would seem most likely that the sensitive area is the stretch-sensitive paramedian region under the floor of the fourth ventricle. Unilateral ischemic lesions of the NTS appear to be exceptional and case histories of patients with bilateral vascular lesions of the NTS have, to our knowledge, never been described. This must probably be explained by the fact that the NTS in man is extremely well-vascularized and that acute bilateral destruction of the NTS is not compatible with survival. Most authors (Tyler and Dawson, 1961; Marshall, 1966; Sandok and Whisnant, 1974) agree that there is so far no sufficient reason for assuming that vertebro-basilar ischemia can cause longer lasting hypertension and in a recent publication, Dickinson (1976) has apparently come to the same conclusion.

It has been known since the classical experiments of Karplus and Kreidl (1909, 1910) in the beginning of this century that an increase of blood pressure can be produced by electrical stimulation of the hypothalamus. The pressor areas have been more clearly defined in later years by Hess (1969) and by Ranson and Magoun (1939). As was to be expected, these vasopressor structures appear to have a more differentiated function than those in the medulla, as was shown by Folkow and Rubinstein (1965).

Hypertension has also been caused by experimental lesions in the hypothalamus. Contrary to lesions of the NTS they involve, depending on the site of the lesion, either the adrenal cortex or the adrenal medulla. To our knowledge no clear syndromes of arterial hypertension have been described which can be attributed to hypothalamic destructive or irritative lesions in man.

As far as the cerebral hemispheres are concerned, electrical stimulation of various parts of the so-called limbic system has been shown to produce a transient increase of arterial pressure. In our opinion this has been documented most clearly by Van Buren (1958, 1961), who observed short-lasting periods of hypertension sometimes associated with tachycardia, during early stages of spontaneous and induced temporal lobe seizures. A similar effect was obtained on electrical stimulation of the amygdala when this led to a minor seizure. However, hypertension never occurred as an isolated phenomenon but always as part of a more complex symptomatology. The same observation was made by Chapman (1960). Lesions of the cerebral hemispheres are not associated with an increase of the blood pressure unless they are associated with a marked increase of intracranial pressure. Usually this is due to uncal herniation and displacement or distortion of the lower brain stem. However, Weinstein et al. (1964) have also produced a vasopressor response with intracerebral balloon injections of minute quantities of fluid with only moderate elevation of the intracranial pressure and free communication throughout the cranio-spinal axis.

As we have seen there are only few neurological diseases which have been known to produce arterial hypertension, and this only in a small proportion of patients suffering from such diseases. Apart from these diseases there are certain syndromes such as the Cushing response and loss of baroreceptor control, which are also characterized by transient or labile hypertension. This seems to be characteristic of neurogenic hypertension. Whereas humoral factors appear to be mainly responsible for the long-term regulation of blood pressure, nervous mechanisms apparently serve mainly to make rapid and transient adjustments.

SUMMARY

The literature concerning neurological disorders which may be associated with an increased blood pressure has been reviewed.

Three types of neurogenic hypertension have been discussed. In each of these types a particular structure of the medulla oblongata appears to be affected. For the Cushing response a stretch-sensitive area under the floor of the fourth ventricle is essential. This area is probably also sensitive to a reduction of capillary flow. The original Cushing response only occurs when the intracranial pressure reaches the level of the arterial blood pressure. But the same response can be elicited by a transaxial distortion of the lower brain stem and the threshold of the Cushing response is lowered substantially in cases of space-occupying lesions, when there is a pressure gradient between the supratentorial space and the posterior fossa due to obstruction of the CSF flow across the tentorial incisura.

Experimental evidence has demonstrated that loss of baroreceptor control with labile hypertension without a change of the heart rate can be produced in chronic experiments in the cat by bilateral destruction of the nucleus tractus solitarii (NTS). Such bilateral chronic lesions are apparently extremely rare in man. Two previously published case histories of patients with syringomyelia and syringobulbia, who suffered from labile hypertension and loss of baroreceptor control, have been briefly presented. A renewed examination of the microscopic preparations of the medulla oblongata, made after one of these patients had died, showed that the syringobulbar lesion had caused serious bilateral damage to the NTS. The same syndrome was also present in a case of tabes dorsalis with gastric crises. At present we do not have an explanation for this observation.

A third type of hypertension, associated with tachycardia, has been described in patients with bulbar poliomyelitis. Neuropathological studies by several authors all lead to the same conclusion that the cardio-vascular disturbances are due to damage to the magnocellular nucleus in the medial part of the bulbar reticular formation. Together with the NTS this region receives considerable baroreceptor input. It is not yet understood how the activities of these three centers are integrated. There is not sufficient evidence for the assumption that ischemia of the vertebro-basilar system can cause neurogenic hypertension.

Superimposed on the medullary centers are various vaso-active centers of higher levels, notably in the hypothalamus and the limbic system. Lesions in these parts of the brain are not known to cause systemic hypertension in man. But a short-lasting increase of blood pressure has been reported in temporal lobe seizures and after electrical stimulation in the region of the amygdala in man.

No evidence has been found for the assumption that an organic brain disorder can cause chronic arterial hypertension in man.

REFERENCES

Andy, O.J., Bonn, P., Chinn, R.McC. and Allen, M. (1959) Blood pressure alterations and periamygdaloid afterdischarges. *J. Neurophysiol.*, 22: 51—60.

216

Baker, A.B., Matzke, H.A. and Brown, J.R. (1950) Poliomyelitis. III. Bulbar poliomyelitis. A study of medullary function. *Arch. Neurol. Psychiat. (Chic.)*, 63: 257—281.

Baker, A.B. and Watson, C.J. (1945) The central nervous system in porphyria. *J. Neuropath. exp. Neurol.*, 4: 68—77.

Bennett, I.L. and Heyman, A. (1948) Paroxysmal hypertension associated with tabes dorsalis. *Amer. J. Med.*, 5: 729—735.

Browder, J. and Meyers, R. (1936) Observations on behavior of the systemic blood pressure, pulse and spinal fluid pressure, following craniocerebral injury. *Amer. J. Surg.*, 31: 403—426.

Browder, J. and Meyers, R. (1938) Behavior of the systemic blood pressure, pulse rate and spinal fluid pressure associated with acute changes in intracranial pressure artificially produced. *Arch. Surg.*, 36: 1—19.

Cameron, S.J. and Doig, A. (1970) Cerebellar tumours presenting with clinical features of phaeochromocytoma. *Lancet*, 1: 492—494.

Chapman, W.P. (1960) Depth electrode studies in patients with temporal lobe epilepsy. In *Electrical Studies on the Unanesthetized Brain*, E.R. Ramey and D.S. O'Doherty (Eds.), Hoeber, New York, pp. 334—350.

Cushing, H. (1901) Concerning a definite regulatory mechanism of the vasomotor centre which controls bloodpressure during cerebral compression. *Bull. Johns Hopk. Hosp.*, 12: 290—292.

Cushing, H. (1902a) Physiologische und anatomische Beobachtungen über den Einfluss von Hirnkompression auf den intrakraniellen Kreislauf und über einige hiermit verwandten Erscheinungen. *Mitt. Grenzgeb. Med. Chir.*, 9: 773—808.

Cushing, H. (1902b) Some experimental and clinical observations concerning states of increased intracranial tension. The Mütter Lecture for 1901. *Amer. J. med. Sci.*, 124: 375—400.

Cushing, H. (1903) The blood pressure reaction of acute cerebral compression illustrated by cases of intracranial hemorrhage (a sequel to the Mütter lecture for 1901). *Amer. J. med. Sci.*, 125: 1017—1044.

De Jong, W., Zandberg, P. and Bohus, B. (1975) Central inhibitory noradrenergic cardiovascular control. In *Hormones, Homeostasis and the Brain, Progr. in Brain Res. 42*, W.H. Gispen, Tj.B. van Wimersma Greidanus, B.Bohus and D. de Wied (Eds.), Elsevier, Amsterdam, pp. 285—298.

De Jong, W., Zandberg, P., Palkovits, M. and Bohus, B. (1977) Acute and chronic hypertension after lesions and transections of the rat brain stem. In *Hypertension and Brain Mechanisms, Progr. in Brain Res., Vol.47*, W. De Jong, A.P. Provoost and A.P. Shapiro (Eds.), Elsevier, Amsterdam, pp. 189—197.

Dickinson, C.J. (1965) *Neurogenic Hypertension*, Blackwell, Oxford, 274 pp.

Dickinson, C.J. (1976) How far do animal models of neurogenic hypertension resemble the human predicament. In *The Nervous System in Arterial Hypertension*, S. Julius and M.D. Esler (Eds.), Thomas, Springfield, Ill., pp. 99—118.

Doba, N. and Reis, D.J. (1972) Localization within the lower brain stem of a receptive area mediating the pressor response to increased intracranial pressure (The Cushing response). *Brain Res.*, 47: 487—491.

Doba, N. and Reis, D.J. (1973) Acute fulminating neurogenic hypertension produced by brainstem lesions in the rat, *Circulat Res.*, 32: 584—593.

Duret, H. (1878) *Etudes Expérimentales et Cliniques sur les Traumatismes Cérébraux*, V. Adrien Delahaye, Paris.

Evans, J.P., Espey, F.F., Kristoff, F.V., Kimbell, F.D. and Ryder, H.W. (1951) Experimental and clinical observations on rising intracranial pressure. *Arch. Surg.*, 63: 107—114.

Evans, Ch.H., Westfall, V. and Atuk, N.O. (1972) Astrocytoma mimicking the features of pheochromocytoma. *New Engl. J. Med.*, 286: 1397—1399.

Fallert, M. und Bucher, V.M. (1966) Lokalisation eines blutdruckactiven Substrats in der Medulla oblongata des Kaninchens. *Helv. Physiol. Acta*, 24: 139—163.

Fisher, C.M., Karnes, W.E. and Kubik, C.S. (1961) Lateral medullary infarction. The pattern of vascular occlusion. *J. Neuropath. exp. Neurol.*, 20: 323—379.

Folkow, B. and Rubinstein, E.H. (1965) Behavioural and autonomic patterns evoked by stimulation of the lateral hypothalamic area in the cat. *Acta. physiol. scand.*, 65: 292—299.

Folkow, B. and Rubinstein, E.H. (1966) Cardiovascular effects of acute and chronic stimulation of the hypothalamic defense area in the rat. *Acta. physiol. scand.*, 68: 48—57.

Greenfield, G. (1963) Syringomyelia and syringobulbia. In *Greenfield's Neuropathology*, 2nd ed., W. Blackwood, W.H. McMenemey, A. Meijer, R.M. Norman and D.S. Russell (Eds.), Arnold, London, pp. 331—335.

Grimson, K.S. (1950) Role of sympathetic nervous system in hypertension, as revealed by the action of sympatholytic and depressor drugs. In *Factors Regulating Blood Pressure, Transact. Third Conf. (1949)*, Jos. Macy Jr. Found., New York.

Hauw, J.-J., Der Agopian, P., Trelles, L. et Escourolle, R. (1976) Les infarctus bulbaires. Etude systématique de la topographie lésionelle dans 49 cas. *J. neurol. Sci.*, 28: 83—102.

Hering, H.E. (1927) *Die Karotis Sinus Reflexe auf Herz und Gefässe*, Steinkopf, Leipzig.

Hess, W.R. (1969) *Hypothalamus and Thalamus. Experimental Documentation*, Thieme, Stuttgart.

Heymans, C., Bouckaert, I.J. et Regniers, P. (1933) *Le Sinus Carotidien*, Doin, Paris.

Hoff, J.T., Nishimura, M. and Pitts, L. (1975) Effect of raised intracranial pressure in pulmonary function in cats. In *Intracranial Pressure, II*, N. Lundberg, U. Pontén and M. Brock (Eds.), Springer, Berlin, pp. 293—297.

Hoff, J.T. and Reis, D.J. (1970) Localization of regions mediating the Cushing response in CNS of cat. *Arch. Neurol. (Chic.)*, 23: 228—240.

Ionesco-Sisesti, N. (1932) *La Syringobulbie*, Masson, Paris.

Ito, A., Omae, T. and Katsuki, S. (1973) Acute changes in blood pressure following vascular diseases in the brain stem. *Stroke*, 4: 80—84.

Karplus, J.P. und Kreidl, A. (1909) Gehirn und Sympathicus. Zwischenhirnbasis und Halssympathicus. *Pflügers Arch. ges. Physiol.*, 129: 138—144.

Karplus, J.P. und Kreidl, A. (1910) Gehirn und Sympathicus. Ein Sympathicus Zentrum im Zwischenhirn. *Pflügers Arch. ges. Physiol.*, 135; 401—406.

Kemp, E. (1957) Arterial hypertension in poliomyelitis. *Acta med. scand.*, 157: 109—118.

Kezdi, P. (1954) Neurogenic hypertension in man in porphyria. Transient hypertension and tachycardia caused by disruption of the carotid sinus; review of buffer nerve mechanism. *Arch. intern. Med.*, 94: 122—130.

Kocher, T. (1901) Hirnerschütterung, Hirndruck und chirurgische Eingriffe bei Hirnerkrankungen. In *Nothnagels specielle Pathologie und Therapie*, Holder, Wien, pp. 81—290; 325—367.

Koster, M. (1952) *Bloeddrukschommelingen bij aandoeningen van het ruggemerg (poikilopiësis spinalis)*. Thesis Univ. of Amsterdam.

Koster, M. and Bethlem, J. (1961) Paroxysmal hypertension and hypotension in patients with spinal cord lesions (Poikilopiësis spinalis). *Acta psychiat. neurol. scand.*, 36: 347—368.

Lachmund, H. (1950) Hochdruck bei Poliomyelitis. *Dtsch. med. Wschr.*, 75: 450—452.

Löblich, H.J. (1950) Lage und Funktion des blutdruckregulierenden Zentrums in der Medulla oblongata (nach Befunden bei Poliomyelitis). *Virchows Arch. path. Anat.*, 318: 211—233.

Marshall, J. (1966) Evidence upon the neurogenic theory of hypertension. *Lancet*, 410—412.

McDowell, F.H. and Plum, F. (1951) Arterial hypertension associated with acute anterior poliomyelitis. *New Engl. J. Med.*, 245: 241—245.

McGillicuddy, J.E., Kindt, G.W., Miller, C.A. and Raisis, J.E. (1975) The interrelations between intracranial pressure, cerebral ischemia, cerebral hypoxia and cerebral hypercapnia on the Cushing response. In *Intracranial Pressure, II*, N. Lundberg, K. Pontén and M. Brock (Eds.), Springer, Berlin, pp. 303—306.

Meyer, B.C. (1941) Neoplasm of the posterior fossa simulating cerebral vascular disease. Report of five cases with reference to the role of the medulla in the production of arterial hypertension. *Arch. Neurol. Psychiat. (Chic.)*, 45: 468—480.

Miura, M. and Reis, D.J. (1969) Terminations and secondary projections of carotid sinus nerve in the cat brain stem. *Amer. J. Physiol.*, 217: 142—153.

Montgomery, B.M. (1961) The basilar artery hypertensive syndrome. *Arch. intern. Med.*, 108: 115—125.

Nathan, M.A. and Reis, D.J. (1975) Fulminating arterial hypertension with pulmonary edema from release of adrenomedullary catecholamines after lesions of the anterior hypothalamus in the rat. *Circulat. Res.*, 37: 226—235.

Naunyn, B. and Schreiber, J. (1881) Ueber den Hirndruck. *Arch. exp. Path. Pharmak.*, 14: 1—112.

Nosuka, S. (1966) Hypertension induced by extensive medial anteromedian hypothalamic destruction in the rat. *Jap. Circulat. J.*, 30: 509—523.

Okamoto, K., Nosuka, S. and Yamori, Y. (1964) Experimental hypertension and hypotension induced by hypothalamic destruction in the rat, *Jap. Circulat. J.*, 29: 251—261.

Pal, J. (1903) Ueber Gefässkrisen und deren Beziehungen zu den Magen und Bauchkrisen der Tabetiker. *Münch. med. Wschr.*, 50: 2135.

Pal, J. (1905) *Gefässkrisen*, Hirzel.

Penfield, W. (1929) Diencephalic autonomic epilepsy. *Arch. Neurol. Psychiat. (Chic.)*, 22: 358—374.

Ranson, S.W. and Magoun, H.W. (1939) Hypothalamus. *Ergebn. Physiol.*, 41: 56—163.

Reis, D.J. and Doba, N. (1974) The central nervous system and neurogenic hypertension. *Progr. Cardiovasc. Dis.*, 17: 51—71

Reis, D.J., Doba, N., Snyder, D.W. and Nathan, M.A. (1977) Brain lesions and hypertension: Chronic lability and elevation of arterial pressure produced by electrolytic lesions and 6-hydroxydopamine treatment of nucleus tractus solitarii (NTS) in rat and cat. In *Hypertension and Brain Mechanisms, Progr. in Brain Res., Vol. 47*, W. De Jong, A.P. Provoost and A.P. Shapiro (Eds.), Elsevier, Amsterdam, pp. 169—188.

Rowan, J.O. and Johnston, I.H. (1975) Blood pressure response to raised CSF pressure. In *Intracranial Pressure, II*, N. Lundberg, U. Pontén and M. Brock (Eds.), Springer, Berlin, pp. 298—302.

Sandok, B.A. and Whisnant J.P. (1974) Hypertension and the Brain. *Arch. intern Med.*, 133: 947—954.

Spencer, W. and Horsley, V. (1892) On the changes produced in circulation and respiration by increase of the intra-cranial pressure or tension. *Phil. Trans. B*, 182: 201—254.

Thompson, R.K. and Malina, S. (1959) Dynamic axial brain stem distortion as a mechanism explaining the cardio-respiratory change in increased intracranial pressure. *J. Neurosurg.*, 16: 664—675.

Tyler, H.R. and Dawson, D. (1961) Hypertension and its relation to the nervous system. *Ann. intern. Med.*, 55: 681—694.

Van Buren, J.M. (1958) Some autonomic concomitants of ictal automatism. A study of temporal lobe attacks. *Brain*, 81: 505—528.

Van Buren, J.M. (1961) Sensory, motor and autonomic effects of mesial temporal stimulation in man. *J. Neurosurg.*, 18: 273—288.

Weinstein, J.D., Langfitt, T.W. and Kassell, N.F. (1964) Vasopressor response to increased intracranial pressure. *Neurology (Minneap.)*, 1118—1131

Weinstein, J.D., Langfitt, T.W., Bruno, L., Laren, H.A. and Jackson, J.L.F. (1968) Experimental study of patterns of brain distortion and ischemia produced by an intercranial mass. *J. Neurosurg.*, 28: 513—521.

Weinstein, L. (1957) Cardiovascular disturbances in poliomyelitis. *Circulation*, 15: 735—756.

Yamori, Y. (1967) Hypothalamic hyper- and hypotension induced by the destruction of the tubero-mamillary regions in the rat. *Jap. Circulat. J.*, 31: 743—780.

Pathogenic Mechanisms and Prevention of Stroke in Stroke-prone Spontaneously Hypertensive Rats

Y. YAMORI, R. HORIE, I. AKIGUCHI, Y. NARA, M. OHTAKA and
M. FUKASE

*Japan Stroke Prevention Center, Izumo, Departments of Pathology, Neurosurgery and
Internal Medicine, Kyoto University, Kyoto and The Center for Adult Diseases, Osaka
(Japan)*

INTRODUCTION

One of the great causes of death in acculturated people is stroke, i.e.,
cerebral hemorrhage and infarction. However, extensive experimental studies
on the pathogenesis of stroke have not been available, because there have been
no adequate models for stroke in man. But since a stroke-prone substrain of
the spontaneously hypertensive rat (SHRSP) was established in 1974 (Okamoto
et al., 1974; Yamori et al., 1974a), it has become possible to study the
pathogenesis. Thus various systemic and local factors of stroke have been
analyzed experimentally, so that the pathogenic mechanisms, having been
only speculated in man, are being rapidly clarified in this model (Yamori
et al., 1975b, 1976c).

DEVELOPMENT OF THE STROKE-PRONE SHR

Spontaneously hypertensive rats (SHR), selectively bred and established as
an inbred strain at our laboratory (Okamoto and Aoki, 1963), are now in the
F_{40} generation and used all over the world as good animal models for essential
human hypertension (Yamori and Okamoto, 1974). However, the incidence of
cerebrovascular lesions, so called stroke, was relatively low averaging about 10%
before the F_{20} generation. Therefore, attempts were made to increase the
incidence of stroke by changing environmental factors or by selecting genetic
disposition. Chronic loading of stress or high salt diet aggravated hypertensive
complications (Yamori et al., 1969). However, the effect of high salt intake, for
example, was clearly different within the SHR substrains; in the A substrain the
incidence of stroke was significantly higher and the life span was clearly shorter
than in the B substrain (Okamoto et al., 1973). These results indicate that not
only environmental factors but also the genetic disposition is greatly
responsible for the development of stroke.

Therefore, selective breeding was attempted to obtain SHR which would
spontaneously develop a high incidence of stroke; young candidates were
selected from some families with a high incidence of stroke, and mated with
each other to obtain the offspring in advance. Only the offspring of SHR, one

220

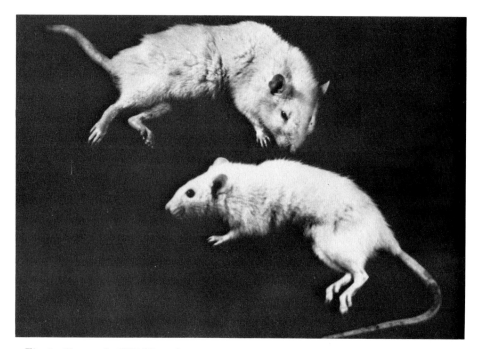

Fig. 1. Two male SHRSP at the age of 8 months, showing paresis in the hindlimbs.

or both parents having died of stroke, were maintained. Thus we selectively obtained offspring from parents who had stroke for the past 14 generations. The incidence of stroke in adult males in these selectively bred offspring was greatly increased, from an averaged 39% up to nearly 90% at present. When the selection seemed to be nearly completed, these selectively bred SHR were called "stroke-prone SHR" (SHRSP) (Okamoto et al., 1974; Yamori et al., 1974a). However, the offspring of SHR with a low incidence of stroke averaging about 7% have also been maintained. These SHR were named "stroke-resistant SHR" (SHRSR).

SHRSP show various symptoms such as irritability, paralysis (Fig. 1), general weakness, urinary incontinence and an attack of stroke; they die at the average ages of 8 and 13 months, in males and females, respectively. Autopsy of SHRSP shows cerebrovascular lesions such as massive or small hemorrhage with or without subarachnoid effusion as well as cerebral softening with or without cystic formation (Fig. 2).

PATHOGENIC FACTORS OF STROKE

The establishment of SHRSP by selective breeding itself indicates the importance of heredity in the development of stroke. After stroke was observed in the parents for 3 successive generations, the incidence of stroke was clearly increased in the offspring and their life span was shortened. The

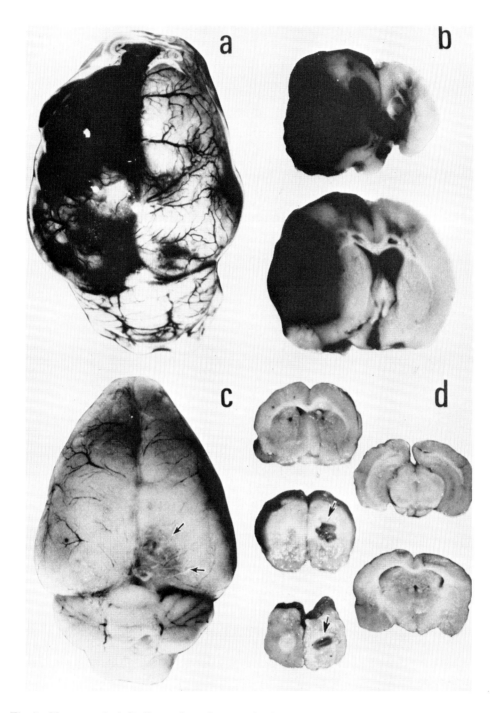

Fig. 2. Macroscopical findings of cerebrovascular lesions in SHRSP. a: massive hemorrhage with subarachnoid effusion in the left cortex. b: massive hemorrhage in the left basal ganglia observed in the coronal sections. c: infarction in the right occipital cortex (indicated with arrows). d: cystic softening in the right basal ganglia.

222

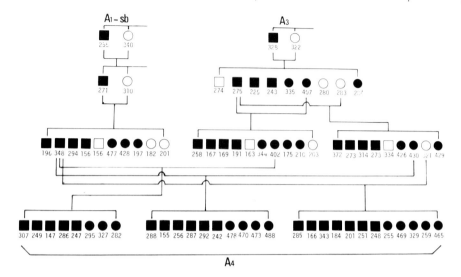

Fig. 3. Incidence of stroke in the offspring (A_4) obtained from cross between A_{1-sb} and A_3 substrains. ■, males with stroke; □, males without stroke; ●, female with stroke; ○, females without stroke. Numbers indicate life span.

incidence of stroke was high in the offspring of parents, where both had had cerebral lesions confirmed at autopsy. By crossing the A_3 and A_{1-sb} substrains, where both had an approximate 80% incidence of stroke, we obtained the substrain A_4. In this strain the incidence of stroke became nearly 100% (Fig. 3). These findings validated the important role of heredity in stroke. On the other hand, stress, salt-loading or low-protein diet increased the incidence of stroke, while high-fat cholesterol diet or high-protein diet clearly decreased the incidence. These findings indicate the importance of gene—environment interaction in stroke (Yamori, 1976).

We have further analyzed systemic and local factors which are involved in the development of stroke. As for the *systemic factors* of stroke, the importance of hypertension was statistically analyzed in 8 substrains of SHR. Highly significant correlations were noted between the incidence of stroke and the severity, age, or speed of the development of hypertension; rapidly developing severe hypertension at a young age was closely related to a high incidence of stroke (Okamoto et al., 1974; Yamori et al., 1974b).

Secondly, the systemic factors involved in the disposition of stroke seem to be related to the alteration of the physical characteristics of the vascular wall. The aortas of stroke-prone SHR, stroke-resistant SHR, and normotensive Wistar—Kyoto rats were first comparatively studied morphologically. In the aortas of SHR, the number of elastic lamellae was increased and the interlamellar spaces were widened with hyperplasia and hypertrophy of smooth muscle cells. However, neither a clear morphological nor histometrical difference was noted between stroke-prone and -resistant SHR (Yamori and Sasagawa, 1975). On the other hand, the stress-elongation curve of the aorta of

TABLE I

LOCALIZATION OF CEREBROVASCULAR LESIONS IN STROKE-PRONE SHR — ANALYSIS OF 1740 LESIONS

	Anteromedial cortex	Lateral cortex	Occipital cortex	Basal ganglia	Thalamus	Total (%)**
Softening (%)*	437 (33.6%)	78 (6.0%)	419 (32.3%)	296 (22.8%)	69 (5.3%)	1299 (74.7%)
Bleeding (%)**	51 (39.5%)	7 (5.4%)	20 (15.5%)	41 (31.8%)	10 (7.8%)	129 (7.4%)
Hemorrhagic infarction (%)	98 (31.4%)	19 (6.1%)	84 (26.9%)	90 (28.8%)	21 (6.7%)	312 (17.9%)
Total (%)	586 (33.7%)	104 (6.0%)	523 (30.1%)	427 (24.5%)	100 (5.7%)	1740 lesions (1278 cases)

*% in the localizations of softening, bleeding, hemorrhagic infarction and sum of them, respectively.
** % of softening, bleeding and hemorrhagic infarction in total cases.

stroke-prone SHR was clearly different from that of stroke-resistant SHR or of the normotensive Wistar—Kyoto strain. The maximum stress required to cause ductile failure of the aorta was clearly less in stroke-prone SHR. Moreover, this difference in the elasticity was already noted in the aorta of stroke-prone SHR even 3 months after birth. The difference between stroke-prone and -resistant SHR was greatest at the age of 10 months (Yamori and Sasagawa, 1975).

Thirdly, other systemic factors of stroke might be related to some humoral factors or blood platelets (Okuma and Yamori, 1976). As for the renin—angiotensin system, plasma renin concentration was determined by sampling the minimum amount of blood through an aortic canule implanted in unanesthetized rats. Plasma renin was usually not increased in stroke-resistant SHR as compared with Wistar—Kyoto. However, it tended to increase in stroke-prone SHR at 5 months of age and it significantly increased at over 6 months of age when vascular lesions such as arterionecrosis, hemorrhage of softening were noted (Matsunaga et al., 1975). Therefore, plasma renin appears to be one of the indices which indicate the degree of vascular damage.

In order to analyze the *local factors* of stroke, we studied the predilection sites of stroke in 1200 SHR (Yamori et al., 1976e). The incidence of stroke was highest in the anteromedial and occipital cortex (about 34% and 30%, respectively), and about 25% of the total lesions were noted in the basal ganglia (Table I). However, in humans, more than 60% of all cerebral lesions are noted in the basal ganglia, thus the distribution of lesions is somewhat different from that in stroke-prone SHR. We also studied angiographically the localization of pre-stroke lesions in stroke-prone SHR. We confirmed that these predilection sites corresponded to the boundary zone between the two areas receiving blood supply from different cerebral arteries, that is, the middle cerebral artery and anterior or posterior cerebral artery (Yamori et al., 1976e).

Our detailed comparative studies on the angioarchitecture of rat and human brains revealed that the anteromedial or occipital cortex of the rat — the predilection sites of stroke, were fed by recurrent arteries branching from the anterior or posterior cerebral artery. Such recurrent arteries were not observed in human telencephalon, probably because of the difference in phylogenetic development of the human telencephalon. On the other hand, such recurrent branchings are commonly noted in the basal ganglia of both rats and humans. These findings indicate that the common feature in the predilection sites of stroke of both man and rat is the presence of recurrent arteries (Yamori et al., 1976e).

MECHANISMS OF STROKE

The mechanisms involved when these systemic and local factors cooperatively induce cerebrovascular lesions were further examined by various approaches. First, blood supply through such recurrent arteries is thought to be less in amount and poor in erythrocyte content, especially under conditions of severe hypertension. This idea was confirmed rheologically by observing flow dynamics in tubes with current and recurrent branches. That is, low oxygen supply to the area fed by recurrent arteries may cause damage in the vascular wall.

In addition to these angioarchitecturally determined local factors, functional vasoconstriction of arterioles may also be another important factor for inducing local hemodynamic impairment. Ophthalmoscopic observation revealed that arterioles of the ocular fundi showed marked irregular narrowing, even in young (3-month-old) SHRSP with severe hypertension (Fig. 4). Such vasoconstriction is thought to occur in intracerebral arterioles or arteries (Yamori et al., 1976j).

Our recent studies using the hydrogen clearance method confirmed that regional cerebral blood flow decreased especially in the area fed by recurrent arteries in severe hypertensive states over 200 mm Hg (Fig. 5) (Yamori et al., 1976a,f). These findings support the view that recurrent branching is the important local factor for stroke, and that the impairment of regional cerebral blood flow (rCBF) in severe hypertensive states precedes the development of vascular damage. As stroke in rats and humans is caused by similar mechanisms at the predilection sites fed by recurrent branches, it can be concluded that stroke-prone SHR is a good pathogenetic model for stroke in man (Yamori et al., 1976e).

Fluorescence microscopic observation was done on the brain specimen prepared by Falck–Hillarp's technique (1962), and especially by Kimura and Tohyama's modification of glyoxylic acid–formaldehyde fixation (Kimura et

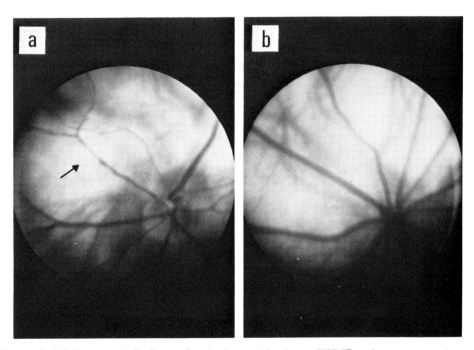

Fig. 4. Ophthalmoscopic findings of retinal arterioles in an SHRSP and a normotensive rat of Wistar–Kyoto (WK). a: optic fundus of a 9-month-old male SHRSP after an attack of stroke (blood pressure, 260 mm Hg). Arrow points to irregular narrowing. b: optic fundus of a 9-month-old male WK (blood pressure, 142 mm Hg).

226

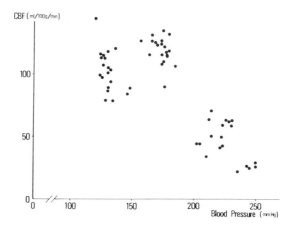

Fig. 5. Relationship between blood pressure and cerebral blood flow in the frontal region of normotensive and spontaneously hypertensive rats.

al., 1976). It was shown that intracerebral arteries such as those in the cortex also had noradrenergic terminals with augmented fluorescence in SHR. At the sites of infarction or hemorrhage noradrenergic fluorescence was reduced in the center and was sometimes augmented within a few thicker fibers at the periphery of these lesions (Fig. 6). Noradrenaline appears to be released from nerve terminals around the lesioned areas. It may be possible that this noradrenaline accelerates the vasoconstriction of arteries and further decreases the blood supply to these areas. Thus, noradrenaline might be involved in the vicious circle of inducing vascular lesions.

In the areas fed by recurrent arteries, such as the cortex and basal ganglia, vascular permeability was increased at the advanced stage of hypertension, as

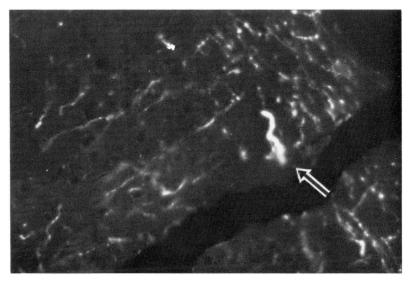

Fig. 6. Fluorescent microscopical findings in the brain of SHRSP, showing an abnormal noradrenergic fiber (arrow) with intensified fluorescence near a lesioned area in the cortex.

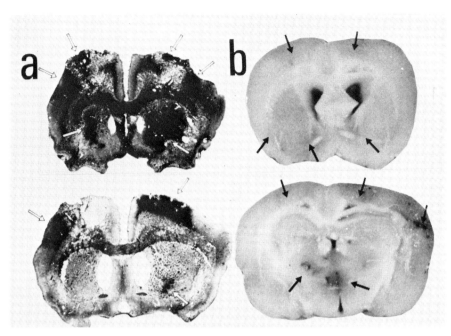

Fig. 7. Increased vascular permeability in SHRSP in the advanced stage of hypertension. a: leakage of peroxidase, mainly observed in the area fed by recurrent arteries. b: leakage of trypan blue, noted not only around minute bleeding but also at the area fed by recurrent arteries.

detected by the leakage of trypan blue or peroxidase injected intravenously (Fig. 7) (Yamori et al., 1975b). Extensive increase in permeability induces arterionecrosis, which was later histologically observed in SHRSP with severe hypertension (Fig. 8a). Arterial walls with arterionecrosis became thin and dilated, forming microaneurysms. Hemorrhage was observed around the ruptured microaneurysms. On the other hand, infarction or softening was observed around the arteries or microaneurysms occluded with thrombi (Fig. 8b). Arterionecrosis and microaneurysms were the basic arterial lesions inducing thrombogenesis.

In summary, the mechanisms of stroke are speculated from these findings as follows (Fig. 9): hypertension is the most important systemic factor for stroke, and physicochemical alteration of vascular walls or some humoral factors may also be involved in the pathogenesis of stroke, whether primarily or secondarily. As for the local factors, recurrent branching and boundary zone of arterial supply, these seem to be the angioarchitectural basis for the insufficiency of rCBF, which is intensified under severe hypertension states rheologically with vasoconstriction. The long-standing impairment of rCBF causes vascular damage due to hypoxia or through further intensified vasoconstriction induced by released noradrenaline around the lesioned areas; it finally increases vascular permeability or induces arterionecrosis. Arterionecrosis is the common basic vascular lesion both for hemorrhage and softening. Therefore, stroke in these rats can be called "arterio-necro-thrombogenic stroke".

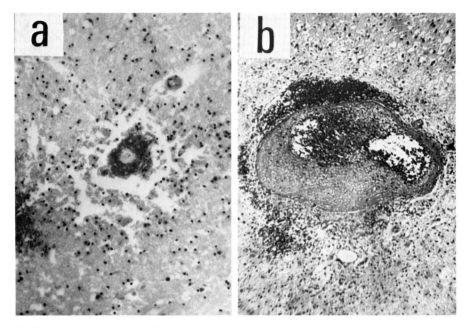

Fig. 8. Basic vascular lesions for hemorrhage and infarction. a: arterionecrosis, common basic lesions for microaneurysms, hemorrhage and thrombus formation. b: microaneurysm with thrombus formation.

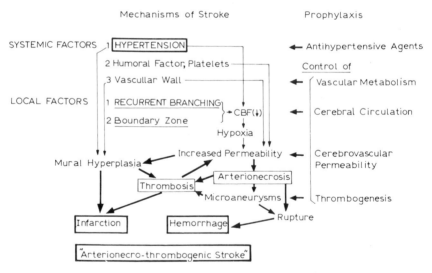

Fig. 9. Proposed pathogenic mechanisms of stroke and prophylaxis.

RELATION TO ATHEROSCLEROSIS

SHRSP was confirmed to be a good model for stroke, especially arterionecro-thrombogenic stroke. Our recent studies have revealed that SHR is also a good model for atherogenesis, although rats are not generally regarded as a suitable model for experimental atherogenesis. SHR fed on a high-fat cholesterol (HFC) diet containing 20% suet, 5% cholesterol and 2% cholic acid quickly develop hypercholesterolemia within a week, and concomitantly ring-like fat deposits in mesenteric and cerebral arteries within a few weeks (Fig. 10) (Yamori, 1974, 1977; Yamori et al., 1975a, 1976b). These responses

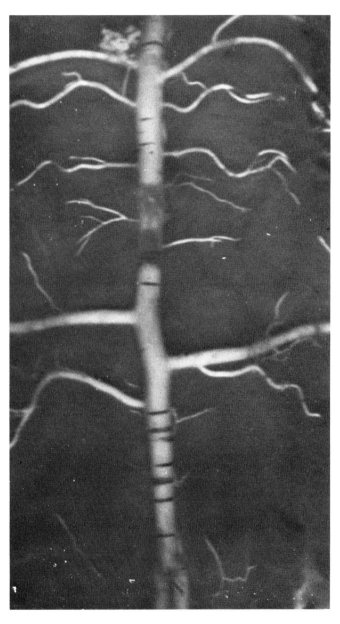

Fig. 10. Ring-like fat deposits at the basilar artery in an SHR fed on a high-fat cholesterol diet for 3 weeks.

230

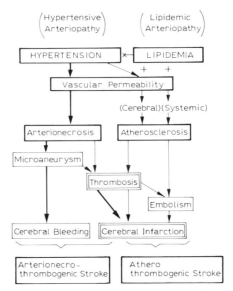

Fig. 11. Proposed pathogenic relation between stroke and cerebral atherogenesis.

were especially marked in SHR which had been selected for greater reactive hypercholesterolemia for the past 6 generations, and these SHR were named "arteriolipidosis-prone SHR" (Yamori, 1977). Among various models, fat deposits in cerebrobasal arteries were only observed in SHR and experimental hypertensive rats. Such deposits were greatly delayed in anti-hypertensive agents-treated SHR, and never noted in normotensive rats (Yamori et al., 1976d). Therefore, hypertension was confirmed to be very important for arterial fat deposition, especially in the cerebral arteries. However, the incidence of stroke was clearly decreased in these SHR in spite of hypercholesterolemia (Yamori et al., 1976h). This marked reduction of the incidence is thought to be due to the attenuation of severe hypertension in SHR or renal hypertensive rats fed on an HFC diet.

To summarize the relationship between stroke and atherogenesis, hypertension is the common important factor for stroke and atherogenesis (Fig. 11). While hypertension is a direct cause of arterionecro-thrombogenic stroke, it accelerates atherogenesis in cerebral arteries when accompanied with lipidemia. Lipidemia causes atherogenesis, but it also attenuates the development of severe hypertension and decreases the incidence of arterio-necro-thrombogenic stroke (Yamori et al., 1976b). Although the incidence of stroke was apparently reduced by a HFC diet in so far as observed during the life span of rats, long-standing lipidemia is thought to finally increase athero-thrombogenic stroke.

PROPHYLACTIC APPROACH TO THE PATHOGENESIS OF STROKE

Since the pathogenesis of stroke was partly clarified, various procedures against these pathogenic mechanisms were theoretically used as the prophylaxis of stroke. The control of severe hypertension from a critical level of about 200 mm Hg was confirmed statistically to be the most reliable prophylaxis of stroke (Yamori and Horie, 1975). The litter of stroke-prone SHR with the same genetic disposition was divided into treated and non-treated groups so that the blood pressure of the treated group was kept under 200 to 210 mm Hg, at a similar level to that in stroke-resistant SHR. The prophylactic control of blood pressure was so effective that no stroke was observed in the treated group, but 80% of the non-treated group developed stroke. Although the life-long prophylactic control of hypertension was very effective for preventing stroke, temporary treatment of hypertension at the initial stage or at the advanced stage of hypertension was not effective, as shown by the high incidence of stroke and reduced life span ($P < 0.05$) in these groups (Fig. 12). These experiments offered the first experimental evidence indicating that prophylactic control of blood pressure is important in the prevention of stroke.

On the other hand, there are epidemiological data showing differences in the incidence of stroke between males and females or between Japan and western countries. These data offer useful information about the prophylaxis of stroke. If the prophylaxis of stroke is experimentally possible according to these epidemiological data, we also have some insight as to the undetermined pathogenesis of stroke.

Preponderant occurrence of stroke in males, especially at a young age, was observed in both man and SHRSP. Experimentally, in SHRSP, estrogen treatment decreased the incidence and androgen treatment increased the incidence of stroke (Yamori, 1975; Yamori et al., 1976i). The prophylactic effect of estrogen was proven to be related to the attenuation of severe hypertension, probably because of the reduction of vascular collagenous protein synthesis (Yamori et al., 1976i).

Another epidemiological study shows a clear difference in the incidence of stroke among various countries; the incidence is very high in Japan in comparison with European countries and U.S.A. As such an environmental factor as nutrition may be related to this marked difference in the incidence of stroke. We have been observing the effect of various nutritional conditions on

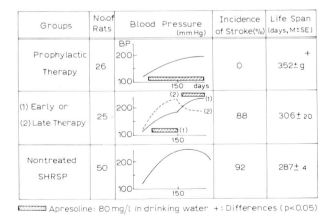

Fig. 12. Importance of prophylactic control of hypertension for the prevention of stroke.

232

the incidence of stroke in stroke-prone SHR. As mentioned previously, a hypercholesterolemic diet dramatically decreased the incidence of stroke, and such a marked decrease in the incidence seems to be related to the attenuation of severe hypertension in stroke-prone SHR fed on a hypercholesterolemic diet (Yamori et al., 1976g,h). The worst nutritional condition was a low protein diet plus salt water, which clearly increased the incidence of stroke within a short period. On the other hand, a high protein diet was confirmed to be very effective, as no stroke was observed in stroke-prone SHR fed on a diet containing 50% protein (Yamori et al., 1976c). We further observed that a high protein diet of different sources had a different effect on hypertension; fish protein decreased the blood pressure but soybean protein did not affect the development of severe hypertension. Although SHRSP fed on a high soybean protein diet did develop severe hypertension like those fed on a normal diet, stroke was not observed in them. These data indicate that some factors other than the blood pressure-lowering effect may be important for this prophylactic mechanism, and they suggest the possible involvement of the vascular wall factor in the pathogenic mechanisms of stroke (Yamori et al., 1976b).

In conclusion, an animal model for stroke research is now available, so that, it has become possible for us to study the pathogenic mechanisms of stroke. As far as extensively studied up to the present, the mechanisms seem to be very similar to those in humans. Some of our experimental attempts to prevent stroke in this model were successful enough both to indicate that stroke is preventable, and also to offer a new insight into the pathogenesis of stroke.

SUMMARY

The establishment of stroke-prone spontaneously hypertensive rats (SHRSP), of which more than 80% died of stroke, has enabled us to extensively study the mechanisms of cerebrovascular lesions. Our studies have revealed that hypertension is the most important systemic factor for stroke. Other possible factors are the alteration of the physical characteristics of the arterial wall, and involvement of humoral factors such as renin. Further, our angioarchitectural studies have clarified that the predilection sites of stroke are the boundary zone of the 3 main cerebral arterial supplies and also the areas fed by recurrent arteries. Therefore, using implanted electrodes at these sites, we measured the regional cerebral blood flow (rCBF) by the hydrogen clearance method without anesthesia. We then assayed norepinephrine in the brain quantitatively or by fluorescent histochemical methods.

rCBF tended to increase under hypertensive state below 200 mm Hg, but it decreased abruptly in SHRSP with severe hypertension over 220 mm Hg. Such a reduction lasted for several months before SHRSP died of stroke. Antihypertensive agents improved this decrease and prevented the development of stroke. Norepinephrine was markedly depleted at the site of cerebrovascular lesions.

The impairment of rCBF, which is induced at angioarchitectural "minor loci" probably by rheological mechanisms plus vasoconstriction in severe hypertensive states, is thought to be the basis for increasing vascular permeability as well as for releasing norepinephrine to decrease further rCBF. Increased vascular permeability results in arterionecro-thrombogenic stroke. On the other hand, various prodecures against these mechanisms have been proven to be effective for preventing stroke.

ACKNOWLEDGEMENTS

This study was supported by grants from the Science and Technology Agency of the Government of Japan, the Japan Ministry of Education NHLBI of NIH, U.S.A. (HL 1775), and Japan Tobacco and Salt Public Corporation.

REFERENCES

Falck, B., Hillarp, N.A., Thieme, G. and Torp, A. (1962) Fluorescence of catecholamines and related compounds condensed with formaldehyde. *J. Histochem. Cytochem.*, 10: 348—354.

Kimura, H., Tohyama, M., Maeda, T. and Shimizu, M. (1976) A stable modified histofluorescence method using glyoxylic acid (GA). *Acta Histochem. Cytochem.*, 9: 98.

Matsunaga, M., Yamamoto, J., Hara, A., Ogino, K., Yamori, Y. and Okamoto, K. (1975) Plasma renin and hypertensive vascular complications: an observation in the stroke-prone spontaneously hypertensive rats. *Jap. Circulat. J.*, 39: 1305—1311.

Okamoto, K. and Aoki, K. (1963) Development of a strain of spontaneously hypertensive rats. *Jap. Circulat. J.*, 27: 282—293.

Okamoto, K., Yamori, Y., Nosaka, S., Ooshima, A. and Hazama, H. (1973) Studies on hypertension in spontaneously hypertensive rats. *Clin. Sci. molec. Med.*, 45: 11S—14S.

Okamoto, K., Yamori, Y. and Nagaoka, A. (1974) Establishment of the stroke-prone spontaneously hypertensive rats (SHR). *Circulat. Res.*, 34, 35, Suppl. 1: 143—153.

Okuma, M. and Yamori, Y. (1976) Platelet survival studies in the stroke-prone spontaneously hypertensive rats (SHRSP). *Stroke*, 6: 60—64.

Yamori, Y. (1974) Metabolic pathology of vasculartures in hypertension and vascular lesions in spontaneously hypertensive rats. *Trans. Soc. Pathol. Jap.*, 63: 226—227.

Yamori, Y. (1975) Neural and vascular systems in hypertension. *Proc. 19 Gen. Assembly of Jap. Med. Soc.*: 866—868.

Yamori, Y. (1977) Hypertensive strains of rat. In *Gene-Environment Interaction in Common Diseases*, E. Inoue and M. Higure (Eds.), Tokyo Univ. Press, Tokyo, in press.

Yamori, Y. and Horie, R. (1975) Experimental studies on the pathogenesis and prophylaxis of stroke in stroke-prone spontaneously hypertensive rats (SHR). (2) Prophylactic effect of moderate control of blood pressure on stroke. *Jap. Circulat. J.*, 39: 607—611.

Yamori, Y. and Okamoto, K. (1974) Spontaneous hypertension in the rats; a model of human "essential" hypertension. *Proc. 80th Congr. Germ. Soc. intern. Med.*: 168—170.

Yamori, Y. and Sasagawa, S. (1975) Physico-morphological characteristics of aorta in stroke-prone and -resistant spontaneously hypertensive rats. *Jap. Heart J.*, 16: 293—353.

Yamori, Y., Matsumoto, M., Yamabe, H. and Okamoto, K. (1969) Augmentation of spontaneous hypertension by chronic stress in rats. *Jap. Circulat. J.*, 33: 399—409.

Yamori, Y., Nagaoka, A. and Okamoto, K. (1974a) Importance of genetic factors in hypertensive cerebrovascular lesions; an evidence obtained by successive selective breeding of stroke-prone and -resistant SHR. *Jap. Circulat. J.*, 38: 1095.

Yamori, Y., Tomimoto, K., Ooshima, A., Hazama F. and Okamoto, K. (1974b) Developmental course of hypertension in the SHR-substrains susceptible to hypertensive cerebrovascular lesions. *Jap. Heart J.*, 15: 209—210.

234

Yamori, Y., Hamashima, Y., Horie, R., Handa, H. and Sato, M. (1975a) Pathogenesis of acute arterial fat deposition in spontaneously hypertensive rats. *Jap. Circulat. J.*, 39: 601—609.

Yamori, Y., Horie, R., Sato, M., Sasagawa, S. and Okamoto, K. (1975b) Experimental studies on the pathogenesis and prophylaxis of stroke in stroke-prone spontaneously hypertensive rats (SHR). (1) Quantitative estimation of cerebrovascular permeability. *Jap. Circulat. J.*, 39: 611—615.

Yamori, Y., Horie, R., Hand, H., Nara, Y., Ohtaka, M. and Fukase, M. (1976a) Cerebral circulation and electroencephalographical approach to stroke in stroke-prone SHR. In *Spontaneous Hypertension*, DHEW Publ. No. (NIH) 77-1179, NIH, Bethesda, Md., pp. 208—215.

Yamori, Y., Horie, R., Ohtaka, M., Nara, Y., Ohta, K., Okamoto, K., Handa, H. and Fukase, M. (1976b) Pathogenic approach to the prophylaxis of stroke and atherogenesis in SHR. In *Spontaneous Hypertension*, DHEW Publ. No. (NIH) 77-1179, NIH, Bethesda, Md., pp. 198—207.

Yamori, Y., Horie, R., Sato, M., Akiguchi, I., Ohtaka, M., Nara, Y. and Fukase, M. (1976c) New models of SHR for studies on stroke and atherogenesis. *Clin. exp. Physiol. Pharmacol.*, in press (also reported at 21. Fall Meeting of Jap. Pathol. Soc., 1975).

Yamori, Y., Horie, R. and Sato, M. (1976d) Hypertension as an important factor for cerebrovascular atherogenesis in rats. *Stroke*, 7: 120—125.

Yamori, Y., Horie, R., Sato, M. and Handa, H. (1976e) Pathogenetic similarity of stroke in stroke-prone SHR and humans. *Stroke*, 7: 46—53.

Yamori, Y., Horie, R., Sato, M. and Handa, H. (1976f) Regional cerebral blood flow in stroke-prone SHR; a preliminary report. *Jap. Heart J.*, 17: 384—386.

Yamori, Y., Horie, R., Sato, M., Ohtaka, M., Nara, Y. and Fukase, M. (1976g) Effect of hypercholesterolemic diet on the incidence of cerebrovascular and myocardial lesions in spontaneously hypertensive rats. *Clin. Sci. molec. Med.*, in press.

Yamori, Y., Sato, M. and Horie, R. (1976h) Blood pressure and vascular lesions in SHR fed on a high-fat-cholesterol diet. *Jap. Heart J.*, 17: 396—398.

Yamori, Y., Sato, M., Horie, R. and Ohta, K. (1976i) Prophylactic trials for stroke in stroke-prone SHR; effect of sex hormones. *Jap. Heart J.*, 17: 410—412.

Yamori, Y., Yoshida, M., Yoshida, H. and Horie, R. (1976j) Photographic findings on ocular fundus of the stroke-prone spontaneously hypertensive rat. In *Spontaneous Hypertension*, DHEW Publ. No. (NIH) 77-1179, NIH, Bethesda, Md.,

On the Pathogenesis of Hypertensive Encephalopathy as Revealed by Cerebral Blood Flow Studies in Man

ERIK SKINHØJ

Department of Neurology, Rigshospitalet, Copenhagen (Denmark)

In the treatment of acute hypertensive encephalopathy it is important to have the integrity of the medical specialist fields preserved since the symptoms of the disease are of a neurological nature while its causes are of internal medical origin. Occasionally the underlying hypertension has to be surgically treated. Finally, the pathogenesis can hardly be comprehended except on the basis of circulatory physiology and biochemistry.

Instantaneous institution of a rational therapy could save lives and prevent disablement in about 100% of the cases. If such rational treatment is to be accomplished, the prerequisite is a thorough insight into the pathogenesis and dynamics involved in the various phases of the syndrome. It is especially in this field that Scandinavian scientists in recent years have contributed valuable propositions.

If the matter is to be fully comprehended it is of primary necessity to study in detail cerebal autoregulation, one of the fundamental principles involved in cerebral haemodynamics. Mogens Fog (1937, 1939), on the basis of findings in animal experiments, first described the cerebal autoregulation. The physical perfusion equation reads as follows:

$$CBF = \frac{P_{a-v}}{CVR}$$

thus denoting that cerebral blood flow (CBF) is directly proportional to blood pressure (P_{a-v}) and inversely proportional to cerebral vascular resistance (CVR). Autoregulation implies the presence of a biological relationship between numerator and denominator in the perfusion equation; consequently changes in blood pressure (BP) by way of a reflex, result in similar changes in cerebrovascular resistance. Autoregulation is a highly vulnerable mechanism, globally as well as focally, and it may be affected by almost any type of organic injury to the nerve tissue, for instance, infarction, trauma, inflammation, acidosis, etc. Thus, a study of autoregulation is found to be a very sensitive method for evaluating morphological or metabolic cerebral disturbances. For instance, we have managed in several cases to unveil and localize epileptic foci or tumours which escaped detection by other methods and procedures such as EEG, scanning, angiography, etc. In other words, this type of examination is aimed primarily at an evaluation of the function rather than the structure and morphology of autoregulation. Various theories have been advanced to explain whether the autoregulation is myogenic, metabolic, or neurogenic in origin, or a combination of these. According to the original theory, it is of a myogenic nature. This theory, further elaborated by Folkow (1964), holds the dilatation of vessels to be the specific irritant responsible for the contraction of the smooth muscles, especially of arterioles (the Bayliss reflex). If true, a rise in BP and the resulting vasodilatation would by way of reflex intensify the resistance, whereas a fall in BP would result in a reduced resistance and CBF would thus remain constant. It has been observed, however, that autoregulation does not merely apply to changes in BP, rather it applies equally to changes in intracranial pressure. The hypothesis therefore had to be altered and it has been suggested that it is not the dilatation, but rather the transmural pressure in the vascular wall which determines the degree of contraction of the smooth muscles. By now it is well-established that the theory in this form holds true though it does not represent the exclusive explanation of cerebral auto-regulation or overall cerebral haemodynamics. Once the CBF could be assessed it was also realized that CO_2 and the hypoxic O_2 values in tissue are of essential importance since the result of a high pCO_2 as well as of a low pO_2 level is an increased CBF. As regards CO_2 it is, within a broad interval (arterial pCO_2 20—70 mm Hg), an almost linear correlation of considerable steepness. A change in arterial pCO_2 by 1 mm Hg results in a change in flow by approximately 4%. As a rule, the assessment and control of CO_2 should be a sine qua non in all determinations of CBF. A factor common to a rising pCO_2 and a falling pO_2 is the intracerebral shifting of pH towards acidity. In the presence of hypoxia this is due to a formation of lactic acid. Because of the presence of high arterial pCO_2, CO_2 passes the blood—liquor barrier as easily as indifferent gases, whereas normally this barrier is only passed slowly by the HCO_3^- ion. As pH is ascertained by the ratio of HCO_3^- to CO_2, the factor primarily determining the intracerebral pH is arterial pCO_2. If the change in arterial pCO_2 persists, the intracerebral HCO_3^- adjusts itself in accordance with arterial pCO_2 thereby resulting in a normalization of pH. The subtlety of this mechanism, which terminates within 24—26 min (Christensen et al., 1973), even outmatches that of homeostatic pH-regulation in the blood, irrespective of the fact that a buffer capacity is nearly absent in the cerebrospinal fluid. We have observed, for instance, that pH might be completely compensated in the cisternal fluid in the presence of severely incompensated acidosis or baseosis in the blood.

About 10 years ago, these studies prompted us to formulate a theory proposing cerebral interstitial pH as the factor determining the CVR and thus, also CBF. The correctness of this hypothesis was later completely corroborated and it seems now to be generally accepted that pH represents the mediating link in the metabolic regulation of CBF. The role of metabolic regulation for autoregulation per se, however, is still under discussion. Presumably auto-regulation is of a myogenic nature, despite the fact that the level to which it is adjusted is contingent on the pH or on metabolic factors.

Opinions are highly divergent towards the theory that autoregulation is of a neurogenic origin, and particularly the theory that the sympathetic nervous system may be involved. This is mainly because the results obtained in individual studies are very conflicting. Russian scientists propose that the autonomous nervous system is of essential importance in these mechanisms. American research workers, relying on animal experiments and anatomical studies hold that the sympathetic nervous system is involved. From a review of the numerous reports on conditions in man and our own studies we conclude that neither blocking nor stimulation of the alpha- and/or beta-adrenergic systems has any effect on CBF in man or on its regulation (Skinhøj, 1972, 1975).

To outline discussions on the role of the autonomous system in the cerebral haemodynamics is beyond the scope of the present paper as are the criticisms raised against the experimental criteria on which individual opinions are based. Murray Harper comes probably nearest to the truth when he theorized that the degree of contraction of large cerebral arteries may be subject to a vegetative nervous regulation is not manifested in the course of flow-examinations. His theory assumes that intact autoregulation may involve a compensation of the overall cerebrovascular resistance at the level of the arterioles which are not subject to autonomous nervous control, or at least only to minor degree.

These introductory comments are necessary for the comprehension of the subject at issue, but we shall now proceed to the topic of current interest; acute hypertensive encephalopathy.

Acute hypertensive encephalopathy is in its classical form, rarely encountered in our days. It was previously seen in connection with glomerulonephritis, mainly in children, and with eclampsia. At present it is usually observed in cases where hypertension remains undetected, especially if the hypertension is of a paroxysmal nature, or in cases of maltreated hypertension, for example, in patients who discontinue their treatment because of side effects. The symptoms are multiform: headache, disturbed consciousness, various forms of disturbed eyesight, convulsions, pareses (which only rarely are purely hemiform as those seen to develop in connection with apoplexia), varying degrees of disturbed coordination and afferent phenomena. If left untreated, the rate of mortality is high. At autopsy, brains may be found to be oedematous, major or minor haemorrhages or extravasations of blood may be evidenced as well as dispersed infarctions, provided of course that the disease has run a sufficiently protracted course to result in patho-anatomically demonstrable infarctions.

The diagnosis is established primarily by measuring blood pressure; still, blood pressure at levels sufficiently high to release hypertensive crises may vary widely in the individual patients, and may even vary in the same subject, depending on the rate at which BP is elevated and on the actual arterial pCO_2. Other types of hypertensive manifestations, mainly in the form of fundic changes, are almost obligatory findings. One exception to the rule is the purely paroxysmal rise in BP occurring in the presence of phaeochromocytoma; another exception is the rise in BP due to medication, as seen for instance in cases of amphetamine intoxication, especially if the vasoactive amines are combined with MAO-inhibitors.

The present paper is concerned primarily with the pathogenesis of hypertensive encephalopathy. Fundamental studies are ascribable to Byrom (1969) who, in the brains of hypertensive mice, observed phenomena similar to those otherwise seen in the retina of hypertonic subjects namely, alternating calibres of small arteries such that the lesion resembles a sausage-string. Such areas may be surrounded by minor haemorrhages or exudates and microcirculation may be compromised. Quite naturally, Byrom as well as other investigators interpreted these findings as arterial spasms provoked by hypertension and resulting ischaemic changes. Theoretically, it seemed reasonable to therapeutically administer spasmolytic drugs and vasodilating substances.

We approached these problems in a rather awkward and arbitrary way. In clinical studies, and particularly in pharmacological studies, it is essential to ensure that autoregulation is intact; it may be accomplished by determining CBF at various levels of blood pressure in the presence of controlled hypertension or hypotension. During the first procedure we observed some patients whose blood pressure was elevated to a point where a global rise in CBF might suddenly set in although the autoregulation otherwise was well-preserved. Häggendal and Johansson (1972) observed that the same phenomenon may occur in hypercapnic dogs while it cannot be provoked in normocapnic animals. Consequently we decided to embark on a systematic study of these problems.

The intra-arterial ^{133}Xe-method introduced by Lassen and Ingvar does not seem to be particularly well-fitted for studies of this type since an interval of about 15 min between the individual measurements is required making it difficult to define the exact relationship between CBF and BP. It is therefore preferred (Strandgaard et al., 1973) to use the indirect procedure in which CBF is evaluated on the basis of arterial and venous O_2 difference ($(a - v)O_2$). Assuming that the cerebral metabolic rate of oxygen remains constant, $(a - v)O_2$ expresses the reciprocal CBF values. The patient to be examined is placed on a tilting table. A catheter, guided by X-ray, is introduced into the bulbus vena jugularis interna, and another catheter is introduced into a peripheral artery. Hypertension is induced by drop-wise application of angiotensin while hypotension is induced by means of the ganglion blocking agent Arfonad® combined with tilting. Intrinsically, these drugs do not affect the CBF. $(a - v)O_2$ is determined by photospectrometry. The BP in the artery is continuously checked and all measurements include an assessment of pCO_2 (Fig. 1). The curves uppermost in the figure apply to hypertonic subjects while those lowermost in the figure apply to normotensive subjects. The most characteristic feature observed in both groups is the horizontal plateau expressed by preserved autoregulation. If blood pressure falls below a certain level, the lower limit of autoregulation is achieved and CBF is gradually reduced. At early stages, this phenomenon does not involve any metabolic or clinical consequences as it is compensated by an increased extraction of O_2 from the blood. In addition, the reserves of phosphate compounds rich in energy contribute to maintain the required development of energy for a few minutes. It is not until a low level of the declining curve is reached that the insufficiency becomes clinically manifest in the form of restlessness, perspiration, anxiety, and hyperventilation, occasionally in the form of lipothymia. Owing to this interval of compensation, EEG monitoring is not suitable as a means of determining the lowermost limit of a therapeutic BP level in hypertonic patients. In the situation of current interest, it is the uppermost

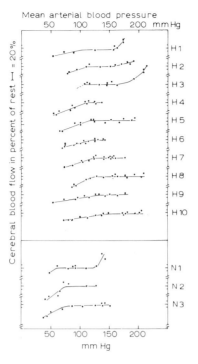

Fig. 1. Cerebral perfusion at different, controlled levels of blood pressure in hypertonic subjects (uppermost) and normotonic subjects.

limit of the autoregulation which attracts the greatest attention. It appears from the curves that the elevated BP does not in any case bring about a fall in CBF as otherwise is expected according to the theory on spasm. In some cases, however, a sudden rise in CBF may occur. A conspicuous feature in the figure is a shifting of the lower and the upper limits of autoregulation in hypertonic subjects to the right. This phenomenon is later studied more systematically and verified by Strandgaard (1976). For one thing, it explains why hypertensive crises rarely occur in chronically hypertonic patients; secondly, it supports the phenomenon often observed in the clinical routine that hypertonic patients may not always tolerate an acute normalization of blood pressure. In experiments with hypertensive animals it is observed by Folkow et al. (1971) that the phenomenon is morphologically associated with hypertrophy of the muscle layer in arterioles and that the process is reversible if the blood pressure is kept at normal levels for a certain length of time. Strandgaard (1976) demonstrates that this may also be the case in man, namely that hypertensive cerebral vascular changes may be reversible, at least functionally, during adequate anti-hypertensive treatment.

Objections to conclusions based on investigations using the $(a - v)O_2$ method are primarily that the method assumes cerebral metabolism to remain constant even while BP is elevated and secondly, the method only reflects average CBF values. From a purely theoretical viewpoint it is reasonable to assume that CBF may be elevated in certain areas at the same time as a fall in other areas may be

240

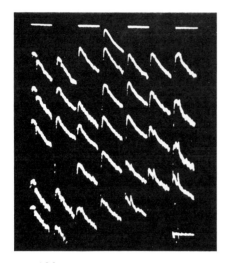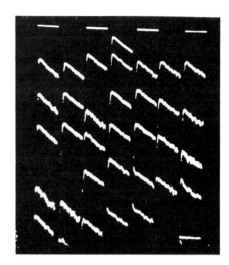

Fig. 2. ^{133}Xenon clearance curves from different brain areas during controlled hypertension. To the right: mean arterial blood pressure: 145 mm Hg, CBF 37 ml/100 g/min. To the left: 155 mm Hg, CBF 62 ml/100 g/min. Steepness of the curves denotes the cerebral blood flow (Skinhøj and Strandgaard, 1973).

provoking symptoms. Both of these objections are refuted by direct CBF measurements which reveal that the rise in CBF is even and generalized at the time that the point of penetration is achieved (Fig. 2) (Skinhøj and Strandgaard, 1973).

Rises in blood pressure to the level of breakthrough are often observed in man as a physiological phenomenon, for instance, during extreme bodily efforts. The same applies to the "cold pressure test" where the subject jumps directly from a sauna into cold water. As a rule, this results in a feeling of well-being. In this context it is essential to emphasize that the haemodynamic changes provoked by extreme acute hypertension as well in the baboon (Strandgaard, 1973) as in the cat (Johansson, 1974) are completely reversible if the hypertension lasts for less than 1 hr. If the hypertension persists for a longer period they saw a clinical as well as a pathological picture comparable with that known from the acute hypertensive encephalopathy in man. In this connection, it is necessary to consider in greater detail the patho-anatomical changes provoked by excessive perfusion of cerebral vessels during episodes of hypertension. These problems have been studied in particular by Johansson (1974) in animal experiments. Having experimentally induced hypertension, she demonstrates a multifocal extravasation of tracers such as Evans blue, fluorescein-labelled albumin, and fluorescein-sodium which ordinarily do not penetrate the blood-liquor barrier (Fig. 3). At the same time, the fluid content is found to be increased, in other words, oedema develops. Strictly focal CBF-measurements by means of implanted hydrogen-electrodes show beyond a doubt that extravasation occurs primarily in foci where CBF is at a high level. This confirms earlier findings obtained by Giese in a study of the mesenterial vessels. During induced hypertension, carbon particles are seen to penetrate into the tissue at sites corresponding to dilated areas in the sausage-string, but

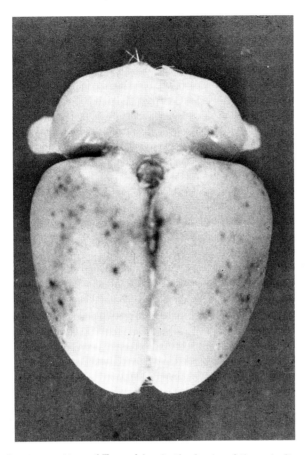

Fig. 3. Sporadical extravasation of Evans-blue in the brain of the rat after acute rise in blood pressure (Johansson, 1974).

not at sites corresponding to contracted areas. Furthermore, Johansson (1974) observes that patho-anatomical phenomena occur whether hypertension is induced by compression of the thoracic aorta or by drugs, thus indicating that the rise in BP is exclusively responsible. She also demonstrates that a co-incident vascular dilatation, for instance in the presence of hypercapnoea, intensifies the phenomenon; as if the blood-liquor barrier has been damaged by preceding irradiation.

It may be obviously concluded from these findings that the macro- and microscopic pictures of the small arteries and arterioles obtained during an acute rise in BP do not reflect pathological spasms resulting in ischaemia. Rather the "spasms" represent extreme efforts on the part of the organism to maintain autoregulation and dilatation of the sausage-string is moreover an expression of pathological decompensation.

Furthermore, Farrar et al. (1976) have demonstrated, that all vessels in animals, even those in the sausage-string which are contracted during the early phase, would be dilated if blood pressures were maintained at 180—220 mm Hg.

Although the results obtained in experiments carried out in recent years are clear as to the occurrence of haemodynamic phenomena during acute rises in BP, it remains to be conclusively established whether this model also applies to the pathogenesis of hypertensive encephalopathy in man.

Direct CBF-examination during hypertensive crises in man is not ethically permissible unless the clinical picture suggests the presence of well-defined haematomas or points to other differential diagnosis. If so the rCBF findings will be difficult to interpret, because the stage is a mixture of a possible previous hyperperfusion and hypoperfusion because of oedema formation. The closest we have come to a longitudinal study is when we observed the development of severe hypertension in a middle-aged patient during an attack of migraine. This patient had been hospitalized on several occasions, and other causes of paroxysmal hypertension were ruled out each time. When the patient was admitted on the present occasion he had an attack of migraine; the blood pressure was found to range at 185/120 and examination of CBF showed extremely high values: 140 ml/100 g/min. A few hours later the clinical symptoms resembled those encountered in the presence of acute hypertensive encephalopathy specifically convulsions, changed muscular tonus, bilateral Babinski, and coma. At this stage, the CBF was found to be greatly reduced: 26 ml/100 g/min. The intra-cranial pressure had risen up to 210 mm H_2O, and increased protein content and moderate plecytosis in the spinal fluid suggested that the blood-liquor barrier had been damaged. The therapy otherwise applied to hypertensive crises was instituted and the patient recovered completely.

It seems justifiable to consider the course of this disease as parallel to that of acute hypertensive encephalopathy. An acute rise in BP in which cerebral autoregulation is decompensated while the pressure of perfusion in the brain is intensified, results in damage to the blood-liquor barrier and the development of oedema. As a secondary result, the oedema is seen to compromise CBF leading to ischaemia and transitory or permanent damage.

It seems equally justifiable to draw certain therapeutic conclusions on the basis of this pathological model, despite the lack of controlled clinical investigations. As the primary pathogenetic manifestation, elevated BP has to be normalized immediately, using for example quick-action diuretics, such as furosemide (Lasix®), alpha blockers or dihydralazine (Nepresol®) even though the latter are not the drugs of choice at later stages. It is important, however, to test in advance possible specific cerebral haemodynamic action of the drugs.

The action of dihydralazine for example is found to be highly complex (Overgaard and Skinhøj, 1975). An almost instantaneous rise in intracranial pressure is followed by a fall in BP, a combination markedly reducing perfusion pressure. Even so, CBF is observed to be elevated. This apparently paradoxical phenomenon can hardly be explained unless we accept the existence of "resistance" as well as "capacitance" vessels within the brain. In fact, it must be assumed that hydralazine exerts its primary action on the capacitance vessels and much later exerts a greatly intensified action on the resistance vessels. The same applies to histamine. A model of this type does not simplify the study of the cerebral haemodynamics, however, it is urgently required, especially in pharmacological studies.

Cerebral vasodilating agents are contra-indicated as are morphinic drugs and procedures tending at hypoventilation. Active hyperventilation may occasionally be of value. Ischaemic damages may develop during the final phase and, if a development of permanent sequelae is to be prevented it is of essential importance to reduce the demands for oxygen in cerebral tissue; by for example keeping patients under hypothermal conditions or at least under normothermal conditions.

SUMMARY

The "breakthrough" phenomenon, namely a sudden increase in global cerebral blood flow at certain levels of induced controlled hypertension, is demonstrated in man. Its possible pathogenetic role in the hypertensive crisis is discussed. It seems related to the arterial pCO_2. Blockade of the sympathetic system does not influence the blood pressure level needed for a "breakthrough". The complicated cerebral haemodynamic effect of dihydralazine is described.

REFERENCES

Byrom, F.B. (1969) *The Hypertensive Vascular Crisis*, Heinemann, London.

Christensen, M.S. (1973) Cerebral apoplexy treated with or without prolonged artificial hyperventilation. 2. Cerebrospinal fluid acid-base balance and intracranial pressure. *Stroke*, 4: 620—631.

Farrar, J.K., Jones, J.V., Graham, D.I., Strandgaard, S. and MacKenzie, E.T. (1976) Evidence against cerebral vasospasm during occultly induced hypertension. *Brain Res.*, 104: 176—180.

Fog, M. (1937) Cerebral circulation. I. The reaction of the pial arteries to a fall in blood pressure. *Arch. Neurol. Psychiat. (Chic.)*, 37: 351—358.

Fog, M. (1939) Cerebral circulation. II. Reaction of pial arteries to increase in blood pressure. *Arch. Neurol. Psychiat. (Chic.)*, 41: 260—268.

Folkow, B. (1964) Description of the myogenic hypothesis. *Circulat. Res.*, 14—15, Suppl. I: 279—287.

Folkow, B., Hallbäck, M., Lundgren, Y. and Weiss, L. (1971) The effect of intense treatment with hypotensive drugs on structural cardiovascular changes after reversal of experimental renal hypertension in rats. *Acta physiol. scand.*, 83: 280—282.

Häggendal, E. and Johansson, B. (1972) On the pathophysiology of the increased cerebrovascular permeability in acute arterial hypertension in cats. *Acta neurol. scand.*, 48: 265—270.

Johansson, B. (1974) *Blood—Brain Barrier Dysfunction in Acute Arterial Hypertension*, Thesis, Göteborg.

Overgaard, J. and Skinhøj, E. (1975) A paradoxical cerebral haemodynamic effect of hydralazine. *Stroke*, 6: 402—404.

Skinhøj, E. (1972) The sympathetic nervous system and the regulation of cerebral blood flow in man. *Stroke*, 3: 711—716.

Skinhøj, E. (1975) The upper limit of autoregulation and the sympathetic system. In *Cerebral Circulation and Metabolism*, T.W. Langfitt et al. (Eds.), Springer, New York, pp. 487—488.

Skinhøj, E. and Strandgaard, S. (1973) Pathogenesis of hypertensive encephalopathy. *Lancet*, 3: 461—462.

Strandgaard, S. (1976) Autoregulation of cerebral blood flow in hypertensive patients. *Circulation*, 53: 720—727.

Strandgaard, S., Skinhøj, E. and Lassen, N.A. (1973) Autoregulation of brain circulation in severe arterial hypertension. *Brit. med. J.*, 159: 507—510.

SESSION IV

INTEGRATED BRAIN FUNCTION AND HYPERTENSION

Chairmen: D. De Wied (Utrecht)
A.P. Shapiro (Pittsburgh, Pa.)

A Longitudinal Study of the Hypertensive Process in Man

W.H. BIRKENHÄGER, T.L. KHO, M.A. SCHALEKAMP, G.A. ZAAL,
A. WESTER, P.W. DE LEEUW, R. VANDONGEN, T.D. FAWZI-MEININGER
and A.Th. VAN EDIXHOVEN

Department of Internal Medicine, Zuiderziekenhuis, Rotterdam (The Netherlands)

Recently we completed a cross-sectional study of 120 patients with uncomplicated essential hypertension. When the physiological-biochemical profile was related to age, we were struck by the finding that it tended to be altered rather abruptly in the fifth decade. At that point a very high vascular resistance pattern became detectable, particularly as far as renal circulation was concerned. Moreover the cluster of low renin levels we encountered in that decade was dissolved beyond the age of 50. Such findings call for a longitudinal investigation.

Studies of this kind are scarce and limited to systemic haemodynamics. In an earlier study we have shown that both total peripheral and renal vascular resistance tend to increase in the course of the hypertensive process, whilst blood volume does not show consistent changes (Birkenhäger et al., 1972). The present investigation is an extension of the previous one, its main purpose being the assessment of trends in plasma renin levels in relation to possible changes in blood pressure, plasma volume and renal haemodynamics.

Twenty-three hypertensive patients (11 men, 12 women), aged 22—60 years, were studied for an average period of 4.7 years (1—7.1 years). The diagnosis of essential hypertension was made after screening the patients for endocrine or renal disorders. At the onset none of them presented signs of organ damage. Patients had two characteristics in common: they were willing to be recruited for periodical investigations, but they disliked drugs and were definitely undertreated. The drugs they eventually used were stopped 10 days before the initial and follow-up investigations. The investigations were carried out under metabolic ward conditions. Sodium intake was 60 mmoles daily and this was checked by urinary sodium excretion. Measurements of plasma renin concentration (PRC) were carried out according to Skinner's method (Skinner, 1967). Although for routine purposes we have switched to radioimmunoassay of PRC, we took care to avoid intraindividual switches in method: those patients whose initial PRC was assessed by bioassay were restudied by the same method.

As to the other investigational methods we refer to earlier studies from our laboratory (Birkenhäger et al., 1968; Schalekamp et al., 1970). Glomerular filtration rate (GFR) was determined originally by means of cyanocobalamin

248

clearance, but from 1973 onwards we used inulin clearance following a period of duplicate measurements.

There appeared to be a case for dividing patients into two groups: those who continued to remain free of cardiovascular complications throughout the follow-up period (group 1; 17 subjects) and those who did not (group 2; 6 patients with myocardial infarction). It should be stressed that the latter group was restudied after clinical recovery under the conditions of the protocol. The subjects received no pharmacotherapy except for anticoagulant treatment.

Group 1: The follow-up period averaged 5.2 years (2—7 years). Ten patients were studied twice, 5 patients 3 times, and 2 patients 4 times or more. The group average of mean arterial pressure remained unaltered throughout the study (130 mm Hg and 133 mm Hg at the initial and final studies). Average plasma volume also did not change (2600 ml and 2700 ml respectively). GFR declined slightly from 111 ml/min to 102 ml/min (N.S.). Renal vascular resistance (RVR) calculated from mean arterial pressure and renal blood flow (RBF) increased from 14,600 to 17,800 dyne/sq. cm^{-5} (N.S.). The initial PRC was 5.3 ± 1.9 ng/ml/hr. Changes in PRC are presented in Figs. 1 and 2.

Although in some patients a decrease in PRC was observed during the first years of follow-up, the long-term change with a few exceptions was found to be a consistent rise in PRC, even in those subjects who exhibited a slight decrease in the first years. The average PRC increased ultimately from 5.3 ± 1.9 to 7.3 ± 2.9 ng/ml/hr ($P < 0.01$).

Group 2: The follow-up period in this group averaged 4 years (1—6.1 years). In these subjects mean average blood pressure declined from 140 to 130 mm Hg (N.S.). Plasma volume did not change significantly. Both GFR and RBF showed a greater decrease and RVR a greater increase (from 14,900 to 19,600

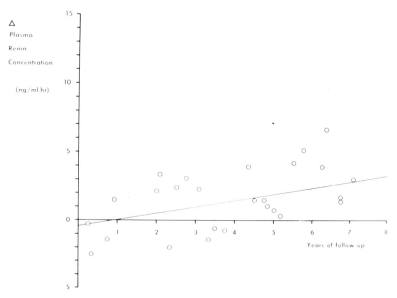

Fig. 1. Changes in plasma renin concentration (ng/ml/hr) observed in 17 essential hypertensives who remained free of complications.

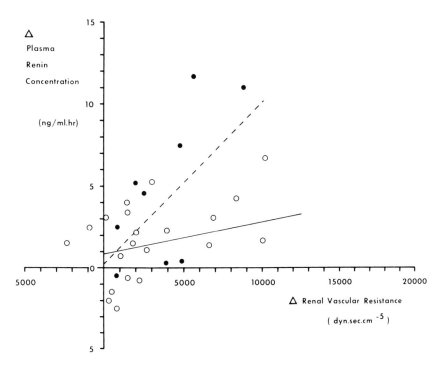

Fig. 2. Relationships between changes in plasma renin concentration and renal vascular resistance in group 1 (○) and group 2 (●). Group 1: $r = +0.34$, $P < 0.025$, y = 0.0002X + 0.85. Group 2: $r = +0.67$, $P < 0.0025$, y = 0.001X + 0.25.

dynes/sq. cm^{-5}) than in group 1. PRC at the start of the observation averaged 5.0 ± 3.2 ng/ml/hr. Four patients were in the low-renin group. PRC did not change uniformly, but the group average increased from 5.0 ± 3.2 to 11.8 ± 6.1 ng/ml/hr. This rise is substantially greater than in group 1. In both groups the rise in renin was unrelated to changes in blood pressure or plasma volume. A positive relationship was found with changes in RVR.

The dynamism of this relationship confirms the biphasic pattern we observed in a previous study (Schalekamp et al., 1973). These results appear to negate the current practice of labeling hypertensives in terms of low-, normal- or high-renin hypertension, particularly because some individuals were shown to pass through all stages of the classification of renin levels. As a corollary, it was observed that patients with low-renin hypertension may meet with myocardial infarction after a short lapse of time and only exhibit high-renin levels afterwards. By this finding alone retrospective studies on renin as a risk factor appear to be invalidated.

REFERENCES

Birkenhäger, W.H., Van Es, L.A., Houwing, A., Lamers, H.J. and Mulder, A.H. (1968) Studies on the lability of hypertension in man. *Clin. Sci.*, 35: 445—456.

250

Birkenhäger, W.H., Schalekamp, M.A.D.H., Krauss, X.H., Kolsters, G. and Zaal, G.A. (1972) Consecutive haemodynamic patterns in essential hypertension. *Lancet*, 1: 560—564.

Schalekamp, M.A.D.H., Schalekamp-Kuyken, M.P.A. and Birkenhäger, W.H. (1970) Abnormal renal haemodynamics and renin suppression in hypertensive patients. *Clin. Sci.*, 38: 101—110.

Schalekamp, M.A., Krauss, X.H., Kolsters, G., Schalekamp, M.P.A. and Birkenhäger, W.H. (1973) Renin suppression in hypertension in relation to body fluid volumes, patterns of sodium excretion and renal haemodynamics. *Clin. Sci. molec. Med.*, 45: 283S—286S.

Skinner, S.L. (1967) Improved assay methods for renin "concentration" and "activity" in human plasma. *Circulat. Res.*, 20: 391—402.

Patterns of Neurogenic Involvement in Borderline and Essential Hypertension

STEVO JULIUS and MURRAY ESLER

Division of Hypertension, Department of Internal Medicine, University of Michigan Medical School, Ann Arbor, Mich. 48109 (U.S.A.)

INTRODUCTION

Considerable evidence points toward a substantial neurogenic involvement in borderline hypertension (Julius and Esler, 1975). Borderline hypertension is an early predictor of future established essential hypertension (Julius and Schork, 1971). However, whereas in borderline hypertension the risk for future hypertension is higher than in the general population, not all patients will later develop hypertension. This poses an interpretative problem: are the signs of neurogenic involvement observed in borderline hypertension characteristically present in subjects who will develop future hypertension or are they unrelated to later hypertension. Since the incidence of future hypertension is relatively low (Julius and Schork, 1971), a prospective study to evaluate the prognostic significance of the autonomic abnormality in borderline hypertension would require a large number of patients and a long period of observation. Cross-sectional comparison of groups of patients with borderline hypertension and with established hypertension offers another more practical, though less direct, approach.

In this report we will show that similar aberrations in the autonomic nervous control of the circulation occur in some patients with borderline hypertension and mild established hypertension. Inferences will be drawn regarding the importance of autonomic nervous dysfunction in the development of essential hypertension.

MATERIAL AND METHODS

All subjects were males and had a minimum of 3 casual sitting blood pressure readings taken in the preceding year. In paid healthy volunteer control subjects all blood pressures were in the normotensive range. In patients with borderline hypertension, at least one diastolic reading was in excess of 90 mm Hg and at least one reading was below that value. In patients with established hypertension, all the diastolic readings were in excess of 90 mm Hg. Every patient had a thorough clinical examination and in none was there evidence that the hypertension was secondary. The overall characteristics of the 3 groups

TABLE I

GENERAL CHARACTERISTICS OF SUBJECTS

Mean and standard deviations are given. Blood pressure was measured intra-arterially after 10 min of rest. Asterisks (*) denote significance of difference from controls; daggers (†) denote significance of difference, borderline hypertension vs. essential hypertension.*** or ††† $P < 0.001$.

	N	Age	Blood pressure (mm Hg)	
			Systolic	Diastolic
Control subjects	86	24.7 ± 4.8	113 ± 12	63 ± 8
Borderline hypertension	145	26.4 ± 6.8	133 ± 14***	75 ± 10***
Established hypertension	16	36.2 ± 4.7***,†††	164 ± 6***,†††	95 ± 3***,†††

of patients are given in Table I. None of the patients had abnormal urine, elevated serum creatinine, signs or a history of congestive heart failure, and grade III or IV hypertensive retinopathy.

In all cases the cardiac output was determined by dye dilution (indocyanine green) with withdrawal of the blood through a Gilford densitometer. The blood pressure was measured through a brachial artery catheter introduced percutaneously. Resting values were obtained in recumbency 10 min after all the catheters were introduced. Values after propranolol, atropine or regitine were obtained 7 min after the completion of the intravenous injections.

Plasma renin activity measurement was performed by the method described by Haber et al. (1969). Twenty-four hour urine was collected in a metabolic ward. Control subjects and patients with borderline hypertension were on their usual diet, whereas patients with established hypertension were on a standard 160 mEq. sodium intake. In all cases blood for plasma renin activity determination was drawn after 1 hr of standing at approximately the same time of the day (9:00 a.m.). Results in patients were referred to a plasma renin activity-urinary sodium nomogram (Esler et al., 1975) developed from 35 male normotensive subjects (aged 18—50). This allowed the classification of patients into high, normal and low renin categories.

Plasma catecholamines were measured by the method described by Renzini et al. (1970) and performed in Dr. Vincent De Quattro's laboratory in Los Angeles. Samples for catecholamine levels were drawn in recumbency on the day of the hemodynamic procedure.

RESULTS

Autonomic regulation of the cardiac output in borderline hypertension

An elevation of the cardiac output in borderline hypertension has been repeatedly reported (Eich et al., 1962; Finkielman et al., 1965; Sannerstedt, 1966; Julius and Conway, 1968; Lund-Johansen, 1967; Frohlich et al., 1970). In our overall material (Fig. 1), it can be seen that the mean cardiac index in

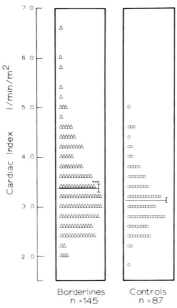

Fig. 1. Distribution of the cardiac index in patients with borderline hypertension (△) and in control subjects (○). Mean is denoted by the horizontal line; vertical bars represent the standard errors of the mean. Measurements taken in recumbency ten minutes after all catheters were introduced. Significance of difference tested by a *t*-test: ***$P < 0.001$, **$P < 0.01$, *$P < 0.05$. (Courtesy of the American Heart Association, Inc., Julius et al., 1975a.)

patients is elevated (3388 ± 69 ml/min/sq. m in patients versus 2991 ± 46 in control subjects, $P < 0.001$), but that there is also a wide overlap (Julius et al., 1975a). Many patients exhibited clearly normal values. In order to specifically investigate the pathophysiology of the elevation of the cardiac output, patients

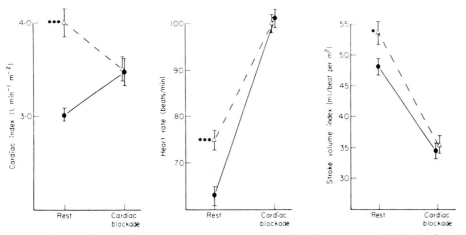

Fig. 2. Cardiac index and its components at rest and after autonomic blockade with 0.2 mg/kg propranolol and 0.04 mg/kg atropine i.v. Patients were selected for an elevated resting cardiac index (one standard deviation above the control's mean value). There were 25 patients (△) and 28 control subjects (●) in this experiment. Symbols as in Fig. 1. (From *Clin. Sci. molec. Med.*, by permission, Julius et al., 1975b.)

whose resting cardiac index exceeded one standard deviation of the mean of control subjects were considered as a separate group (Julius et al., 1975b). The effect of a combined autonomic blockade with propranolol (0.2 mg/kg i.v.) and atropine (0.04 mg/kg i.v.) is shown in Fig. 2. It can be seen that the resting cardiac index in these patients was elevated through a larger stroke volume and a faster heart rate. After the autonomic blockade, heart rate and stroke volume fell into the normal range and the large elevation of the cardiac index in patients (1200 ml/min/sq. m above the mean value for control subjects) was abolished. It was therefore concluded that the elevation of the heart rate and stroke volume in these patients with borderline hypertension is mediated by a neurogenic mechanism.

Autonomic nervous correlates of plasma renin activity in borderline hypertension

The initial work using hemodynamic criteria delineated the cardiac autonomic abnormality in borderline hypertension. Our recent efforts have been focused upon further exploration of the earlier impression (Esler and Nestel, 1973) that the state of plasma renin activity may be a helpful tool in differentiating between "neurogenic" and "non-neurogenic" hemodynamic mechanisms in borderline hypertension. In recent studies plasma renin activity was related in particular to the degree of neurogenic maintenance of peripheral vascular resistance in borderline hypertension. There are two lines of evidence that peripheral resistance in borderline hypertension is not normal. First, if the apparently "normal" mean peripheral resistance in patients with borderline hypertension (Julius et al., 1971) is analyzed with reference to the levels of cardiac output, it becomes evident that the peripheral resistance in patients is inappropriately high for the prevailing level of cardiac output (blood flow) (Julius et al., 1971). The second line of evidence comes from the experiments with cardiac blockade in patients with a high cardiac output (Julius et al., 1975b). In Fig. 3, patients with borderline hypertension are divided into a high and a normal cardiac output group. In the normal output group the pressure elevation was maintained by high peripheral resistance, both at rest and after autonomic cardiac blockade. In the high output group, the resistance was decreased, and at rest the blood pressure elevation was maintained by an elevation of the cardiac output. After cardiac blockade with atropine and propranolol the cardiac output fell into the normal range, but the blood pressure remained elevated. At this point the peripheral resistance increased and the blood pressure elevation was maintained by a predominantly resistance-related mechanism.

In order to assess the neurogenically maintained component of total peripheral vascular resistance in borderline hypertension, the alpha-adrenergic antagonist phentolamine was injected intravenously, in a dose of 15 mg i.v., after prior cardiac blockade with propranolol and atropine (Esler et al., 1975). It can be seen in Fig. 4 that after such a "total" autonomic blockade, the blood pressure in control subjects and patients changes in a similar fashion, but through somewhat different mechanisms. In addition to the decrease in cardiac output, which was observed in both groups, the patients exhibited a small but

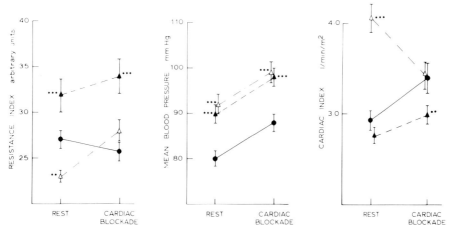

Fig. 3. Hemodynamics in two groups of patients. Patients were divided into two groups based on the mean of the control group (●). The "high-output group" (△) had a resting cardiac output one standard deviation above the controls. The rest of the patients comprised the "normal output" group (▲). Dosage as in Fig. 2. There were 54 patients and 27 control subjects in this experiment.

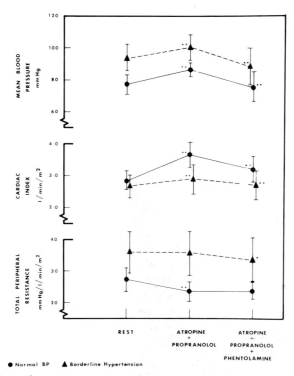

● Normal BP   ▲ Borderline Hypertension

Fig. 4. General hemodynamics at rest, after atropine plus propranolol, and after "total" autonomic blockade in patients with borderline hypertension (▲) and normal subjects (●). Mean values ± one standard deviation are shown. The significance levels of the changes from resting values with atropine plus propranolol ("cardiac autonomic blockade") and the subsequent changes with phentolamine (15 mg i.v.) are indicated for both groups of subjects (*$P < 0.05$, **$P < 0.01$; paired t-test). (Courtesy of the *Amer. J. Cardiol.*, Esler et al., 1975.)

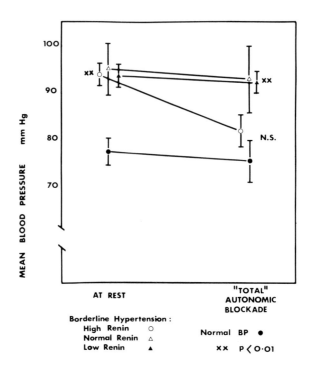

Fig. 5. The effect of "total" autonomic blockade on mean blood pressure (diastolic blood pressure + 1/3 pulse pressure) in normal subjects and renin subgroups of patients with borderline hypertension. Means ± one standard deviation are shown. The significance level refers to the difference in mean blood pressure between the normal subjects and each group with borderline hypertension (Student's *t*-test). After total autonomic blockade mean blood pressure in normal subjects and patients with high-renin borderline hypertension was not significantly different (82 ± 6.6 mm Hg compared with 76 ± 9.2 mm Hg). (Courtesy of the *Amer. J. Cardiol.*, Esler et al., 1975.)

significant decrease in the peripheral resistance. This decrease of peripheral resistance in borderline hypertension was not uniform and largely depended on the patient's renin status. All patients with high renin values exhibited a decrease of the peripheral resistance, whereas in low-renin cases such a decrease of peripheral resistance could not be demonstrated (Esler et al., 1975). Only in patients with high renin did the hypertension appear to be mediated by a neurogenic mechanism; after cardiac *and* alpha-adrenergic blockade, their blood pressure fell into the normal range (Fig. 5).

In addition to signs of an abnormal alpha-adrenergic mechanism, evidence of increased cardiac beta-adrenergic activity is also found in high-renin borderline hypertension; beta-adrenergic blockade with propranolol caused an excessive decrease of the heart rate in such patients (Esler et al., 1976).

In summary, patients with the high-renin type of borderline hypertension exhibit signs of increased alpha- and beta-adrenergic sympathetic drive, and their blood pressure elevation is entirely mediated through a neurogenic mechanism.

Autonomic nervous correlates of plasma renin activity in established
hypertension

In the study of patients with established hypertension, it was possible to compare plasma norepinephrine levels with various hemodynamic indices of cardiac sympathetic activity. One of the most frequently used indices in our previous research was the heart rate and cardiac output response to propranolol. The assumption was always made that a larger response to beta-adrenergic blockade is indicative of a greater beta-adrenergic drive. However, this indirect assessment of the "net" beta-adrenergic drive to the heart is influenced both by the sympathetic discharge rate and by the cardiac responsiveness to beta-adrenergic stimulation. Increased beta-adrenergic responsiveness has been described in some patients with borderline hypertension (Frohlich et al., 1969; Kuchel et al., 1972) although this is probably not the case in the majority of patients (Frohlich et al., 1970; Julius et al., 1975b). Results on the present series of patients with established hypertension indicate that the response to propranolol indeed offers a measure of cardiac sympathetic tone. There was a significant positive correlation between plasma norepinephrine concentration at rest and the heart rate response to propranolol ($r = 0.48$, $P < 0.05$, n = 19).

The utility of plasma renin status, as an indirect index of sympathetic nervous involvement in hypertension, was further investigated in patients with established hypertension. Patients with high-renin values (n = 7) were compared to low-renin patients (n = 9). The heart rate in patients with high renin was significantly elevated. After cardiac autonomic blockade with propranolol and atropine, the difference in heart rate between the two groups of patients was abolished (Fig. 6). Thus the heart rate elevation in high-renin established hypertension was of a similar neurogenic origin to that in borderline hypertension (see Fig. 2).

A strong sympathetic involvement in high-renin established hypertension is further supported by plasma norepinephrine levels. The plasma norepinephrine

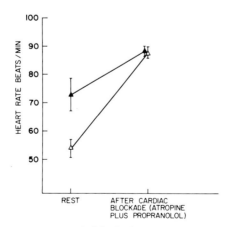

Fig. 6. Heart rate response to autonomic blockade in patients with established hypertension. High-renin hypertension (▲, n = 7), low-renin hypertension (△, n = 9). Dosages as in Fig. 2.

level in high-renin hypertension was 241 ± 56 ng/l whereas in patients with low renin the value was 103 ± 62 ng/l ($P < 0.01$).

DISCUSSION

Similarities of the autonomic nervous aberrations in borderline and established hypertension

The problem of transition from borderline to established hypertension is perplexing. A large number of patients with borderline hypertension will indeed "cross the border" and evolve established hypertension (Julius and Schork, 1971), but many patients will remain in the borderline range and a substantial proportion will become normotensive. Unfortunately it is not known which of the abnormalities observed in borderline hypertension are associated with the later development of established hypertension. Certain physiologic abnormalities, such as elevation of the cardiac output, are common in borderline hypertension but are rare in established hypertension. Elevation of the cardiac output, therefore, could be either unrelated to established hypertension or the elevation could precede the later normal cardiac output of established hypertension. Consequently similarities between the pathophysiology of borderline hypertension and established hypertension are of specific interest. If similar pathophysiological abnormalities were to be found in borderline hypertension and established hypertension, it might be inferred that these abnormalities are pathogenically significant in the transition from borderline to established hypertension.

We have found a number of similarities between borderline and established hypertension. Whereas in borderline hypertension one can find elevation of both the cardiac output and heart rate and in established hypertension only the heart rate is elevated, the underlying mechanism of the tachycardia is the same; an increased net sympathetic drive to the heart prevails. The plasma renin distribution in borderline hypertension and established hypertension is abnormal; a substantial proportion of cases have either low- or high-renin values. In both borderline hypertension and established hypertension the high-renin group exhibits more and the low-renin group less sign of sympathetic activity. By using propranolol in the high-renin borderline hypertensives, we were able to demonstrate an excessive beta-adrenergic chronotropic drive to the heart; the same was the case in high-renin established hypertension. In established hypertension the use of the cardiac response to propranolol as an index of sympathetic drive was cross-validated against plasma norepinephrine as another index of sympathetic tone; a positive correlation between the two existed. Finally, patients with established high-renin hypertension had significantly elevated plasma norepinephrine levels.

As stated earlier, pathophysiologic similarities between borderline and established hypertension are of general interest for the understanding of the "transition" from borderline to established hypertension. We chose to view these similarities as an expression of a commonly shared pathophysiologic mechanism. Direct evidence for this view does not exist, but the known facts about the natural history of borderline hypertension justify the hypothesis. Within the framework of this hypothesis the similarities of autonomic dysfunction in borderline and established hypertension attain specific significance. The nervous abnormalities in borderline hypertension are frequently viewed as an expression of "innocent" anxiety, whereas in established hypertension it is held that the autonomic abnormality may be secondary to pressure-related resetting of baroreceptors (McCubbin et al., 1956). The existence of similar autonomic abnormalities in some patients with borderline and established hypertension (those with elevated plasma renin activity) suggests that the autonomic dysfunction may well play an integral role in the development, via a stage of borderline hypertension, of certain cases of established hypertension. Further, the existence of the autonomic abnormality in patients with minimal and transient blood pressure elevation speaks against a secondary pressure-related resetting of the autonomic control as the mechanism of the sympathetic nervous overactivity.

Origin of the autonomic nervous aberrations

The increased cardiac sympathetic drive observed in borderline hypertension and essential hypertension theoretically could result from (a) increase in sympathetic tone only; (b) a combination of an increase in sympathetic stimulation and decreased vagal inhibition; or (c) from an increased sensitivity of adrenergic receptors. Increased arteriolar sympathetic drive observed in high-renin hypertension could reflect (a) increased sympathetic tone, and (b) increased vascular reactivity. In a recent publication (Julius and Esler, 1975), the evidence supporting each of these possibilities was reviewed. Our work suggests that the abnormality stems from the higher areas of cerebral integration of autonomic cardiovascular function. The evidence for this view will now be presented.

In Fig. 7 a stepwise injection of propranolol and atropine was given to patients with borderline hypertension and control subjects. The slope of the change of heart rate from rest to propranolol corresponds to the amount of sympathetic beta-adrenergic drive which has been removed by beta-receptor blockade. The patients in Fig. 7 exhibit a larger amount of cardiac beta-adrenergic drive; there is a substantially larger reduction of heart rate after propranolol. However, it can also be seen from the figure that removal of the excessive beta-adrenergic drive in patients did not result in a fully normal heart rate. Only with removal of the parasympathetic influence on the heart by atropine was heart rate normalized. After atropine, patients' heart rate decreased less; thus they exhibited a lesser degree of parasympathetic inhibition than control subjects. In short, Fig. 7 conveys evidence (a) that both sympathetic and parasympathetic abnormalities are involved in the maintenance of the elevated cardiac output, and (b) that there is more sympathetic stimulation and less vagal inhibition of the heart. Such a reciprocal relationship, where increased sympathetic stimulation is coupled with decreased vagal inhibition, is typical of the functional organization of the integrative areas of cardiovascular control. An abnormal but *integrated*

260

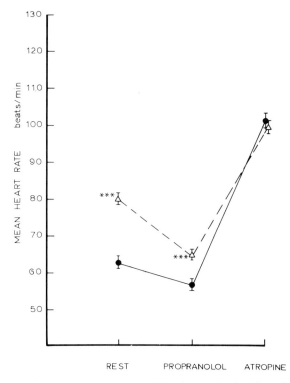

Fig. 7. Response of the heart rate to propranolol and atropine in 28 patients with borderline hypertension (△) and 29 control subjects (●). Dosage schedule as in Fig. 2. Patients were selected for an elevated resting heart rate (one standard deviation above the mean of control subjects).

response is obtained. The site of the abnormal integration is most likely in the medulla oblongata.

An additional argument for the central origin of the autonomic abnormality can be found in its *wide distribution*. Thus, there is evidence of increased adrenergic drive to both the heart and the resistance vessels (arterioles) in patients with high-renin hypertension. In such patients the elevation of the plasma renin activity in itself appears to be just another expression of increased sympathetic drive to yet another target organ, the kidney. Such a widespread and integrated pattern of autonomic abnormality speaks against possible receptor or organ hypersensitivity as its cause.

SUMMARY

Borderline hypertension is a predictor of essential hypertension, but it is not known which aspects of the pathophysiology of borderline hypertension are pathogenically related to the later development of established hypertension. Comparison of the hemodynamic characteristics of borderline hypertension and essential hypertension may yield some useful information on this question.

Hemodynamics and indices of neurogenic tone are compared in 145 patients with borderline hypertension, 21 patients with essential hypertension, and 86 normal subjects.

Some patients with borderline hypertension have an elevation of cardiac output which is fully neurogenic: cardiac output becomes normal after beta-adrenergic and parasympathetic cardiac blockade with intravenous propranolol and atropine. Sequential administration of propranolol and atropine in these patients reveals more sympathetic cardiac stimulation and less vagal inhibition which points toward an altered integration of autonomic cardiac control. Analysis by renin status provides further insight. Based on the hemodynamic responses to propranolol and alpha-adrenergic blockade with phentolamine, borderline hypertensives with high plasma renin show evidence of increased adrenergic drive to the heart and resistance vessels. In these patients the hypertension is entirely neurogenic, since a combined cardiac and vascular autonomic blockade elicits normotension. In borderline hypertensives with low plasma renin activity there is no evidence of increased sympathetic tone.

In mild established essential hypertension renin categorization allows a similar differentiation. Essential hypertensives with high plasma renin activity have a faster heart rate, which is related to excess beta-adrenergic drive (assessed by propranolol). Plasma norepinephrine concentration in these patients is elevated. Patients with low-renin essential hypertension show neither abnormality.

It is concluded that subcategories of borderline and mild established essential hypertension (high-renin hypertension) exhibit a similar pattern of autonomic nervous abnormality. Sympathetic nervous system overactivity present in some patients with borderline hypertension may lead to the later development of established hypertension.

ACKNOWLEDGEMENT

This work was supported in part by a grant-in-aid from the Michigan Heart Association.

REFERENCES

Eich, R.H., Peters, R.J., Cuddy, R.P., Smulyan, H. and Lyons, R.H. (1962) Hemodynamics in labile hypertension. *Amer. Heart J.*, 63: 188—195.

Esler, M.D. and Nestel, P.J. (1973) Renin and sympathetic nervous system responsiveness to adrenergic stimuli in essential hypertension. *Amer. J. Cardiol.*, 32: 643—649.

Esler, M.D., Julius, S., Randall, O.S., Ellis, C.N. and Kashima, T. (1975) Relation of renin status to neurogenic vascular resistance in borderline hypertension. *Amer. J. Cardiol.*, 36: 708—715.

Esler, M., Julius, S., Randall, O., De Quattro, V. and Zweifler, A. (1977) High-renin essential hypertension: adrenergic cardiovascular correlates. *Clin. Sci. molec. Med.*, in press.

Finkielman, S., Worcel, M. and Agrest, A. (1965) Hemodynamic patterns in essential hypertension. *Circulation*, 31: 356—368.

Frohlich, E.D., Tarazi, R.C. and Dustan, H.P. (1969) Hyperdynamic β-adrenergic circulatory state: increased β-receptor responsiveness. *Arch. intern. Med.*, 123: 1—7.

Frohlich, E.D., Kozul, V.J., Tarazi, R.C. and Dustan, H.P. (1970) Physiological comparison of labile and essential hypertension. *Circulat. Res.*, 26, Suppl. I: 55—69.

Haber, E., Koerner, T., Page, L.B., Kliman, B. and Purnode, A. (1969) Application of a radioimmunoassay for angiotensin I to the physiologic measurements of plasma renin activity in normal human subjects. *J. clin. Endocrinol.*, 29: 1349—1355.

Julius, S. and Conway, J. (1968) Hemodynamic studies in patients with borderline blood pressure elevation. *Circulation*, 38: 282—288.

Julius, S. and Esler, M. (1975) Autonomic nervous cardiovascular regulation in borderline hypertension. *Amer. J. Cardiol.*, 36: 685—696.

Julius, S. and Schork, M.A. (1971) Borderline hypertension — a critical review. *J. chron. Dis.*, 23: 723—754.

Julius, S., Pascual, A., Sannerstedt, R. and Mitchell, C. (1971) Relationship between cardiac output and peripheral resistance in borderline hypertension. *Circulation*, 43: 382—390.

Julius, S., Randall, O.S., Esler, M.D., Kashima, T., Ellis, C.N. and Bennett, J. (1975a) Altered cardiac responsiveness and regulation in the normal cardiac output type of borderline hypertension. *Circulat. Res.*, 36—37, Suppl. I: I-199—I-207.

Julius, S., Esler, M.D. and Randall, O.S. (1975b) Role of the autonomic nervous system in mild human hypertension. *Clin. Sci. molec. Med.*, 48: 243S—252S.

Kuchel, O., Cuche, J.L., Hamet, P., Boucher, R., Barbeau, A. and Genest, J. (1972) The relationship between adrenergic nervous system and renin in labile hyperkinetic hypertension. In *Hypertension '72*, J. Genest and E. Koiw (Eds.), Springer, New York, pp. 118—125.

Lund-Johansen, P. (1967) Hemodynamics in early essential hypertension. *Acta med. scand.*, Suppl. 482: 1—105.

McCubbin, J.W., Green, J.H. and Page, I.H. (1956) Baroreceptor function in chronic renal hypertension. *Circulat. Res.*, 4: 205—210.

Renzini, V., Brunori, C.A. and Valori, C. (1970) A sensitive and specific fluorimetric method for the determination of noradrenaline and adrenaline in human plasma. *Clin. chim. Acta*, 39: 587—594.

Sannerstedt, R. (1966) Hemodynamic response to exercise in patients with arterial hypertension. *Acta med. scand.*, Suppl. 458: 1—83.

The Social Environment and Essential Hypertension in Mice: Possible Role of the Innervation of the Adrenal Cortex

JAMES P. HENRY and PATRICIA M. STEPHENS

University of Southern California School of Medicine, Department of Physiology, Los Angeles, Calif. 90033 (U.S.A)

INTRODUCTION

For some years we have been using complex population cages stocked with CBA mice to test the hypothesis that psychosocial interaction which produces aversive behavioral conditioning will lead to prolonged elevations of systolic blood pressure (Henry et al., 1967, 1975). In the control situation, the animals are brought up together from birth with resulting minimal emotional arousal, despite social interaction. In the experimental condition, adult males and females which had been isolated since weaning are placed together in a design that induces sustained competition for territory. Our hypothesis has been that the repeated confrontations lead to repeated arousal of the sympathetic adrenal-medullary and the pituitary adrenocortical neuroendocrine response patterns (Henry, 1976a; Henry and Ely, 1976). The use of this technique has established that the CBA strain, which is not spontaneously hypertensive, develops sustained elevations of systolic blood pressure. In addition, there is significant aortic arteriosclerosis and myocardial fibrosis (Henry et al., 1971) together with renal failure (Henry, 1976a). These pathophysiological changes and the high blood pressure persist, despite prolonged return to isolation (Henry et al., 1975).

FURTHER EVIDENCE OF THE SEPARATION OF THE SYMPATHOADRENAL AND PITUITARY ADRENOCORTICAL SYSTEMS

The focus of this report is on the status of a continuing effort to disentangle the social stimuli and behavioral patterns that lead to arousal of the sympathoadrenal-medullary system from those involving the hypothalamoadrenal-cortical system and to continue with the problem of relating these to low renin essential hypertension (Henry et al., 1974).

Arousal of the sympathetic fight-flight reaction is triggered by the urge to protect access to valued goals and is dependent on the integrity of the amygdalar nuclear complex (Rolls, 1975). Perception of loss of relevant feedback with control of status and expectancies leads to hippocampal arousal. The conservation-withdrawal, depressive "hopeless" response that ensues

264

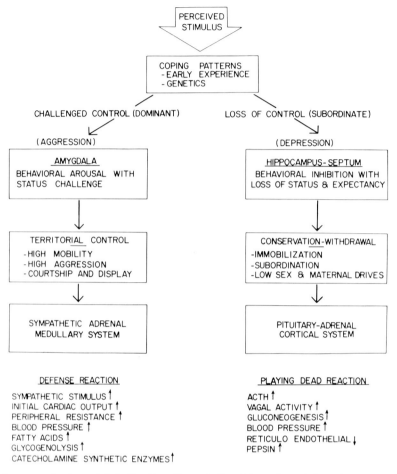

Fig. 1. A conceptual model indicating the relationships of social environmental stimuli, behavioral patterns, and modes of activation of the neuroendocrine system. The relationship of the amygdala, sympathoadrenal-medullary system, and the defense reaction are contrasted with that of the hippocampus-septum, pituitary adrenocortical system, and the reaction of playing dead. For further details see *Advanc. vet. Sci.*, (1976) 20: 115—145. (From Henry 1976a.)

stimulates the pituitary adrenocortical system. The evidence on which these conclusions were based have been reviewed elsewhere (Henry and Ely, 1976; Henry, 1976b) and Fig. 1 summarizes the concepts. Therefore attention will be drawn only to some relevant new work.

Russo et al. (1976) have shown that despite the passive-avoidance learning deficit, which develops after destruction of the amygdala, the pituitary-adrenal response to the stress of active avoidance of foot shock remains unimpaired. This implies independence of the pituitary-adrenal mechanism from the amygdala fight-flight complex. On the other hand, Weiss et al. (1976) show that if paired rats can engage in active aggression with fighting behavior, their exposure to foot shock will not induce as severe a lesion as if they had received equal shock in isolation. Weiss suggests that the act of aggression (with its amygdalar arousal) acts as a relevant feedback and in effect the animal perceives itself as achieving its expectations. This decreases the intensity of the hypothalamoadrenal-cortical response which leads to stomach ulceration (Weiss et al., 1976). The studies of Carroll (1976) fit here, for he has established that the limbic system hypothalamopituitary-adrenal dysfunction with elevated cortisol that occurs in primary depressive illness is not found in secondary depression. He also showed that there is an impaired response to dexamethasone. The stimulus for primary depression, as both Weiss et al. (1976) and Seligman (1975) observe, is the failure to achieve relevant feedback as it occurs when control is attained over the environment. This is effectively demonstrated in the rhesus monkey by the studies of Hanson et al. (1976). Working at the Wisconsin Regional Primate Research Center, they demonstrated the results of giving the animals control over a high intensity noise that would otherwise induce an elevation of plasma cortisol. Primates that can control the noise have no significant elevation, but those exposed to the noise without any possibility or expectation of being able to turn it off show significant diminution of social contact and a marked cortisol response. Animals that were deprived of a control method after successfully learning to use it responded with aggression and had an even greater response. It is compatible with a theory that the hippocampus and the adrenocorticotropic hormone (ACTH) are related to depression which a conservation-withdrawal mode should have developed in subjects that were without expectations. There is a clear contrast here with the aggressive, i.e., amygdalar fight-flight, arousals of subjects whose expectations are so recently denied that they continue to perceive the possibility of regaining control.

This recent work is compatible with the hypothesis that the limbic response patterns of the challenged dominant differ from those of the defeated animal with constricted expectations. We have earlier suggested that as the formerly isolated mice in one of our socially disturbed colonies age, they progress from the dominant to the subordinated pattern: that is, they start with the sympathetic adrenal-medullary fight-flight response in which the renin-angiotensin-catecholamine system is highly activated (Henry et al., 1974). As they age in a socially abrasive situation, they gradually change from aggression toward avoidance. This shift would be associated with neuroendocrine changes which could relate to the incidence of low renin essential hypertension. For if the sympathetic adrenal-medullary system can be aroused by the fight-flight response while the adrenal cortical mechanism is triggered by depression, we may expect different responses from the adrenal cortex as the organism experiences different emotions.

EVIDENCE OF NEURAL CONTROL OF THE ADRENAL CORTEX

The new work of Friedman et al. (1975) indicates that Funkenstein's (1956) early subdivision into anger for norepinephrine and fear for epinephrine may have been correct. They have shown that when the fight response is aroused in a Type A personality, the behavior suggests anger rather than fear; with this there is an increase in norepinephrine. On the other hand, as Mason (1972) notes, epinephrine is associated with generally arousing situations and with the threat of loss of desiderata, such as social status and the access to territory, food and water, and to the attachment figures that go with it. Recently Henry et al. (1976) have shown that in groups of formerly isolated mice that were fighting vigorously because they had never been confronted with other mice, bilateral and even unilateral adrenal denervation led to a failure of the plasma corticosterone to rise. Such animals responded with a normal rise of corticosterone after dosage of adrenocorticotropic hormone (ACTH). Corticosterone response was also normal in mice that had been socialized and then placed in a communal cage where they had to establish a hierarchy. After repeated experiments it appears that the difference was due to the fact that formerly isolated mice are more aroused and fight more vigorously than socialized animals. It is possible that the amygdalar fight-flight response, which involves activation of sympathetic fibers to the adrenal, was more strongly elicited in these formerly isolated groups.

A review of the literature by Kross (1975) showed that the most recent anatomical work on the controversial question of the innervation of the adrenal cortex by Mikhail and Amin (1969) and Unsicker (1971) points to a rich nerve supply. Furthermore, in addition to our own observations (Henry et al., 1976), Paul et al. (1971) present biochemical evidence of the influence of the nerves. For they show that adrenal cortical adenosine 3,5-monophosphate (cyclic AMP) production is reduced following splanchnic denervation. Very recently Ciaranello et al. (1976) have reported that the combination of the foregoing work with the results of their own studies of the regulation of both phenylethanolamine N-methyltransferase (PNMT) and dopamine-β-hydroxylase have led them to conclude that there is autonomic regulation of adrenal corticoidogenesis. Indeed the Axelrod group proposes that steroidogenesis and the delivery of glucocorticoids to the medulla may depend on the action of a permissive receptor at the cortical cell synapse which allows the ACTH to regulate corticoid synthesis. This is a process in which cyclic AMP plays a critical role. The anatomist Mikhail had pointed to the rich nerve supply to the inner zones and suggested that this represents an important factor in the control of the gland in addition to ACTH (Mikhail and Amin, 1969). The biochemical evidence just cited supports this hypothesis.

The fact that there is an active innervation of the adrenal cortex which modifies control by ACTH provides a mechanism by which subtle changes in steroidogenesis might develop, especially if they acted over a long period. Thus it opens a new path to the study of low renin essential hypertension.

ABNORMALITIES OF THE ADRENAL CORTEX AND LOW RENIN ESSENTIAL HYPERTENSION

The evidence that the adrenal cortex may be involved in low renin essential hypertension has been given a suggestive pathophysiological basis by Russell and Masi's (1973) study of 35,000 autopsies at Johns Hopkins Medical School which yielded 870 with adrenal cortical abnormalities. They found evidence of some progression with age, for adenomas were more frequent in the group over

60 years. They established that there was a greater chance ($P < 0.001$) for a hypertensive to have adrenal cortical abnormalities than a matched normotensive control. Gunnells et al. (1970) submitted a group of 32 severe low renin essential hypertensives with a high incidence of plasma sodium-potassium ratio abnormalities to operative intervention. They found that 80% had adenoma or hyperplasia or both. Spark (1972) has pointed out that the effectiveness of a variety of maneuvers directed at the adrenal cortex, such as adrenalectomy, inhibition of steroidogenesis, and peripheral inhibition of mineralocorticoid action by spironolactone all point to the cortex as important in low renin essential hypertension, and Liddle (1973) has discussed the type of mineralocorticoid that may be involved. He, too, was struck by the fact that the mineralocorticoid antagonist spironolactone is only effective in low renin essential hypertension. As Rapp et al. (1973) point out in their study of genetic control of blood pressure and corticosteroid production in rats, an excess of 18-hydroxy-desoxycorticosterone (18-OH-DOC) is found in the adrenals of their salt-sensitive rats. Since these inner zone corticosteroids are not responsive to the feedback loops suppressing the outer zone aldosterone, increases would be particularly serious at high levels of salt intake. The lack of a feedback suppressing the abnormal mineralocorticoid would mean that excessive salt retention might occur despite suppressed aldosterone.

Messerli et al. (1976) have shown that the urinary and plasma levels of 18-OH-DOC were significantly ($P > 0.001$) higher in patients with low plasma renin-angiotensin. In addition, plasma aldosterone was significantly higher in their low renin essential hypertensives than in their controls. Also there was evidence of close interdependence in the secretion of the three mineralocorticoids, i.e., 18-OH-DOC, corticosterone, and desoxycortico-sterone acetate (DOCA) in patients with low renin, but not in normal controls. Interestingly, their patients with low renin essential hypertension were ten years older. They suggest that in essential hypertension there is a biosynthetic variation of the mineralocorticoid pathways but withhold judgment whether these changes are related to the low renin state. These results recall those of Kornel et al. (1975) who show that in essential hypertension the corticosteroid-metabolizing enzymes have aberrant activity. This point is also made by Kittinger and Wexler (1965) in their studies of the hyper-adrenocorticism that develops in rapidly aging breeder rats. They found abnormal dehydrogenase activity in the hyperplastic adrenal cortices of their animals.

LOW RENIN ESSENTIAL HYPERTENSION AS A VARIANT OF CLASSIC PRIMARY ALDOSTERONISM

Recently Grim (1973) has argued that the so-called normal levels of aldosterone in the plasma and urine of low renin essential hypertensives are in fact inappropriately high for the low levels of plasma renin activity. A significant percentage of his patients with low renin had bilateral adrenal hyperplasia. In a clean-cut study, Shade and Grim (1975) have given DOCA and have thus increased extracellular fluid volume and suppressed plasma renin.

268

Their data suggest that the level of aldosterone is unduly elevated in low renin essential hypertension. In an editorial Grim (1975) proposes that the condition is in fact a variant of classic primary aldosteronism. He argues that excessive mineralocorticoid is coming from either an adenoma or as a result of the deranged metabolism of a small group of cells in the inner zones of the cortex.

These observations that aldosterone is in effect increased in low renin essential hypertension would answer the criticism voiced by Dunn and Tannen (1974) in their thoughtful review. They were puzzled by the normal or even high levels of aldosterone reported by Gunnells in his study. The answer, according to Grim, would be that low renin essential hypertension with normal aldosterone actually represents an inappropriate excess that may precede the development of full blown primary aldosteronism.

The adrenal cortex of the low renin essential hypertensive appears to be undergoing progressive disturbance morphologically and biochemically. In his editorial, Grim (1975) proposes that further research should be directed at understanding the primary disturbances leading to an abnormal growth pattern of adrenal cells. One may ask whether it is the combination of intense and sustained autonomic drive together with the endocrine drive operating over the years that eventually leads to the low renin state as a precursor of hyperaldosteronism.

The autonomic input to the adrenal cortex may be a critical factor that has not been considered thus far. We would link it to increasing activation of the depressive conservation-withdrawal pattern in addition to or in place of the sympathetic adrenal-medullary response.

THE CONCORDANCE OF RENIN AND CATECHOLAMINE VALUES IN ESSENTIAL HYPERTENSION

It is relevant that Esler and Nestel (1973) show that with low renin essential hypertension the norepinephrine response to tilting was also decreased. Berglund et al. (1975) report similar results relating low renin to low urinary norepinephrine. Collins et al. (1970) also found that catecholamine excretion was less in low renin hypertensives. By contrast the depressed patients of Louis et al. (1975) had lower blood pressure but higher plasma norepinephrine than low renin hypertensives. Thus in the low renin group, the level of catecholamines does not parallel blood pressure but tends to be depressed. This too would point to a preponderance of the pituitary adrenocortical-depressive over the sympathetic adrenal-medullary response in this type of essential hypertension.

The viewpoint of the Glasgow group as expressed recently by Padfield et al. (1975) is compatible with the previous suggestion of adrenal cortical dysfunction and would help to explain why renin levels can be so low in the aging severe hypertensive. They suspect that it may be due to a progressive failure of the kidney to produce renin. They found no evidence of a separate subpopulation with low renin levels in a group of hypertensives. But the low renin patients were older and there was a significant negative correlation between renin and age. They concluded that plasma renin normally falls with age in essential hypertension and that low renin hypertension is not a separate entity.

EXPERIMENTAL STUDIES WITH COLONIES OF CBA MICE

We may ask at this stage whether our study of socially interacting colonies has thrown any light on this question of a change in the neuroendocrine response patterns and in the type of hypertension as the aging animal changes its perception of the environment. Two areas of observation have provided suggestive clues. The one concerns the changes that develop as mice pass through their life-span in a situation of enhanced social stress. The other is related to neuroendocrine changes that develop as a formerly dominant animal is subordinated and loses control.

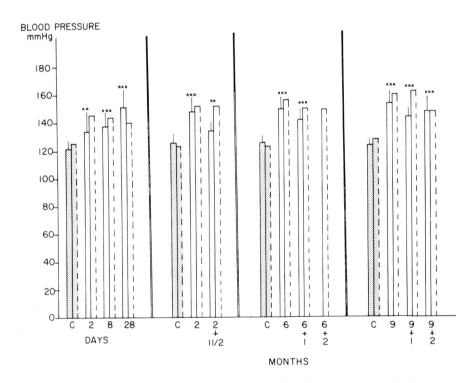

Fig. 2. Average systolic blood pressures of socially disordered colonies of mice terminated after progressively increasing periods of social interaction. The open histograms with solid lines refer to a group of 10 colonies; those to the right with broken lines, to a second study run a year later with 11 colonies. The abscissa represents the number of days or months each of the colonies was exposed to social stimulation in a standard seven-box population cage. The hatched histograms labeled C represent the blood pressures of control groups of mice remaining as siblings in plastic shoe box cages. The different controls approximate the ages of the different subgroups of colonies; +1 and +2 indicate that the males were returned to isolation one or two months before the end of the experiment. The vertical lines represent standard error of the mean, * = $P < 0.05$; ** = $P < 0.01$; *** = $P < 0.001$.

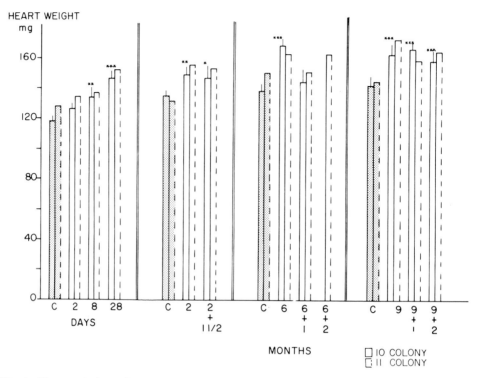

Fig. 3. Heart weights of males in the same two sets of socially disordered colonies whose blood pressures are shown in Fig. 2. The hatched columns represent appropriately aged control groups. As in Fig. 2, they were terminated at 4, 8, 10 and 15 months, respectively. The abscissa and statistical details are the same as in Fig. 2.

We have completed 2 year-long studies of groups of 10 and 11 progressively older colonies. We terminated them after 2, 8, and 21 days and 2, 6, and 9 months of social interaction, respectively. Since the colonies are initiated with fully adult 4-month-old mice, when the 9-month colony is terminated the animals are 13 months old. Since the breeders are considered old at 8—9 months, this represents much of the active life-span. Death from old age occurs between 24 and 30 months. In addition to the 2-, 6- and 9-month colonies, there were 2 + 1, 6 + 1, and 9 + 1 and 9 + 2 colonies in which for a further month or two months the mice were returned to isolation to see if the changes that occurred were reversible.

The results of the blood pressure, heart and adrenal weight observations are presented side by side so that it can be seen how much variability there is from experiment to experiment. Fig. 2 is of the blood pressure. The results of the second study duplicate data that were obtained on the previous occasion except that the pressures are higher, suggesting more intense interaction. The heart weights show similar changes in the two sets of colonies (Fig. 3). Adrenal weights also show the same trends but in keeping with the higher blood pressures were more severely affected in the second study (Fig.4). The adrenals of these aging, competing mice in colonies were significantly increased at the later

271

stages of life. Since 80% of the weight of an adrenal is cortex, this implies that there is adrenal cortical hypertrophy in the older colonies. The question of hyperplastic changes has yet to be answered but work to this end is in progress. A single study has been made of the levels of the catecholamine-synthesizing enzyme tyrosine hydroxylase in the adrenal medulla (Fig. 5). The data suggest high levels of activity at 21 days and at 6 months, but not at 2 months and 9 months. According to the evidence from bites and scarring, there was less fighting when tyrosine hydroxylase was lower. The reason that fighting fell at the 2-month period may have been because the females were breeding actively. It may have risen again at 6 months because the females were now past their reproductive prime. This may have affected the males by making them more prone to fight. Finally at 9 months the mice were fighting less despite the continuing social disorder because they were aging rapidly. Further work is needed and it is anticipated that the results of a second set of tyrosine hydroxylase measurements will be available shortly.

Preliminary observation of renin-angiotensin activity in the socially interacting colonies indicates an increase in the early stages and the rise is

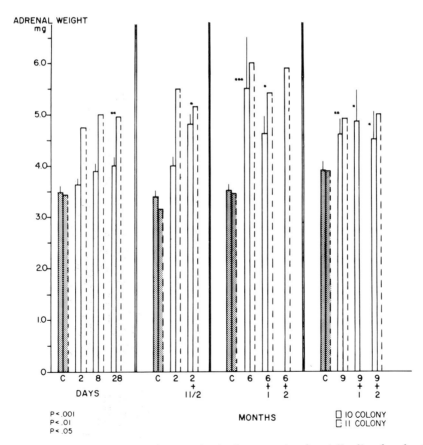

Fig. 4. Absolute adrenal weights of the males in the two sets of socially disordered colonies whose blood pressures are shown in Fig. 2 and heart weights in Fig. 3.

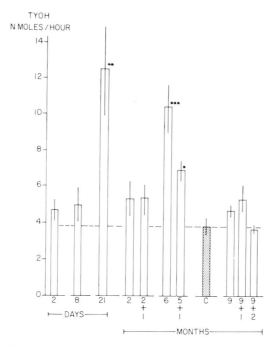

Fig. 5. The tyrosine hydroxylase activity (TYOH) of an n = 8 random sample of the male members of each of the 10 colonies described in Figs. 2—4. The abscissa and statistical details are as before. C represents a control value taken from an n = 15 group of mice that had been isolated for 10 months.

proportional to the intensity of social arousal. Further work is planned, including determination of whether renin-angiotensin activity parallels catecholamine synthesis and whether both become lower as the mutually competitive colonies age. If this is so, then the colonies will be following the pattern shown by aging humans in whom low renin essential hypertension is more frequent.

If the hypertension found in aging mouse colonies is of the low renin type and if it is related to a conservation-withdrawal response by animals that no longer perceive themselves as getting relevant feedback, an increase of the pituitary adrenocortical response can be expected. We have some supporting evidence for this. Two separate assays of adrenal medullary PNMT showed an increase with aging (Fig. 6). This enzyme depends on cortical activity and is responsible for epinephrine biosynthesis. Since the single study of plasma corticosterone showed the same trend (Fig. 7), the combined data support the adrenal weights obtained and point to changes in the cortex as these hypertensive socially disturbed mice age.

Thus our current observations of aging colonies, incomplete as they are, are compatible with the hypothesis that as time goes on the mice could well be developing a low renin essential hypertension and with it a depressive conservation-withdrawal response.

As sketched out previously, Ely's observations of the biochemical changes accompanying the subordination of a former dominant animal support these conclusions (Henry et al., 1974). The corticosterone level in the plasma of a newly subordinated animal rises while there is a fall in the adrenaline-synthesizing enzyme PNMT. His tyrosine hydroxylase, which is important in norepinephrine synthesis, remains elevated. Meanwhile the blood pressure of the now passively avoiding depressed animal rises still further from the elevated value held as a dominant when he was successfully protecting his territory. Plasma renin data unfortunately are not available.

The picture emerging from the studies accomplished to date is compatible with the hypothesis that hypertension in the young animal exposed to challenge has elevated plasma renin and catecholamines and is associated with an aggressive fight-flight behavioral pattern. As CBA mice age they fight less vigorously. At the same time the increase of adrenal weight suggests cortical hypertrophy. There is increased adrenal medullary PNMT and plasma corticosterone is elevated. It remains to be seen whether these aging hypertensive mice that have changed their behavior from an aggressive fight-flight pattern to one of avoidance fit the pattern of low renin essential hypertension.

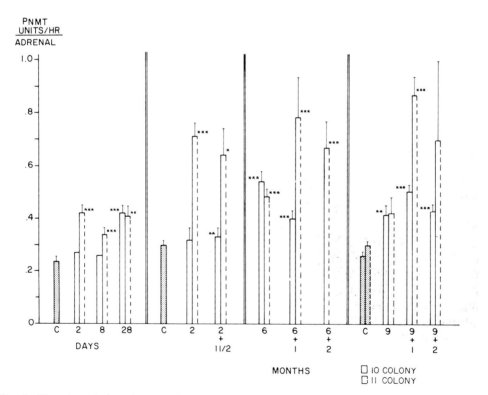

Fig. 6. The phenylethanolamine-N-methyltransferase (PNMT) activities of the same males of the 10 colonies as shown in Fig. 5 (left, solid columns) and of an n = 8 sample of the males in the 11 colonies described in Figs. 2—4 (right, broken columns). Abscissa and statistics are as shown in previous figures.

274

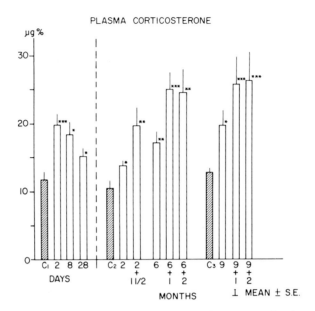

Fig. 7. Plasma corticosterone levels of all males in the group of 11 socially disordered colonies of mice. The abscissa, statistical details, and controls follow the design used in previous figures.

SUMMARY

A distinction is drawn between social stimuli that lead to arousal of the sympathoadrenal medullary as opposed to the hypothalamoadrenocortical system. The former plays a critical role in the mechanism of high renin-high catecholamine hypertension. The latter may be involved in the development of low renin essential hypertension. The recently discovered evidence that autonomic innervation of the adrenal cortex plays a part in steroidogenesis may prove related to the abnormalities in adrenal morphology and in the peculiar biochemical correlates of low renin essential hypertension as a possible variant of primary aldosteronism. Studies of our model of psychosocial hypertension with CBA mice living in a population cage indicate that as the chronically conflicting colonies age, the individual members shift away from a state of high catecholamine sympathetic arousal. The older groups develop fixed hypertension and adrenal hypertrophy with increased corticosterone and PNMT levels. They fight far less and avoid confrontations. It is proposed that under the influence of depression plus arousal repeated stimulation of the autonomic innervation of the adrenal cortex in combination with sustained hormonal drives may lead to the peculiar pathophysiology of low renin essential hypertension.

ACKNOWLEDGEMENTS

This work was supported by the U.S. Public Health Service Grant HL17706 from the National Institutes of Health.

We express our appreciation to Dr. Julius Axelrod of the National Institute of Mental Health for his continuing interest and to Dr. Roland D. Ciaranello of Stanford University, Stanford, California for kindly performing the assays of tyrosine hydroxylase and phenylethanolamine N-methyltransferase. Dr. Arthur Vander and Dr. David Mouw of the University of Michigan, Ann Arbor, Michigan are responsible for the preliminary data on plasma renin assays in a collaborative study which our two groups have just initiated.

REFERENCES

Berglund, G., Aurell, M., Wallentin, I., Wikstrand, J. and Wilhelmsen, L. (1975) Plasma renin activity, sodium excretion and organ manifestations in essential hypertension. In *Pathophysiology and Management of Arterial Hypertension*, G. Berglund, L. Hansson and L. Werkö (Eds.), A. Lindgren and Söner AB, Mölndal, pp. 127—150.

Carroll, B.J. (1976) Limbic system-adrenal cortex regulation in depression and schizophrenia. *Psychosom. Med.*, 38: 106—121.

Ciaranello, R.D., Wooten, G.F. and Axelrod, J. (1976) Regulation of rat adrenal dopamine-β-hydroxylase. II. Receptor interaction in the regulation of enzyme synthesis and degradation. *Brain Res.*, 113: 349—362.

Collins, R.D., Weinberger, M., Gonzales, C., Nokes, G. and Luetscher, J.A. (1970) Catecholamine excretion in low renin hypertension. *Clin. Res.*, 18: 167 (abstr.).

Dunn, M.J. and Tannen, R.L. (1974) Low-renin hypertension (editorial review). *Kidney Int.*, 5: 317—325.

Esler, M.D. and Nestel, P.J. (1973) Renin and sympathetic nervous system responsiveness to adrenergic stimuli in essential hypertension. *Amer. J. Cardiol.*, 32: 643—649.

Friedman, M., Byers, S.O., Diamant, J. and Rosenman, R.H. (1975) Plasma catecholamine response of coronary-prone subjects (Type A) to a specific challenge. *Metabolism*, 24: 205—210.

Funkenstein, D.H. (1956) Norepinephrine-like and epinephrine-like substances in relation to human behavior. *J. nerv. ment. Dis.*, 124: 58—68.

Grim, C.E. (1973) Demonstration of elevated plasma aldosterone in low renin hypertension. *Clin. Res.*, 21: 493 (abstr.).

Grim, C.E. (1975) Low renin "essential" hypertension. A variant of classic primary aldosteronism (editorial). *Arch. intern. Med.*, 135: 347—350.

Gunnells, Jr., J.C., McGuffin, Jr., W.L., Robinson, R.R., Grim, C.E., Wells, S., Silver, D. and Glenn, J.F. (1970) Hypertension, adrenal abnormalities, and alterations in plasma renin activity. *Ann. intern. Med.*, 73: 901—911.

Hanson, J.D., Larson, M.E. and Snowdon, C.T. (1976) The effects of control over high intensity noise on plasma cortisol levels in rhesus monkeys. *Behav. Biol.*, 16: 333—340.

Henry, J.P. (1976a) Understanding the early pathophysiology of essential hypertension. *Geriatrics*, 30: 59—72.

Henry, J.P. (1976b) Mechanisms of psychosomatic disease in animals. *Advanc. vet. Sci.*, 20: 115—145.

Henry, J.P. and Ely, D.L. (1976) Biologic correlates of psychosomatic illness. In *Biological Foundations of Psychiatry*, R.G. Grenell and S. Gabay (Eds.), Raven Press, New York, pp. 945—980.

Henry, J.P., Meehan, J.P. and Stephens, P.M. (1967) The use of psychosocial stimuli to induce prolonged systolic hypertension in mice. *Psychosom. Med.*, 29: 408—432.

Henry, J.P., Ely, D.L., Stephens, P.M., Ratcliffe, H.L., Santisteban, G.A. and Shapiro, A.P. (1971) The role of psychosocial factors in the development of arteriosclerosis in CBA mice: observations on the heart, kidney, and aorta. *Atherosclerosis*, 14: 203—218.

Henry, J.P., Ely, D.L. and Stephens, P.M. (1974) The role of psychosocial stimulation in the pathogenesis of hypertension. *Verh. dtsch. Ges. inn. Med.*, 80: 107—111 and 1724—1740.

Henry, J.P., Stephens, P.M. and Santisteban, G.A. (1975) A model of psychosocial hypertension showing reversibility and progression of cardiovascular complications. *Circulat. Res.*, 36: 156—164.

Henry, J.P., Kross, M.E., Stephens, P.M. and Watson, F.M.C. (1976) Evidence that differing psychosocial stimuli lead to adrenal cortical stimulation by autonomic or endocrine pathways. In *Catecholamines and Stress*, E. Usdin, R. Kvetňanský and I.J. Kopin (Eds.), Pergamon Press, New York, pp. 457—468.

Kittinger, G.W. and Wexler, B.C. (1965) Adrenal gland dehydrogenases and corticosteroid production in normal and arteriosclerotic female rats. *Proc. Soc. exp. Biol. (N.Y.)*, 118: 365—367.

Kornel, L., Miyabo, S., Saito, Z., Cha, R.-W. and Wu, F.-T. (1975) Corticosteroids in human blood. VIII. Cortisol metabolites in plasma of normotensive subjects and patients with essential hypertension. *J. clin. Endocr.*, 40: 949—958.

Kross, M.E. (1975) *Neural Modulation of Adrenal Cortical Function in CBA and NZB Mice*, Ph.D. Dissertation, University of Southern California, Los Angeles.

Liddle, G.W. (1973) Blueprints for the solution of three endocrinological enigmas. *J. Endocr.*, 59: 2—9.

Louis, W.J., Doyle, A.E. and Anavekar, S.N. (1975) Plasma noradrenaline concentration and blood pressure in essential hypertension phaeochromocytoma and depression. *Clin. Sci. molec. Med.*, 48: 239—242.

Mason, J.W. (1972) Organization of psychoendocrine mechanisms: a review and reconsideration of research. In *Handbook of Psychophysiology*, N.S. Greenfield and R.A. Sternbach (Eds.), Holt, Rinehart and Winston, New York, pp. 3—117.

Messerli, F.H., Kuchel, O., Nowaczynski, W., Seth, K., Honda, M., Kubo, S., Boucher, R., Tolis, G. and Genest, J. (1976) Mineralocorticoid secretion in essential hypertension with normal and low plasma renin activity. *Circulation*, 53: 406—410.

Mikhail, Y. and Amin, F. (1969) Intrinsic innervation of the human adrenal gland. *Acta anat. (Basel)*, 72: 25—32.

Padfield, P.L., Brown, J.J., Lever, A.F., Schalekamp, M.A.D., Beevers, D.G., Davies, D.L., Robertson, J.I.S., Tree, M. and Titterington, M. (1975) Is low-renin hypertension a stage in the development of essential hypertension or a diagnostic entity? *Lancet*, i: 548—550.

Paul, M.I., Kvetňanský, R., Cramer, H., Silbergeld, S. and Kopin, I.J. (1971) Immobilization stress induced changes in adrenocortical and medullary cyclic AMP content in the rat. *Endocrinology*, 88: 338—343.

Rapp, J.P., Knudsen, K.D., Iwai, J. and Dahl, L.K. (1973) Genetic control of blood pressure and corticosteroid production in rats. *Circulat. Res.*, 32 and 33, Suppl. I: 139—149.

Rolls, E.T. (1975) *The Brain and Reward*, Pergamon Press, Oxford.

Russell, R.P. and Masi, A.T. (1973) Significant associations of adrenal cortical abnormalities with "essential" hypertension. *Amer. J. Med.*, 54: 44—51.

Russo, II, N.J., Kapp, B.S., Holmquist, B.K. and Musty, R.E. (1976) Passive avoidance and amygdala lesions: relationship with pituitary-adrenal system. *Physiol. Behav.*, 16: 191—199.

Seligman, M.E.P. (1975) *Helplessness: on Depression, Development, and Death*, Freeman, San Francisco, Calif.

Shade, R.E. and Grim, C.E. (1975) Suppression of renin and aldosterone by small amounts of DOCA in normal man. *J. clin. Endocr.*, 40: 652—658.

Spark, R.F. (1972) Low renin hypertension and the adrenal cortex. *New Engl. J. Med.*, 287: 343—349.

Unsicker, K. (1971) On the innervation of the rat and pig adrenal cortex. *Z. Zellforsch.*, 116: 151—156.

Weiss, J.M., Pohorecky, L.A., Salman, S. and Gruenthal, M. (1976) Attenuation of gastric lesions by psychological aspects of aggression in rats. *J. comp. physiol. Psychol.*, 90: 252—259.

Pituitary Neuropeptides, Emotional Behavior and Cardiac Responses

BÉLA BOHUS

Rudolf Magnus Institute for Pharmacology, Medical Faculty, University of Utrecht, Utrecht (The Netherlands)

INTRODUCTION

The organisms' adaptation to environmental influences requires a chain of behavioral, autonomic, endocrine and metabolic responses in order to preserve homeostasis. The integration of these adaptive functions is assured through central nervous control mechanisms. The pituitary gland and its target organ hormones serve an important modulatory function in the adaptive processes. It was recognized more than a quarter of a century ago that not only physical or chemical but also merely psychological stress activated the pituitary-adrenal axis (Selye, 1950). Since that time a large number of publications indicate that subtle psychological stimuli present during everyday life and provoking changes in emotionality (fear, anxiety, disappointment, etc.) are among the most potent stressors which elicit the release of ACTH (Mason, 1968), MSH (Sandman et al., 1973), and vasopressin (Thompson and De Wied, 1973). On the other hand, evidence collected during the last decade clearly indicates that the release of these pituitary hormones is not merely a concomitant of emotional behavior. It became increasingly clear that the brain serves as a target organ of pituitary peptide hormones and their central effects result in alterations of behavioral adaptation (see De Wied and Weijnen, 1970; Zimmermann et al., 1973; Gispen et al., 1975). The most prominent feature of the research on endocrine-behavioral interactions is the recognition that the behaviorally active entities of the hypothalamo-pituitary peptides related to ACTH, MSH and vasopressin are practically devoid of target gland effects such as stimulation of the adrenal cortex, melanocyte-stimulating activity or antidiuretic and pressor action, and yet these pituitary gland peptides, designated as neuropeptides, are involved in the formation and maintenance of new behavior patterns subserving adaptation (De Wied, 1969). Recent observations demonstrating opiate-like peptides in the brain originating from pituitary β-LPH (Hughes et al., 1975; Bradbury et al., 1976; Guillemin et al., 1976) reinforce the neuropeptide hypothesis and further suggest that numerous, centrally controlled adaptive functions may be modulated by pituitary neuropeptides.

Changes in cardiovascular function due to psychic (emotional) stress are one of the most prominent reactions of the organism. The relationship between behavior and cardiovascular responses has been the subject of continuing interest, although psychophysiological research on the cardiovascular system is a rather controversial area of neurobiology. Heart rate changes observed during emotional behavior have been viewed as reflections of arousal, motivation, attention or somatic activity related to behavioral coping (Gantt, 1960; Malmo and Bélanger, 1964; Black, 1965; Obrist et al., 1970).

Our interest in cardiovascular changes related to emotional behavior stems from the need to learn about the role and the mechanism of action of pituitary neuropeptides in centrally controlled adaptive processes. A psychophysiological approach provides the means to understand the physiology of the neuropeptides. Moreover, indications of the eventual pathological consequence of increased production or absence of neuropeptides on cardiovascular function may be obtained.

PASSIVE AVOIDANCE BEHAVIOR AND HEART RATE CHANGES IN THE RAT

To study cardiovascular and behavioral relationships demands a precise control of both behavioral and autonomic responses. Accordingly, our first effort was to select a paradigm of emotional behavior in which behavior of the rats is highly predictable and the effect of the psychological stimulus (conditioned fear) can be studied separately from that of the physical stress which leads to the emotional experience. A one-trial learning passive avoidance paradigm in a step-through type situation meets these criteria. This paradigm uses the innate preference of the rat for darkness rather than light (Ader et al., 1972). From the elevated, illuminated platform of the apparatus the rat enters the dark, large compartment within a few seconds. After 4 pre-training trials the rat receives a single unavoidable electric footshock immediately after entering the dark compartment. Learning experience as tested 24 hr later is manifested by readily avoiding re-entering the dark compartment from the platform. In these and subsequent experiments the electrocardiogram of free-moving rats was recorded from transcutaneous electrodes with the aid of radiotelemetry (Bohus, 1974). Electrocardiograms were recorded during the 4th pre-training trial and through the passive avoidance retention test 24 hr after the single learning trial. A PDP-8/I computer was used for off-line analysis which consisted of the measurement of R-R intervals and computation of mean heart rate (HR), R-R interval distribution histogram and the trend of HR changes.

Passive avoidance behavior of the rats depends upon the intensity of the aversive stimulus at the learning trial. The stronger the aversive stimulus, the more time the animal takes to re-enter the dark compartment (latency) at the retention test 24 hr later. This emotional behavior of the rats appears to be accompanied by tonic and phasic changes in cardiac rhythm. Tonic changes are represented by a decrease in mean HR during avoidance behavior relative to pre-learning values. The degree of bradycardia again depends upon the intensity of the aversive stimulus; the more pronounced bradycardia occurs after the higher intensity shock punishment (Table I). A close correlation between

TABLE I

CARDIAC RESPONSES OF RATS DURING PASSIVE AVOIDANCE BEHAVIOR 24 hr AFTER THE LEARNING TRIAL

Aversive stimulus intensity (mA for 1 sec)	0.0	0.25	0.5
Passive avoidance latency (sec)	5.0[§]	17.0[††]	209.0[††]
Tonic HR response (bpm)*	-2.0 ± 2.6[§§]	-18.3 ± 3.8[††]	-28.6 ± 3.2[††]
Phasic HR response (bpm)**	-0.5 ± 0.9	-13.8 ± 1.1[†]	-14.2 ± 0.9[†]
Duration of phasic response***	30.0	25.2	16.8

*Mean heart rate (HR) during passive avoidance behavior minus mean HR during the last pre-shock trial.

**Mean HR during approaching shock compartment minus mean HR during non-approach periods of avoidance behavior.

***Relative duration of approaching shock compartment in % of total avoidance latency.

[§] Median.

[§§] Mean ± S.E.M.

[†] $P < 0.05$.

[††] $P < 0.01$.

individual passive avoidance latencies used as the behavioral measure and mean HR change is, however, absent. Accordingly, tonic change in HR reflects the intensity of punishment leading to emotional experience but in individual rats, it is unrelated to the actual behavioral performance.

Analysis of beat-to-beat changes during passive avoidance behavior shows that phasic changes in HR occur in the form of abrupt bradycardia and arrhythmia which accompany approach-avoidance movements. This locomotor activity is typical of conflict situations. From time to time, the rat approaches or partially enters the dark compartment. Approach behavior regularly coincides with an immediate decrease in HR and sometimes arrhythmia is coupled with this behavior. Computing mean HR for approach and non-approach periods indicates that phasic bradycardia is only present after the aversive learning experience but its magnitude does not correlate with the intensity of punishment during the learning trial.

That these abrupt changes in HR occur only after aversive experience indicates that phasic changes are rather specific signs of conditioned fear. This statement is further supported by the fact that the blocking of approach responses in non-punished rats by lowering the sliding door between the elevated platform and the dark compartment results in phasic increase rather than a decrease in HR.

Phasic changes in HR in the form of arrhythmia occur independently from approach-avoidance movements as well. These changes are however rather infrequent and of short duration. The rat is always motionless in these periods. The appearance of these arrhythmic phases do not relate to any parameters of the passive avoidance paradigm nor to behavioral activities during avoidance behavior.

Recent trends in psychophysiological research concerning the relations between the functioning of heart and behavioral processes claim the importance of cardiac-somatic coupling (Obrist et al., 1974). It is suggested that vagally mediated HR changes are only relevant to behavioral processes to the extent to which these reflect the activity of the muscles. Since both phasic and tonic changes in HR during passive avoidance behavior appear in the form of bradycardia it seemed worthwhile to analyze the somatic activity of the rats during passive avoidance and to compute mean HR for each gross bodily activity. Although somatic activities during passive avoidance behavior such as walking, sniffing, rearing and grooming slightly increase HR, the differences as compared to the motionless state are not significant. In contrast, these somatic activities significantly increase HR when the rat has not had an aversive experience. Accordingly, conditioned emotionality attenuates the somatic influences on the functioning of the heart. These observations further indicate that both the phasic and tonic changes in HR during passive avoidance behavior are due to psychic rather than somatic influences on cardiac rhythm regulation.

Because of the primary importance of psychic mechanisms underlying passive avoidance behavior in the functioning of the heart, regulation of the cardiac rhythm during this emotional behavior has been analyzed by computing R-R interval distribution histograms. In the rat R-R intervals fall in the range of 90—210 msec (270—660 bpm). A class-width of 5 msec was used for the distribution analysis and the proportion of R-R intervals falling within a class is expressed in percentage of the total intervals recorded during the entire avoidance period.

Histograms taken from ECG records during the retention test from non-punished rats or from those receiving low or high shock intensity punishment 24 hr before are depicted in Fig. 1. Aversive experience during the single learning trial results in a shift of the dominant R-R frequency to the right, i.e., the highest percent of the R-R intervals in the rats receiving aversive experience falls into a longer R-R interval class than in the non-punished controls. Although the dominant R-R frequency falls in the same interval class independent of the intensity of shock punishment, the percentage of R-R intervals within this range is lower in rats which had been exposed to a stronger aversive stimulus and a high percentage of intervals appear in the longer interval classes. This indicates that the more pronounced bradycardia after high intensity shock punishment is mainly due to a less regular heart rhythm and the incidence of long R-R intervals is markedly increased.

Taken together, analysis of HR changes in the step-through one-trial learning passive avoidance situation indicates that this conditioned emotional behavior is accompanied by tonic and phasic changes in cardiac rhythm. Tonic changes as represented by a decrease in mean HR are primarily due to a shift of the dominant R-R frequency to the direction of longer R-R intervals and the irregularity of cardiac rhythm is increased with the intensity of punishment. Phasic changes appear as abrupt decrease in HR or arrhythmia and are related to approach-avoidance movements which are relevant behavioral activities in a conflict situation. The rate of phasic changes is independent of the intensity of aversive experience. Accordingly, tonic HR changes reflect conditioned emotionality changes dependent upon the intensity of aversive experience

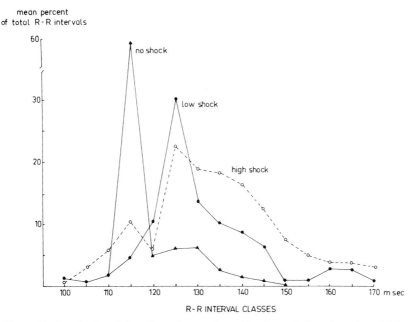

Fig. 1. The effect of the intensity of aversive stimulus at the learning trial on the distribution pattern of R-R intervals during the retention test.

while phasic changes are probably correlates of a more specific discriminative function and reflect the conditioned fear response.

PITUITARY NEUROPEPTIDES AND CARDIAC RESPONSES ACCOMPANYING PASSIVE AVOIDANCE BEHAVIOR

Pituitary neuropeptides related to ACTH or vasopressin influence motivational, learning and memory processes. Behavioral observations indicate that peptides related to ACTH affect motivational processes while vasopressin and its analogs improve consolidation and/or retrieval of memory (De Wied et al., 1975a). Behavioral effect of these peptides is not distinguishable when treatment is given prior to the retention test 24 hr after the single learning trial in the passive avoidance situation. Both $ACTh_{4-10}$ and desglycinamide-lysine vasopressin (DG-LVP), which are practically devoid of classical endocrine activities (De Wied, 1969; De Wied et al., 1972), increase the time the rat takes to re-enter the former shock compartment. Cardiac responses accompanying passive avoidance behavior of peptide-treated rats are, however, different (Bohus, 1975; Bohus et al., 1976). Enhanced passive avoidance in rats treated with $ACTH_{4-10}$ is accompanied by an increase in mean HR relative to pre-learning values. Tonic HR response in rats receiving DG-LVP is bradycardia. The degree of HR decrease is however more pronounced in the peptide treated rats than in controls which received the same punishment during the learning trial (Table II).

282

TABLE II

EFFECTS OF PITUITARY NEUROPEPTIDES ON PASSIVE AVOIDANCE
BEHAVIOR AND ACCOMPANYING CARDIAC RESPONSES IN THE RAT

Treatment*	Saline	$ACTH_{4-10}$	DG-LVP
Passive avoidance latency (sec)	17.0	47.5**	43.0**
Tonic HR response (bpm)	-18.3 ± 3.8	$+20.0 \pm 8.8$***	-32.3 ± 5.4**
Phasic HR response (bpm)	-13.8 ± 1.1	-11.7 ± 2.1	-28.6 ± 1.3**
Duration of phasic response	25.2	27.5	15.8

*Treatment was given subcutaneously 1 hr prior to the retention test in doses of 15 μg
of $ACTH_{4-10}$ and 0.5 μg of DG-LVP (desglycinamide-lysine vasopressin).
**$P < 0.05$.
***$P < 0.01$.

Distribution pattern of R-R intervals, as it is depicted in Fig. 2, is also
differently affected by these neuropeptides. $ACTH_{4-10}$ increases the incidence of shorter R-R intervals but does not cause a shift in the dominant
frequency. In contrast, DG-LVP treatment results in a shift in the dominant
R-R interval in the direction of a longer interval class and the right-hand tail of
the histogram slopes far more gradually, indicating a higher incidence of longer
R-R intervals. Accordingly, $ACTH_{4-10}$ and DG-LVP differentially affect tonic

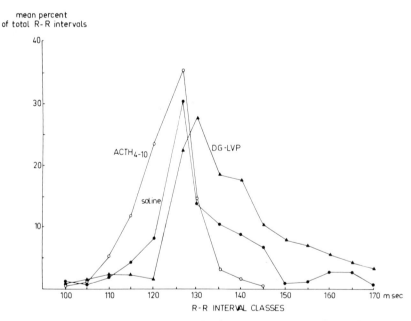

Fig. 2. Distribution pattern of R-R intervals during passive avoidance behavior in rats
treated with $ACTH_{4-10}$ or desglycinamide-lysine vasopressin (DG-LVP)

changes in HR accompanying seemingly identical passive avoidance behavior. Phasic changes in HR are, however, qualitatively the same in the two groups. Approaching the dark compartment is accompanied by abrupt bradycardia as in the controls. The degree of bradycardia, however, is more pronounced in DG-LVP treated rats than in controls or those which received $ACTH_{4-10}$.

These observations indicate that tonic HR responses may differentiate brain mechanisms which are involved in the behavioral effect of peptides related to ACTH or vasopressin. High incidence of short R-R intervals, as observed in rats receiving $ACTH_{4-10}$, suggests that sympathetic influences on HR which are normally minimal are facilitated by this neuropeptide. This suggestion is supported by the observation showing that neonatal chemical sympathectomy prevents the appearance of shorter R-R intervals during passive avoidance behavior in rats treated with $ACTH_{4-10}$ (Bohus et al., 1976). Contemporary psychophysiological research maintains that HR does not provide a simple, unidimensional measure of brain processes underlying behavior such as motivational or affective states. Moreover, it seems that the vagally mediated HR in a mildly stressful behavioral paradigm is related to attentional and expectancy processes while sympathetic influences are evoked by more intense stress in which the organism is actively engaged in the preparation or execution of activities that will cope with the stress (Obrist et al., 1974; Pribram and McGuiness, 1975). Accordingly, increased sympathetic activity in $ACTH_{4-10}$ treated rats may reflect a facilitated arousal state which increases the probability of a given behavioral performance in emotional situations. That the phasic HR response of $ACTH_{4-10}$ treated rats is in the same direction as in the controls (bradycardia) suggests that increased arousal increases the probability of the specific behavioral response which is accompanied by specific phasic HR response. Facilitated arousal by $ACTH_{4-10}$ has also been indicated by electrophysiological studies (Urban and De Wied, 1976) and by observations on HR changes during classical fear conditioning (Bohus, 1973, 1975).

The more pronounced tonic and phasic bradycardiac changes in HR relative to controls in rats receiving DG-LVP suggest that this vasopressin related peptide facilitates memory processes, and these processes exert their cardiac control through vagal innervation. That both the tonic and phasic bradycardia result from a central vagal influence rather than a baroreceptor mediated adjustment of cardiac rhythm, is suggested by observations in neonatally sympathectomized rats. Neonatal chemical sympathectomy attenuates blood pressure increase during classical emotional conditioning (Pappas and DiCara, 1973) and blocks the pressor response to electrical stimulation of the posterior hypothalamus (Provoost et al., 1974), but fails to affect the direction of tonic and phasic changes in HR during passive avoidance behavior (Bohus et al., 1976).

BEHAVIORAL AND CARDIAC CONSEQUENCES OF THE GENETICAL ABSENCE OF VASOPRESSIN

The observations on rats treated with pituitary neuropeptides indicate that the same form of behavioral expression of emotion need not necessarily be accompanied by the same tonic cardiac reaction. One of the alternatives is that the same behavioral expression may occur under different emotional impact. However, it is not unlikely that the behavioral and autonomic changes are under parallel but separate control by the same environmental stimulus events which evoke alterations in emotionality. This alternative may be of primary importance in psychosomatic disorders. Pituitary peptides which are released during the re-appearance of specific environmental cues associated with aversive, "stressful" experience may act as chemical messengers to modify both the expression of behavior and autonomic responses.

Parallel but separate control of behavioral and tonic but not of phasic cardiac response during passive avoidance behavior is indicated by observations on rats with hereditary hypothalamic diabetes insipidus (Bohus et al., 1975a). That vasopressin is physiologically involved in memory processes, has been demonstrated in rats with hereditary hypothalamic diabetes insipidus (De Wied et al., 1975b; Bohus et al., 1975b). Homozygous diabetes insipidus (HO-DI) rats lack the ability to synthetize vasopressin while their heterozygous littermates (HE) have a relatively normal water metabolism (Valtin and Schroeder, 1964). Severe memory impairment was observed in HO-DI rats in a one-trial learning passive avoidance test. Heterozygous rats exhibited full avoidance behavior. Memory impairment of HO-DI rats can be restored by the administration of either arginine vasopressin (AVP) or DG-LVP immediately after the learning trial.

Impairment of passive avoidance behavior in HO-DI rats 24 hr after the learning trial is, however, not associated with an impairment of tonic HR changes. Decrease in mean HR relative to pre-learning values during the passive avoidance test is in the same order of magnitude as in the HE rats in spite of the marked behavioral difference. Phasic changes in HR are however absent in HO-DI rats (Table III). Administration of AVP or DG-LVP immediately after the learning trial or prior to the retention test normalizes behavior and phasic

TABLE III

PASSIVE AVOIDANCE BEHAVIOR AND CARDIAC RESPONSES IN RATS WITH HEREDITARY DIABETES INSIPIDUS; EFFECTS OF VASOPRESSIN TREATMENT

Strain	Treatment*	Passive avoidance latency (sec)	Tonic HR** response	Phasic HR** response
Heterozygous	—	300.0	−19.4 ± 4.7	−22.6 ± 4.1
Homozygous DI	—	15.0	−21.2 ± 12.5	−2.8 ± 4.1
	Arginine VP			
	after learning	300.0	−70.6 ± 4.5	−29.2 ± 3.5
	before retention	300.0	−65.7 ± 4.1	−28.7 ± 6.2
	DG-LVP			
	after learning	300.0	−50.2 ± 8.6	−31.9 ± 4.9
	before retention	227.0	−30.6 ± 3.5	−29.4 ± 6.5

*Both peptides were given subcutaneously in a dose of 1 µg/rat either immediately after the learning trial of 1 hr prior to the retention test.
**In bpm.

changes in HR which accompany passive avoidance behavior. R-R interval distribution histograms indicate that the HR of HO-DI rats is quite irregular. A dominant R-R frequency is almost absent and R-R intervals are distributed in a rather wide range. Administration of AVP but only prior to the retention test partially normalizes the distribution pattern. This suggests that parallel to the neuropeptide function at least, the full vasopressin molecule may play some role in the cardiovascular regulation during emotional stress.

The observations indicate that in the absence of vasopressin and related peptides emotional experience is preserved as indicated by tonic changes in HR, but due to memory deficit, the rat is not able to cope adequately with his behavior to environmental stimuli. The absence of phasic HR changes accompanying inadequate coping behavior and its reappearance during normalised behavior reinforces the notion that phasic changes in HR specifically reflect conditioned fear in this emotional situation.

GENERAL CONCLUSIONS

Subtle aversive experience which only slightly affects cardiovascular function acts as a powerful psychic stressor whenever the specific environmental cues reappear. While tonic changes in HR during emotional behavior in the passive avoidance situation are correlates of a generalized conditioned behavioral change, phasic responses may be viewed as specific signs of a highly discriminative fear response. Pituitary neuropeptides related to ACTH or vasopressin affect emotional behavior and influence HR changes accompanying behavioral adaptation. Tonic changes in HR during emotional behavior differentiate between central nervous mechanisms responsible for the behavioral effects of neuropeptides. Our research does not yet allow conclusions as to whether neuropeptides are involved in the development of pathological cardiovascular changes due to psychic stressor stimuli. It may be noted, however, that both exogenous administration of neuropeptides and the genetic absence of vasopressin appear to increase the irregularity of cardiac rhythm during emotional behavior. Furthermore, psychological stress, which is followed by pituitary peptide release, increases the probability of ventricular fibrillation in the dog (Lown et al., 1973). Removal of the pituitary, on the other hand, which results in learning deficit (De Wied, 1964) prevents the development of sound-withdrawal hypertension in the rat (Marwood et al., 1973). Accordingly, further research on the relation of neuropeptides and psychosomatic disorders has promising perspectives.

SUMMARY

Pituitary neuropeptides related to ACTH or vasopressin affect brain functions and modify behavioral adaptation. The effect of these peptides on cardiac responses accompanying emotional behavior has been studied in the rat in a passive avoidance situation. Passive avoidance behavior is accompanied by tonic and phasic changes in cardiac rhythm. Tonic changes appear as a decrease in mean heart rate as a consequence of emotional experience. Phasic changes are related to approach-avoidance movements in the conflict situation and appear as an abrupt decrease in heart rate or arrhythmias. Pituitary peptides related to ACTH facilitate emotional behavior and tonic HR response appears as tachycardia. Analysis of R-R interval distribution histograms indicate increased arousal and consequent sympathetic activation. Neuropeptides related to vasopressin also facilitate passive avoidance behavior but a more pronounced deceleration of HR accompanies behavior and the irregularity of cardiac rhythm increases. Genetic absence of vasopressin in rats with hereditary hypothalamic diabetes insipidus leads to a deficit in behavioral expression of emotional experience, phasic HR changes are absent but tonic response is present. Vasopressin and related peptides normalise behavioral and cardiac deficits.

ACKNOWLEDGEMENT

A grant from the Dr. Saal van Zwanenbergstichting provided the means for the basic instrumentation used in the present experiments.

REFERENCES

Ader, R., Weijnen, J.A.W.M. and Moleman, P. (1972) Retention of a passive avoidance response as a function of the intensity and duration of electric shock. *Psychon. Sci,*, 26: 125—128.

Black, A.H. (1965) Cardiac conditioning in curarized dogs: the relationship between heart rate and skeletal behavior. In *Classical Conditioning: a Symposium*, W.F. Prokasy (Ed.), Appleton-Century-Crofts, New York, pp. 20—47.

Bohus, B. (1973) Pituitary-adrenal influences on avoidance and approach behavior of the rat. In *Drug Effects on Neuroendocrine Regulation, Progress in Brain Research, Vol. 39*, E. Zimmermann, W.H. Gispen, B.H. Marks and D. De Wied (Eds.), Elsevier, Amsterdam, pp. 407—420.

Bohus, B. (1974) Telemetered heart rate responses of the rat during free and learned behavior. *Biotelemetry*, 1: 193—201.

Bohus, B. (1975) Pituitary peptides and adaptive autonomic responses. In *Hormones, Homeostasis and the Brain, Progress in Brain Research, Vol. 42*, W.H. Gispen, Tj.B. Van Wimersma Greidanus, B. Bohus and D. De Wied (Eds.), Elsevier, Amsterdam, pp. 275—283.

Bohus, B., Van Wimersma Greidanus, Tj.B., De Jong, W. and De Wied, D. (1975) Behavioral, autonomic and endocrine responses during passive avoidance in rats with hereditary hypothalamic diabetes insipidus (Brattleboro strain). *Exp. Brain Res.*, 23, Suppl.: 25.

Bohus, B., Van Wimersma Greidanus, Tj.B. and De Wied, D. (1976) Behavioral and endocrine responses of rats with hereditary hypothalamic diabetes insipidus (Brattleboro strain). *Physiol. Behav.*, 14: 609—615.

Bohus, B., De Jong, W., Provoost, A.P. und De Wied, D. (1976) Emotionales Verhalten und Reaktionen des Kreislaufs und Endokriniums bei Ratten. In *Seelische und körperliche Störungen durch Stress*, A.W. Von Eiff (Ed.), Gustav Fischer Verlag, Stuttgart, pp. 140—157.

Bradbury, A.F., Smyth, D.G., Snell, C.R., Birdsall, N.J.M. and Hulme, E.C. (1976) The C-fragment of lipotropin: an endogenous peptide with high affinity for brain opiate receptors. *Nature (Lond.)*, 260: 793—795.

De Wied, D. (1964) Influence of anterior pituitary on avoidance learning and escape behavior. *Amer. J. Physiol.*, 207: 255—259.

De Wied, D. (1969) Effects of peptide hormones on behavior. In *Frontiers in Neuroendocrinology*, W.F. Ganong and L. Martini (Eds.), Oxford Univ. Press, New York, pp. 97—140.

De Wied, D. and Weijnen, J.A.W.M. (Eds.) (1970) *Pituitary, Adrenal and the Brain, Progress in Brain Research, Vol. 32*, Elsevier, Amsterdam.

De Wied, D., Greven, H.M., Lande, S. and Witter, A. (1972) Dissociation of the behavioural and endocrine effects of lysine vasopressin by tryptic digestion. *Brit. J. Pharmacol.*, 45: 118—122.

De Wied, D., Bohus, B., Gispen, W.H., Urban, I and Van Wimersma Greidanus, Tj.B. (1975a) Pituitary peptides on motivational, learning and memory processes. In *Proc. VIth Int. Congr. Pharmacology, Helsinki, Vol. 3*, J. Tuomisto and M.K. Paasonen (Eds.), pp. 19—30.

De Wied, D., Bohus, B. and Van Wimersma Greidanus, Tj.B. (1975b) Memory deficit in rats with hereditary diabetes insipidus. *Brain Res.*, 85: 152—156.

Gantt, W.H. (1960) Cardiovascular component of the conditioned reflex to pain, food and other stimuli. *Physiol. Rev.*, 40, Suppl. 4: 266—291.

Gispen, W.H., Van Wimersma Greidanus, Tj.B., Bohus, B. and De Wied, D. (Eds.) (1975) *Hormones, Homeostasis and the Brain, Progress in Brain Research, Vol. 42*, Elsevier, Amsterdam.

Guillemin, R., Ling, N. et Burgus, R. (1976) Endorphines, peptides d'origine hypothalamique et neurohypophysaire à l'activité morphinomimétique. Isolement et structure moléculaire d'α-endorphine. *C.R. Acad. Sci. (Paris)*, 282: 1—5.

Hughes, J., Smith, T.W., Kosterlitz, H.W., Fothergill, L.A., Morgan, B.A. and Morris, H.R. (1975) Identification of two related glutapeptides from the brain with potent opiate agonist activity. *Nature (Lond.)*, 258: 557—579.

Lown, B., Verrier, R. and Corbalan, R. (1973) Psychologic stress and treshold for repetitive ventricular response. *Science*, 182: 834—836.

Malmo, R.B. and Bélanger, D. (1967) Related physiological and behavioral changes: what are their determinants? *Res. Publ. Ass. nerv. ment. Dis.*, 45: 288—313.

Marwood, J.F., Ilett, K.F. and Lockett, M.F. (1973) Effects of adrenalectomy and of hypophysectomy on the development of sound-withdrawal hypertension. *J. Pharm. Pharmacol.*, 25: 96—100.

Mason, J.W. (1968) A review of psychoneuroendocrine research on the pituitary-adrenal cortical system. *Psychosom. Med.*, 30: 576—607.

Obrist, P.A., Webb, R.A., Sutterer, J.R. and Howard, J.L. (1970) The cardiac-somatic relationship: some reformulations. *Psychophysiology*, 6: 569—587.

Obrist, P.A., Lawler, J.E. and Gaebelein, C.J. (1974) A psychobiological perspective on the cardiovascular system. In *Limbic and Autonomic Nervous Systems Research*, L.V. DiCara (Ed.), Plenum Press, New York, pp. 311—334.

Pappas, B.A. and DiCara, L.V. (1973) Neonatal sympathectomy by 6-hydroxydopamine: cardiovascular responses in the paralyzed rat. *Physiol. Behav.*, 10: 549—553.

Pribram, K.H. and McGuiness, D. (1975) Arousal, activation, and effort in the control of attention. *Psychol. Rev.*, 82: 116—149.

Provoost, A.P., Bohus, B. and De Jong, W. (1974) Neonatal chemical sympathectomy: functional control of denervation of the vascular system and tissue noradrenaline level in the rat after 6-hydroxydopamine. *Naunyn-Schmiedeberg's Arch. exp. Path. Pharmak.*, 284: 353—363.

Sandman, C.A., Kastin, A.J., Schally, A.V., Kendall, J.W. and Miller, L.H. (1973) Neuroendocrine responses to physical and psychological stress. *J. comp. physiol. Psychol.*, 84: 386—390.

Selye, H. (1950) *Stress. The Physiology and Pathology of Exposure to Stress*, Acta Medica Publication, Montreal.

Thompson, E.A. and De Wied, D. (1973) The relationship between the antidiuretic activity of rat eye plexus blood and passive avoidance behaviour. *Physiol. Behav.*, 11: 377—380.

Urban, I. and De Wied, D. (1976) Changes in excitability in the theta activity generating substrate by $ACTH_{4-10}$ in the rat. *Exp. Brain Res.*, 24: 325—334.

Valtin, H. and Schroeder, H.A. (1964) Familial hypothalamic diabetes insipidus in rats (Brattleboro strain). *Amer. J. Physiol.*, 206: 425—430.

Zimmermann, E., Gispen, W.H., Marks, B.H. and De Wied, D. (Eds.) (1973) *Drug Effects on Neuroendocrine Regulation, Progress in Brain Research, Vol. 39*, Elsevier, Amsterdam.

Stress Reactions of Normotensives and Hypertensives and the Influence of Female Sex Hormones on Blood Pressure Regulation

A.W. VON EIFF and CLAUS PIEKARSKI

Department of Internal Medicine, Bonn Medical School, Bonn University,
5300 Bonn-Venusberg (G.F.R.)

The central nervous system (CNS) has been known for some time to play a certain role in the pathogenesis of essential hypertension. Mostly the CNS has been regarded within multifactorial occurrences, as for instance in Page's Mosaic-Theory (1960).

THEORY OF THE ROLE OF THE HYPOTHALAMUS IN ESSENTIAL HYPERTENSION

Experimental results obtained in the last 10 years have now given us the knowledge to put the CNS into its proper position (Folkow and Rubinstein, 1966; Henry and Cassel, 1969; Henry et al., 1972; Okamoto et al., 1972; Harris and Forsyth, 1973; Brod, 1974; Schaefer, 1974; Richter and Heinrich et al., 1976). In 1957 investigations on stress-response of the autonomic nervous system of normotensives and patients suffering from essential hypertension were started during an interdisciplinary long term study on hypertension (von Eiff et al., 1967). Several different stressors, simulating certain life situations, were used. In order to properly estimate the stress response, comparative tests were carried out under strict basic metabolic conditions in hyper- and normotensive subjects. A number of physiological reactions reflecting the activity of the autonomic nervous system varied proportionately to resting blood pressure in male and female subjects under strict resting conditions. Thus, involuntary muscle activity and the rate of metabolism were likewise proportionate to the blood pressure at rest; they were higher in the group of hypertensives than in the group of normotensives (Fig. 1).

What do these phenomena point out? Up to the present day we regard it to be most probable that this behaviour of the autonomic functions of hypertensives results from an abnormal activity of a cerebral area responsible for blood pressure as well as for muscle tone regulation. The fact that muscle tone was involved excluded a possible localisation in the vasomotor centre of the medulla oblongata. Above all an area in the posterior hypothalamus, first described by W.R. Hess (1947, 1948), seemed to be responsible for these phenomena. He called this area "the dynamogenic zone", which could create

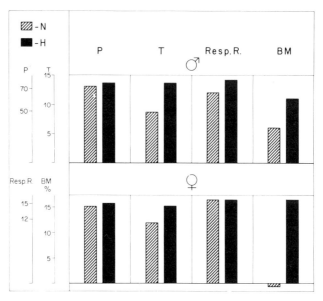

Fig. 1. Reactions of pulse rate (P), muscle tone (T), respiration rate (Resp. R.) and rate of basal metabolism (BM) under strict resting conditions in 65 normotensive (N) and 60 hypertensive (H) subjects.

defence and attack behaviour and accordingly blood pressure and muscle tone rises in the animal experiment.

The following assertions were made on the basis of the above mentioned investigations and other findings (von Eiff, 1972; von Eiff et al., 1967).

(1) Essential hypertension is primarily based on a single pathogenetic mechanism, which consists of a hyperactivity of hypothalamic structures of the sympathetic nervous system.

(2) In this hyperactivity, hereditary and environmental factors, i.e., stressors and personality, play a decisive role.

(3) Hypothalamic hyperactivity may directly provoke (a) hormonal mechanisms in the adrenal gland, (b) reduced renal blood flow with increased production of renin and (c) indirectly produce damages in the vascular system through hypertension itself, especially in the carotid sinus in the very early phase.

These mechanisms suggest that hypertension may exist independently from any central nervous activity. Hypotheses of this kind can only be verified by animal experiments or further conclusions from analogy.

WAYS OF MODIFYING BLOOD PRESSURE REGULATION

Postulating also that stressors were involved in this hypothalamic hyperactivity, our team was interested to find out some factors which may influence stress response of autonomic functions. Some results are reported in the following.

(I) Stress reactions are subject to the individually varying ability of adaptation

Under resting conditions, when a second test was carried out, a reduced activity of various body functions was observed. A reduced response being statistically significant was specified as "effect of adaptation". In a test series (Fig. 2) an effect of adaptation was only statistically significant for systolic blood pressure at rest and during stimulus, which consisted of a simple task of arithmetic. The subjects were normotensives.

More subtle insight into the ability of adaptation was obtained, when some tests on the influence of noise were carried out in our laboratory. Healthy test persons, aged 18—20 years, were exposed on consecutive days at exactly the same time to the noise of a pressure roller at 88 dB (A). The noise was offered in the following manner: (1) continuous noise; (2) noise interrupted in periodic intervals (5 min of noise, 5 min of silence, etc.); (3) noise interrupted in aperiodic intervals. The duration of the test was 65 min each test day. Each test person was exposed to 20 min of continuous noise, then to noise interrupted in periodic intervals and finally to aperiodically interrrupted noise on the first two days. During the last 3 days each person was exposed to only one of the three kinds of noise for 65 min. This variation of single noise conditions was chosen in such a way that effects of series were avoided, and each test person was exposed to all 3 noise qualities in the same frequency. Besides the blood pressure 6 additional autonomic functions were recorded. Concerning the blood pressure, which was of special interest in this study, the following results were obtained: On the first day of the test during the first 5 min of noise a statistically significant rise in systolic and diastolic blood pressure was observed, while in the last 5 min of noise only the diastolic blood pressure rose significantly. On the second day only a rise in diastolic blood pressure was statistically significant during the whole test. An effect of adaptation was seen on the systolic blood pressure. During the last 3 test days the results varied

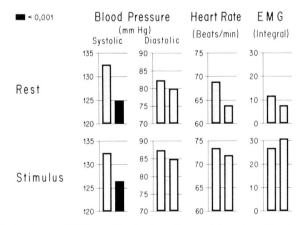

Fig. 2. Average behaviour of different body functions of 6 male subjects on two test days at rest and during stimulus. Systolic/diastolic blood pressure, heart rate and muscle tone (EMG) are recorded. The filled-up rectangles indicate a statistically significant decrease of basic values on the second day (effect of adaptation).

292

according to the noise-conditions. A diastolic blood pressure response during the whole test was only observed during periodically interrupted noise; during continuous noise diastolic blood pressure reaction showed up only at the end of the noise. During the aperiodic noise exposure no blood pressure response could be observed.

(II) Stress reactions are influenced by the quality and intensity of stimuli

The affective component of the stimulus is decisive within a certain degree of intensity. Therefore, different autonomic functions during emotional stresses, comparable in intensity, but not in quality, were recorded from normotensives, from borderline hypertensives and from subjects suffering from essential hypertension (Fig. 3). Analysis of variance of these data showed that autonomic reactions are influenced by three factors: (1) the kind of stressor used; negative affects or the desire to perform well intellectually produced stronger reactions; (2) the relationship to one of the three blood pressure groups defined by WHO; (3) the sex of the subjects in the test.

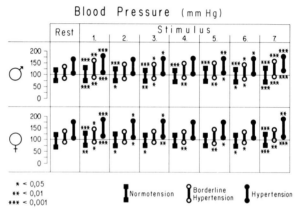

Fig. 3. Blood pressure behaviour of 60 hypertensives, 24 patients suffering from borderline hypertension and 65 normotensives at rest and during 7 different test situations.

(III) Stress reactions are subject to age

Adequate analyses have been made in connection with an interdisciplinary epidemiological study on the influence of aviation noise on a population sample of Munich (von Eiff et al., 1974). The team of investigators consisted of acoustics engineers, ergonomists, psychologists, sociologists and physicians. Besides the investigations in the homes of selected random samples, laboratory tests were carried out on these population groups. The possible influence of age on stress reaction was tested in groups of 191 healthy males and 204 healthy females (Fig. 4). Significant differences in blood pressure response were observed in males and females between the groups of the 3rd and 4th decade and the group comprising subjects in their 6th decade. Moreover, these investigations demonstrated that females of comparative age groups always

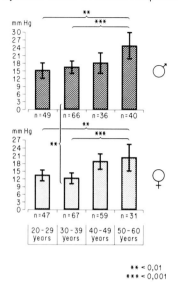

Systolic Blood Pressure Response

Fig. 4. Mean increase of systolic blood pressure of males and females during stimulus (tasks of arithmetic) separated according to life decades in normotensive subjects.

reacted with lower rises in systolic blood pressure than males. This appeared to be statistically significant in the group of the 4th decade (Czernik, 1976).

(IV) Stress reactions are subject to sex

In general, females react to non-sex related stimuli of short duration, for instance simple tasks of arithmetic, with a less distinct rise in blood pressure than males (Fig. 5). Females respond to emotional stimuli specific for them in comparison with males with a more distinct increase of autonomic functions; only blood pressure response is of a lower degree. Men, in contrast, react to sex specific stimuli preferably with systolic blood pressure rises, but not with other autonomic functions (Table I). This means that males react not only more distinctly but also more frequently with blood pressure rises to stress than females (von Eiff, 1970). These results favour the hypothesis that females are in possession of a "protective mechanism" which attenuates stress reactions of the blood pressure.

In order to test this hypothesis the following experiments were performed (von Eiff et al., 1971). In the first experiment we studied the effects of a single injection of a synthetic estrogen ester as well as that of a combination of estrogen and a synthetic progestin on blood pressure regulation in healthy, normotensive women who had undergone bilateral ovariectomy 2—6 years before the test series began. The autonomic functions were recorded at rest and under stress. Stress was elicited by a simple task of arithmetic with and without noise. These subjects were divided at random into 3 groups but each group had the same average age and showed an almost identical estrogen effect on the

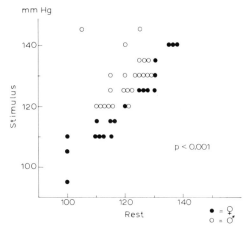

Fig. 5. Systolic blood pressure under resting conditions and during stimulus (simple tasks of arithmetic) in male and female subjects.

vaginal epithelium. Group I received an estrogen ester (20 mg estradiol valerate i.m.), group II was given a combination of the same estrogen plus a progestin (20 mg estradiol valerate plus 250 mg 17 α-hydroxyprogesterone caproate i.m.), and group III received a placebo (0.9% saline solution) only and served as controls. Eight days after the injections, all women were examined again and their circulatory functions were recorded under conditions identical to those of the first part of the experiment. The study was carried out under double-blind conditions.

TABLE I

EFFECTS OF SEX-SPECIFIC STIMULI

DF = degree of freedom; MS = mean squares of differences; RR_s = systolic blood pressure; RR_d = diastolic blood pressure; T = integral of muscle tone; Resp. R. = respiration rate; P = pulse rate. Two films of different themes (jealousy/quarrel) were presented to all subjects. Emotional reactions of male volunteers were stronger during the presentation of the film which showed two colleagues arguing, but only for the systolic blood pressure a statistically significant interaction of sex and stimulus was observed.

Cause	DF	Functions (MS)				
		P	RR_s	RR_d	T	Resp. R.
Sex	1	1250.54***	2338.00***	320.33*	9380.02	7.52
Film	1	88.04	13.00	56.33	1485.20	0.19
Sex x film	1	6.00	2426.08***	147.00	13.03	1.69
Error	44	76.58	100.20	52.41	3245.66	6.93

*$P < 0.05$.
***$P < 0.001$.

The comparison of group I with group III, that is, of the estrogen effect with the placebo effect, shows estrogen to have a distinct effect on all body functions recorded. Specifically, the following has been established as statistically significant: (1) under resting conditions a reduction of pulse rate by an average of 8 beats/min and a reduction of diastolic blood pressure by an average of 6 mm Hg was observed in estrogen-treated subjects; (2) under both forms of stress estrogen treatment led to less pronounced reactions of systolic blood pressure at an average of 16 and 13 mm Hg, respectively; (3) the estrogen effect on all body functions recorded was not greater under stress than at rest — except that on systolic blood pressure. From the results of this experiment we conclude that estrogen exerts a protective mechanism only for the regulation of the systolic blood pressure. Comparing group I with group II, namely, the effect of estrogen with that of the combination of estrogen and progestin, no significant difference was found between the body functions recorded during any phase of the experiment. Only the following trend was noticeable; the combination of estrogen—progestin did not reduce systolic blood pressure response as significantly as did estrogen alone. The combination of both hormones might, therefore, provide less effective protection.

The question remains as to whether the results of this study, in which synthetic estrogens and progestin were used, permit conclusions applicable to hormonal effects during the menstrual cycle under physiologic conditions. Existing literature is limited to studies of various circulatory functions during the menstrual cycle under conditions of rest. To answer this question, the following study was done: Thirty-four normotensive women with normal menstrual cycles were studied during 4 cycles, each under experimental conditions similar to those employed in the group of ovariectomized women. The following results were obtained: (1) there is no distinct difference between the average values of any function recorded during the pre-ovulatory phase and the post-ovulatory phase; (2) systolic and diastolic blood pressure at rest decreased when the estrogen level in the blood increased, and (3) the rise in systolic blood pressure under stress decreased with increasing estrogen level. The estrogen levels were not measured directly in the blood; the hormone levels, however, were estimated from the estrogenic effects on the vaginal smear and on the cervical mucus.

This protective mechanism was even more pronounced in the same proportion as blood pressure response became greater. Therefore, differences in the degree of response between individual groups level off in the pre-ovulatory phase when there is a good estrogen effect, i.e. at the time of ovulation (Fig. 6). A negative correlation between the intensity of estrogen effect and systolic blood pressure response under stress, that is a protective mechanism in both phases of menstrual cycle, became statistically significant only when the average blood pressure response was greater. The effect was barely noticeable when blood pressure responses were less pronounced, but even then a negative correlation was present. Thus, the results we found by administering synthetic hormones to ovariectomized women are indeed applicable to physiological conditions during the normal menstrual cycle. Furthermore, the protective mechanism of blood pressure regulation in women with its possible consequences for the integrity of the vascular system is provided by the estrogen effect.

296

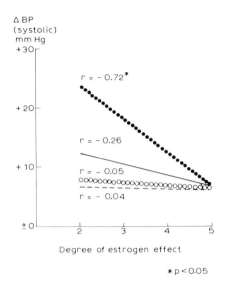

ΔBP
(systolic)
mm Hg

r = − 0.72*

r = − 0.26

r = − 0.05

r = − 0.04

Degree of estrogen effect

*p < 0.05

Fig. 6. Correlation between degree of estrogen effect and change in systolic blood pressure response during stimulus (ΔBP) during preovulatory phase. ——— = all women; — — — = 20—30 years of age; ●●● = 31—40 years of age; ○○○ = older than 40 years of age (von Eiff et al., 1971).

Presently we are continuing these investigations with series of tests on pregnant women. Another group of nonpregnant females in the same age range who are receiving the same anticonceptive drug serves as controls. Up to now 18 pregnant females and 9 nonpregnant controls have been tested. The investigation included a test at the end of each of the trimesters, that is in the 12th, 24th and 36th week of pregnancy. According to our earlier experiments the controls could be tested in a 4-week cycle in order to evaluate the effect of repetition. Even if the sequence of the control tests had been stretched to a

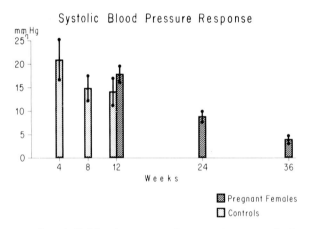

Systolic Blood Pressure Response

Weeks

▨ Pregnant Females
☐ Controls

Fig. 7. Mean increase of systolic blood pressure of pregnant women during stimulus (task of arithmetic) in 12th, 24th and 36th week of pregnancy. Controls were tested in the 4th, 8th and 12th week.

12-week cycle, the effect of repetition would not be intensified in any case, most probably it should be less marked. Besides the registration of body functions of autonomic reactions under resting conditions and stress, analyses of different hormones and their metabolites were carried out. Estradiol, estriol and progestin levels were measured in the blood while in the urine, total estrogens, pregnanetriol and pregnanediol were determined in collaboration with E.T. Plotz et al.

In these test series blood pressure response to stress appeared to decrease during pregnancy parallel to the increase of estrogens and gestagens. In the 3rd trimester a reduced reaction compared with the first trimester was observed (Fig. 7), which was also significant from the reaction of the controls.

(V) Stress response is subject to the relationship to certain blood pressure groups

This fact holds true when hypertensives have again reached the state of normotension. Five groups of subjects being normotensives or borderline hypertensives at the time of investigation have been tested (Fig. 8). The subjects who had a hypertension-anamnesis were divided into 4 groups: group 2 and group 3 had alterations in the ocular fundus, representing a fundus hypertonicus. Group 2 showed normotensive blood pressure at rest, while the systolic blood pressure of group 3 reached borderline hypertension. Groups 4 and 5 still showed no hypertensive damages in the blood vessels of the ocular fundus and differed only in blood pressure at rest, which was normotensive or borderline hypertensive, and group 5 comprised only juvenile hypertensives. The subjects of group 1 were normotensives. The 4 groups with hypertension-anamnesis were set in contrast to group 1 which had no

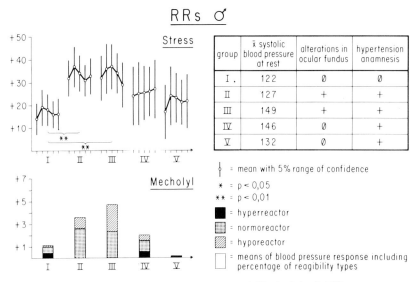

Fig. 8. Systolic blood pressure response to stress and Mecholyl of different groups of male hypertensives being normotensives without direct influence of drug effects at time of test.

hypertension-anamnesis. The groups with alterations in the ocular fundus showed significantly stronger reactions of systolic blood pressure response to stress than the normotensive controls. The mean stress reactions of the group with hypertension-anamnesis, but lacking any alterations in the ocular fundus, were also higher than in the group of normotensive controls, but the difference did not reach statistical significance because of the large variations of the single values. These results demonstrate that more distinct stress reactions can be observed in the group of persons who have had hypertension in their anamnesis and hypertensive alterations in their ocular fundi, even when these subjects are normotensive at the time of the stress test. The influence of age on this phenomenon could be eliminated. The question whether these changes in stress reaction which seem to be important for the pathogenesis of arteriosclerosis are caused by an increased central sympathetic activity, could not be answered in these investigations. The Mecholyl®-test (von Eiff, 1975), as performed on these subjects, gave no answer to this question. Both groups, having had the strongest stress response, showed the weakest reactions in the Mecholyl-test. This can only mean that besides the blood vessels in the ocular fundus also the baroceptors of the carotid sinus had been damaged by earlier hypertension. In cases of that kind nothing precise can be stated about the reactivity of central structures. Therefore the question is still open for discussion, whether electrolytic or arteriosclerotic alterations in the blood vessel walls are responsible for an increased reactivity of this vascular system rather than an increased activity of the central sympathicus (von Eiff, 1976).

CLINICAL IMPORTANCE OF THE "PROTECTIVE MECHANISM" OF ESTROGENS

In respect to clinical relevance, sex is the most important factor which influences blood pressure response to stress. On the other hand, it is still too early to draw conclusions in the field of prophylaxis or therapy.

To avoid premature consequences concerning the prescription of oral contraceptives during menopause the possibility of iatrogenic hypertension should be taken strongly into account. As we all know medication with oral contraceptives may produce hypertension in combination with a certain hereditary susceptibility, especially when there is a high salt intake or the dosage of estrogens is high. On the other hand, we possibly shall be able one day to use steroids for prophylaxis against hypertension and arteriosclerosis. Initial tests to approach the solution of this problem are carried out.

SUMMARY

According to the "hypothalamus theory", essential hypertension is primarily based on one single pathogenetic mechanism, which consists of a hyperactivity of hypothalamic structures of the sympathetic nervous system. In this hyperactivity besides other factors stressors also play an important role. Reactions generated by stressors are influenced by the following factors:

(1) adaptation; (2) intensity and kind of stimuli; (3) age; (4) sex; (5) relationship to certain blood pressure groups.

From the clinical point of view the influence of sex hormones is of central importance.

REFERENCES

Brod, J. (1974) Die Hämodynamik bei der essentiellen Hypertonie und beim emotionellen Stress. *Therapiewoche*, 24: 1737—1749.

Czernik, A. (1976) Körperliche Reaktionen Gesunder auf Lärm. In *Seelische und köperliche Störungen durch Stress*, A.W. von Eiff (Ed.), Fischer, Stuttgart, pp. 178—193.

Eiff, A.W. von (1970) The role of the autonomic nervous system in the etiology and pathogenesis of essential hypertension. *Jap. Circulat. J.*, 34: 147—153.

Eiff, A.W. von (1972) Gegenwärtige Vorstellungen zur Pathogenese der essentiellen Hypertonie. *Hippokrates*, 43: 18—30.

Eiff, A.W. von (1975) Zur Objektivierung der Sympathikusaktivität. In *Kardiale Sympathikolyse als therapeutisches Problem*, H. Lydtin and W. Meesmann (Eds.), Thieme, Stuttgart, pp. 228—237.

Eiff, A.W. von (1976) *Seelische und körperliche Störungen durch Stress*, Fischer, Stuttgart.

Eiff, A.W. von, Quint, A. und Kloska, G. (1967) *Essentielle Hypertonie*, Thieme, Stuttgart.

Eiff, A.W. von, Plotz, E.J., Beck, K.J. and Czernik, A. (1971) The effect of estrogens and progestin on blood pressure regulation of normotensive women. *Amer. J. Obstet. Gynec.*, 109: 887—892.

Eiff, A.W. von, Czernik, A., Horbach, L. und Jörgens, H. (1974) *DFG Forschungsbericht. Fluglärmwirkungen — eine interdisziplinäre Untersuchung über die Auswirkungen des Fluglärms auf den Menschen. Der medizinische Untersuchungsteil*, Boldt, Boppard, Bd. I: pp. 349—424; Bd. II: pp. 149—200.

Folkow, B. and Rubinstein, E. (1966) Cardiovascular effects of acute and chronic stimulations of the hypothalamic defense area in the rat. *Acta physiol. scand.*, 68: 48—57.

Harris, R.E. and Forsyth, R.P. (1973) Personality and emotional stress in essential hypertension in man. In *Hypertension: Mechanisms and Management*, G. Onesti, K.E. Kim and J.H. Moyer (Eds.), Grune and Stratton, New York, pp. 125—132.

Henry, J.P. and Cassel, J.C. (1969) Psychosocial factors in essential hypertension: recent epidemiologic and animal experimental evidence. *Amer. J. Epidemiol.*, 90: 171—200.

Henry, J.P., Ely, D.L. and Stephens, P.M. (1972) Changes in catecholamine-controlling enzymes in response to psychosocial activation of defence and alarm reactions. In *Physiology, Emotion and Psychosomatic Illness, Ciba Found Symp. 8*, Excerpta Medica, Amsterdam.

Hess, W.R. (1947) *Die funktionelle Organisation des vegetativen Nervensystems*, Schwabe, Basel.

Hess, W.R. (1948) *Das Zwischenhirn*, Schwabe, Basel.

Okamoto, K., Yamori, Y., Ooshima, A., Park, C., Haebara, H., Matsumoto, M., Tanaka, T., Okuda, T., Hazama, F. and Kyogoku, M. (1972) Establishment of the inbred strain of the spontaneously hypertensive rat and genetic factors involved in hypertension. In *Spontaneous Hypertension*, K. Okamoto (Ed.), Springer, Berlin.

Page, I.H. (1960) Die Mosaik-Theorie der Hypertonie. In *Essentielle Hypertonie*, K.D. Bock and P. Cottier (Eds.), Springer, Berlin, pp. 1—33.

Richter, H.E., Knust, U., Sprung, H. und Schmidt, K.H. (1976) Psychophysiologische Untersuchungen zur Stress-sensibilität von arteriellen essentiellen Hypertonikern. In *Seelische und körperliche Störungen durch Stress*, A.W. von Eiff (Ed.), Fischer, Stuttgart, pp. 158—177.

Schaefer, H. (1974) Physiologie der Blutdruckregelung und der arteriellen Hypertension. *Therapiewoche*, 24: 1716—1725.

Haemodynamic Responses during Experimental Emotional Stress and Physical Exercise in Hypertensive and Normotensive Patients

J.J. GROEN, B. HANSEN, J.M. HERMANN, N. SCHÄFER, T.H. SCHMIDT, K.H. SELBMANN, Th. V. UEXKÜLL and P. WECKMANN

Departments of Psychosomatics and Internal Medicine and Pediatrics, University of Ulm, Ulm (G.F.R.) and Afdeling Psychobiologie, Jelgersmakliniek, Leyden University, Oegstgeest (The Netherlands)

INTRODUCTION

The etiology and pathogenesis of essential hypertension are still largely unknown. Among the hypotheses which have been proposed, the psychosomatic theory regards the condition as a quantitative exaggeration (in time and intensity) of a physiological response of the circulation to certain environmental situations, which have a threatening, "stressful", meaning for the individual (Groen et al., 1971). Von Uexküll and Wick (1962) have described such a transient "situational hypertension" in normal medical students during examinations and Wolf et al. (1951, 1955) and Van der Valk (1957) have produced temporary rises in blood pressure in normal subjects by involving them in conversations which had an emotional meaning for them. Why such hypertensive responses in normal individuals are only temporary and of moderate magnitude, whereas the high blood pressure in patients with essential hypertension is persistent and mostly on a higher level, is explained by the psychosomatic theory partly by a hereditary propensity, partly by the fact that such patients appear to live continually in what they perceive as a threatening situation, e.g., an unresolved conflict with their marriage partner.

However, more information is needed about the state of the circulation during such periods of transient situational hypertension, compared with essential hypertension, before it is justified to assume that essential hypertension is indeed a permanent or chronic form of situational hypertension. In established essential hypertension the high blood pressure is associated with high peripheral vascular resistance and a normal or even low cardiac output. This is in contrast to, e.g., the high blood pressure which occurs during physical exercise, which is associated with a diminished peripheral vascular resistance and an increased cardiac output.

In the investigation to be reported we have tried to test whether the high blood pressure in situational hypertension is part of the first described "hypertonic" circulatory pattern, as occurs in essential hypertension or part of the "hyperkinetic" pattern, as occurs during exercise. For this purpose we have subjected patients during cardiac catheterisation to an emotional interview aimed to produce situational hypertension and have compared the effects on relevant parameters of the circulation with the effects of physical exercise.

We have examined both normotensive and hypertensive patients because, if the psychosomatic hypothesis that essential hypertension is not a separate disease but only an "exaggeration in intensity and duration" of situational hypertension is correct, it can be predicted that both during physical exercise and emotional stress the behaviour of the blood pressure and the associated parameters of the circulation will be essentially the same (with only quantitative differences) in normotensive and in hypertensive subjects.

METHODS

The following parameters were measured: (1) arterial blood pressure measured directly in the aorta (blood pressure transducers by F. Liechti AG, Bern); (2) right auricular pressure (idem); (3) cardiac output by the thermodilution method (Slaama and Piper) (HZV-Gerät, Fa. Fischer Typ HZV BN 6560); (4) heart rate (ECG).

The following parameters were calculated from the data obtained from these measurements: (1) mean arterial pressure (by automatic integration); (2 mean right auricular pressure (by automatic integration); (3) cardiac index (= cardiac output/body surface); (4) stroke volume index (= cardiac output/heart rate x body surface); (5) index of the peripheral vascular resistance = [(mean arterial pressure − mean auricular pressure) x 60 x 1332]/(cardiac output x body surface).

PROCEDURE

No drugs were administered before or during the test procedures. The parameters were determined during the following experimental conditions:

(1) The patients were instructed about the procedure, asked to lie down comfortably on the couch, after which the probe and catheters were introduced, the adjustments for the measurements made and the apparatus standardised. During the next period of 15—20 min, measurements of the parameters were carried out in 2—5 min intervals, till a steady state was reached; the last 5 measurements (1—5) were used for the calculation.

As the investigations took place in a laboratory situation which can be regarded as by itself emotionally stressing, we do not consider it justified to designate the situation which preceded the other experimental conditions as "rest" or "standard" but prefer to name the period during which measurements 1—5 were made, the "expectancy phase".

Depending on a randomization programme, the examinations proceeded with either exercise or interview.

(2) For the *exercise test* a bicycle ergometer was fixed to the couch and the feet of the patient strapped to the pedals. During the test the patient "rode" the bicycle (remaining in the supine position) against a workload of respectively 40, 60 and 80 W during periods of 4 min successively. Measurements 6—11 were carried out at 2 min intervals in the middle and at

the end of every period. After the test followed a recuperation period of 15 min with measurements 12—17 carried out after 1, 2, 4, 6, 10 and 15 min. Three severely hypertensives and one normotensive patient did not go beyond 60 W during the exercise test.

(3) *Interview*. The patients were subjected to a programmed interview about their previous and present life situations, especially their relations to the keyfigures in their family and their work. The interview lasted about 12—18 min, depending on the duration of the patients' replies. During the interview the following subjects were dealt with, while measurements 18—27 were made every 1 or 2 min: (a) Explanation of the aim of the examination, viz. to find out more about the cause of the hypertension or, in the case of the normotensive patients, of their symptoms. (b) Asking the patient about his symptoms and whether he knew or suspected the cause of these. (c) Questions about his work, his status in the job, his relationships with his boss and colleagues, whether he liked the work, whether it involved him in conflicts, whether it gave him satisfaction or disappointed him. What were his prospects in his present job? (d) Questions about the family, relationships with parents in the past and present, if married about relationships with wife or husband, both in general and sexually. Whether he loved her and she loved him, whether the marriage had brought the patient the happiness he or she had expected from it and whether he (she) believed that the partner had found happiness in the marriage. The relationship to their children and to the parents of the marriage partner. (e) Questions about hobbies, belonging to societies, political and religious affiliations, ideas and problems. (f) Information about what the examination had shown up to now and expression of the hope for a favourable outcome of the treatment.

The interview was followed by a recuperation phase of 4 min at the end of which measurement 28 was made.

SUBJECTS

Eleven patients with essential hypertension (7 males, 4 females) aged 27—45, in whom cardiac catheterisation was carried out in the context of extensive examinations to find out the nature of their hypertension.

Eleven normotensive patients (5 males, 6 females) aged 18—56, in whom for medical reasons cardiac catheterisation was performed but in whom no organic pathology was established. Several of them were finally diagnosed as "neurovegetative vasolability".

There were no significant differences in age or sex between the two groups. All hypertensive patients, besides fulfilling the clinical criteria of essential hypertension, had averaged systolic pressures above 158 mm Hg and diastolic pressures of above 95 during the first phase of the examination; the normotensive patients had averaged systolic and diastolic pressures below 150 and 95 mm Hg. There were no serious impairments of cardiac or renal function in the patients of either group.

RESULTS

Fig. 1 presents the curves of the averaged measurements of the 7 parameters in the hypertensive and normotensive groups. The measurements during the expectancy phase, physical exercise followed by recuperation phase and interview, are given in this sequence, although they were obtained on the subjects in a randomized order. The figure also presents the behaviour of the circulation during some other experimental conditions (looking at pictures of parents and marriage partner, pressing a handergometer) which will not be discussed in this paper.

During *physical exercise* both hypertensive and normotensive patients react with an increase in systolic and diastolic blood pressure. The pressures of the normotensive patients increased further with each increase in work load, the pressures of the hypertensive patients reached a maximum at 60 W, because some of the hypertensive patients had to stop the test at this stage. The resistance index decreased continually during the exercise especially in the hypertensive patients, so that towards the end of the exercise it even approached the non-exercise values of the normotensive patients. Furthermore, it is interesting that while the normotensive patients regained their previous resistance values very quickly during recuperation, the resistance of the hypertensive patients rose more slowly and remained lower for the full 15 min of the recuperation phase. (This may illustrate a possible beneficial effect of physical exercise on the circulation in hypertensive patients.)

Throughout the exercise test the cardiac index and the pulse rate increased continually and equally in both groups; the stroke volume index also increased, although less pronounced, in both groups. The right auricular pressure increased a few millimeters during the beginning of the exercise in both groups; toward the end of the test it was back to the "expectancy" values. It was lowest during the recuperation period.

During the *interview* both groups showed a marked increase in systolic and diastolic blood pressure. The average pulse rate was somewhat higher than during the expectancy phase in both groups. The cardiac index was somewhat higher, the stroke volume index about the same as in the expectancy phase; the resistance index was somewhat higher. In general, whereas both during exercise and interview the blood pressures were high, this was accompanied during the exercise by a large increase in cardiac output and low peripheral resistance, during the interview by small rises in both cardiac output and peripheral resistance. This pattern was the same in both groups.

Fig. 2 summarizes the behaviour of the three main parameters of the circulation (mean blood pressure, cardiac output and peripheral resistance) in the two experimental conditions, exercise and interview, for all subjects. On the left of the figure are illustrated the effects of physical exercise. All subjects show a marked increase in cardiac output, a decrease in peripheral resistance and a moderate increase in mean blood pressure. There is no difference in the behaviour of the parameters between the two groups. On the right of the figure the effects are shown of the interview. It will be seen that there is a much smaller increase and in some cases even a decrease in cardiac output. There is a marked increase in mean blood pressure and, in the majority of cases, an increase in peripheral resistance. Here again there is no obvious difference in circulatory behaviour between the groups. Thus the circulatory reaction pattern under an emotional stress is markedly different compared to that during exercise:

(1) During physical activity the circulatory reaction is characterised in all cases by an increase in arterial pressure with an increase in heart rate and cardiac output and a decrease in vascular resistance (*hyperkinetic reaction*).

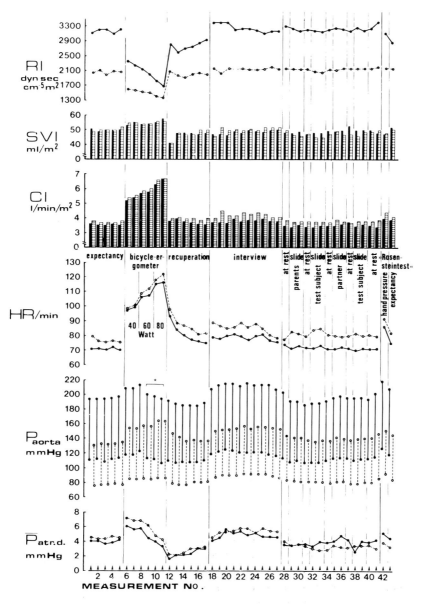

Fig. 1. Averaged values of the circulation parameters of 11 normotensive (●———●, ⊟) and 11 hypertensive patients (○---○, ▉) during all investigative procedures.

306

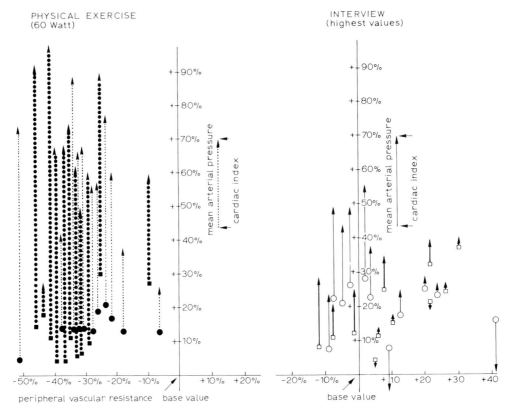

Fig. 2. The percentual changes of the mean arterial pressure, peripheral vascular resistance index and cardiac index of the hypertensive and normotensive patients during the exercise test and the interview. Parameters of hypertensives (fat lines): ■, during exercise; □, during interview. Parameters of normotensives (thin lines): ●, during exercise; ○, during interview.

(2) Under the emotional interview the circulation reacts with an increase in systolic and diastolic blood pressure and, in 15 of the 22 cases, with an increase in vascular resistance, with smaller changes in pulse rate and cardiac output (*predominantly hypertonic reaction*).

The hypertensive patients did not differ fundamentally, only in some respects quantitatively, from the normotensive patients in their circulatory behaviour during both experimental conditions.

DISCUSSION

The finding that the behaviour of the circulation under the experimental conditions was only quantitatively different in hypertensive and normotensive patients confirms Pickering's thesis (1968, 1974) that so-called essential hypertension is only the tail-end of a skewed distribution curve of the blood pressure in the population. This concept is also part of the psychosomatic theory which holds that the level of regulation of the blood pressure is higher in these patients because they experience their psychosocial environment (family and work situation) as threatening. This hypothesis was supported by the finding (like by many others) that normotensive patients also develop a high blood pressure during a stressful "threatening" interview and above all by the demonstration that the mechanism of their experimentally induced situational hypertension is the same as that of the permanently raised blood pressure in hypertensive patients, viz., a rise in peripheral vascular resistance with relatively minor increases in cardiac output.

Another observation also supports this hypothesis. During the expectancy phase, before the beginning of the tests, the average blood pressure in the hypertensives was significantly higher than during the recuperation phase after physical exercise, whereas in the normotensives this was just the reverse. This might indicate that lying down quietly on a couch during an experimental situation was experienced by the hypertensives as more stressful ("threatening") than by the normotensive patients, although they gave no verbal or motoric signal of being apprehensive.

Our findings are in agreement of those of Brod et al. (1959, 1970) who also examined the circulation of normotensive and hypertensive patients during emotional stress and exercise. However they used an "unspecific" psychic stress, mental arithmetics which had to be carried out to the beat of a metronome, at a rate with which the subject was unable to cope. They also found that all normal subjects reacted by a rise in mean blood pressure, which in the majority was caused by a rise in peripheral vascular resistance, and only minor increases in cardiac output, in other words, by the circulation pattern which is characteristic for the permanent situation in essential hypertension. Our subjects showed this pattern when they were asked questions about their family and work situation. This makes our experiment a better test of the psychosomatic hypothesis that patients with essential hypertension experience their relations with marriage partners and keyfigures in the work situation as continuously stressful and react to this by inhibited aggression and the circulatory pattern that goes with this.

SUMMARY

Heart rate, intra-aortal blood pressure, cardiac output and peripheral vascular resistance were determined in 11 hypertensive and 11 normotensive subjects during exercise up to 80 W on a bicycle ergometer and a semi-standardized interview concerning personal life situations. Blood pressure increased during both conditions. During exercise this was associated with increases in heart rate and cardiac output and a decrease in peripheral resistance (hyperkinetic reaction). During the emotional interview the heart rate and cardiac output also increased but less so and in 15 of 22 cases the peripheral resistance rose (predominantly hypertonic reaction). There was no fundamental but only a quantitative difference in the circulatory responses between the two groups. These results support the hypothesis that essential hypertension is not a disease "sui generis" but a quantitative exaggeration of the same processes which regulate blood pressure in different situations in normotensive individuals. The life situations which were discussed during the experimental interview which produced a rise in blood pressure and peripheral resistance of short duration, may have played a role in the pathogenesis of the persistently increased blood pressure in the patients with essential hypertension.

REFERENCES

Brod, J., Fencl, V., Heyl, Z. and Jirke, J. (1959) Circulatory changes underlying blood pressure elevations during acute emotional stress (mental arithmetic) in normotensive and hypertensive subjects. *Clin. Sci.*, 18: 269—279.

Brod, J. (1970) Haemodynamics and emotional stress. In *Psychosomatics in Essential Hypertension*, M. Koster, H. Musaph and P. Visser (Eds.), Karger, Basel, pp. 13—33.

Groen, J.J., Van der Valk, J.M., Welner, A. and Ben-Ishay, D. (1971) Psychobiological factors in the pathogenesis of essential hypertension. *Psychother. Psychosom.*, 19: 1—26.

Pickering, G.W. (1968) *High Blood Pressure*, 2nd ed., Churchill, London.

Pickering, G.W. (1974) *Hypertension, Causes, Consequences, Management*, Churchill-Livingstone, Edinburgh.

Van der Valk, J.M. (1957) Blood pressure changes under emotional influences in patients with essential hypertension and control subjects. *J. psychosom. Res.*, 2: 134—146.

Von Uexküll, Th. und Wick, E. (1962) Die Situationshypertonie. *Arch. Kreisl.-Forsch.*, 39: 236—271.

Wolf, S. and Wolff, H.G. (1951) Experimental evidence relating life stress to essential hypertension. In *Hypertension, a Symposium*, E.T. Bell (Ed.), Univ. of Minnesota Press, Minneapolis, pp. 288—330.

Wolf, S., Cardon, P.V., Shepard, E.M. and Wolff, H.G. (1955) *Life Stress and Essential Hypertension*, Williams and Wilkins, Baltimore, Md.

Behavioral Approaches to the Treatment of Hypertension

ALVIN P. SHAPIRO, GARY E. SCHWARTZ, DONALD C.E. FERGUSON,
DANIEL P. REDMOND and STEPHEN M. WEISS

*(D.C.E.F. and S.M.W.) National Heart and Lung Institute, (D.P.R.) Division of
Neuropsychiatry, Walter Reed Army Institute of Research, Washington, D.C.,
(G.E.S.) Department of Psychology, Yale University and Department of Psychiatry,
Yale University, School of Medicine, New Haven, Conn. and (A.P.S.) Department of Medicine,
University of Pittsburgh, School of Medicine, Pittsburgh, Pa. 15261 (U.S.A.)*

The past decade has seen an increasing interest in the epidemiologic application of newly gained pharmacological knowledge to the management of hypertension. At the same time, non-pharmacologic approaches to the control of blood pressure, particularly those operating through the well-known behavioral influences in hypertension increasingly have been developed and applied.

The non-pharmacological approaches have been considered under 5 major methodological headings. These are: (1) biofeedback techniques; (2) relaxation techniques; (3) psychotherapy; (4) suggestion and placebo effects; (5) environmental modification. Like any new treatment modality, these methods of management should be subject to scrutiny according to an evaluative scheme

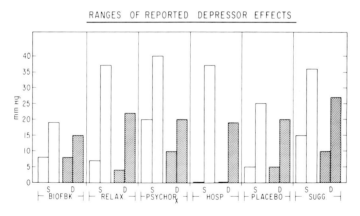

Fig. 1. Indicates the range of reported depressor effects on blood pressure of 6 different behavioral methods of therapy and hypertension, namely, BIOFDK., bio feedback; RELAX., relaxation; PSYCHOR$_x$, psychotherapy; HOSP., hospitalization; PLACEBO., placebo; SUGG., suggestion. The white bars indicate the lowest and highest falls in systolic and the striped bars the lowest and highest falls in diastolic for each technique. These data are gathered from reports in the literature as contained in the various references in the bibliography.

TABLE I

REPORTED METHODS OF BIOFEEDBACK

Study	Reduction (SBP/DPB mm Hg)	No. sessions	No. subject[b]
	I. Normotensives [a]		
(1) Systolic blood pressure biofeedback			
1. D. Shapiro et al. (1969)	5/	1	10
2. D. Shapiro et al. (1970)[b]	5/	1	7
3. Brener and Kleinman (1970)	17/	2	5
4. Fey and Lindholm (1975)	10/	3	5
(2) Systolic blood pressure-heart rate pattern biofeedback			
1. Schwartz (1971)	5/	1	5
2. Schwartz (1972)	6/	1	10
(3) Diastolic blood pressure biofeedback			
1. D. Shapiro et al. (1972)	/2	1	5
(4) Diastolic blood pressure-heart rate pattern biofeedback			
1. Schwartz (1974)	/2	1	10

II. *Hypertensives*[c]

(5) *Systolic blood pressure biofeedback*

1. Benson et al. (1971)	17/	22 (8 − 34)	7
2. Kristt and Engel (1975)	18/8	42	5
3. Goldman et al. (1975)	8/15	9	7
4. Blanchard et al. (1975)	19/	10 (5 − 13)	4

(6) *Diastolic blood pressure biofeedback*

1. Elder et al. (1973)	10%/11%[d]	8	6
2. Elder and Eustis (1975)	8%/9%[e]	10	4
	3%/3%[f]	10	19

[a] Mean reduction of pressure *within* sessions.
[b] Number of subjects given biofeedback for lowering blood pressure.
[c] Mean reduction of pressure *between* baseline and last training session.
[d] Group given biofeedback and verbal praise.
[e] Group given daily (massed) training sessions.
[f] Group given training sessions every few days (spaced).

TABLE II

REPORTED METHODS OF RELAXATION

Study	Reduction (SBP/DBP mm Hg)	No. hypertensives
(1) Progressive relaxation		
1. Jacobson (1939)	17/9	3*
2. Deabler et al. (1973)	16/15	6*
	19/4	5**
3. Shoemaker and Tsato (1975)	10/7	5***
4. Redmond et al. (1974)	14/6	6***
(2) Autogenic training		
1. Luthe (1969)	10—20%/5—10%	—
2. Klumbies and Eberhart (1966)	35/18	26** (of 83 attempted)
(3) Hypnotic relaxation		
1. Deabler et al. (1973)	28/19ᶜ	15*
	25/9ᶜ	15**
(4) Zen meditation		
1. Stone and DeLeo (1976)	14/10	19*
(5) Hatha yoga		
1. Datey et al. (1969)	37/22	10*

(6) *Transcendental meditation*		
1. Benson and Wallace (1972)	7/4	22***
2. Benson et al. (1974)[a]	9/6	22***
3. Benson et al. (1974)[b]	15/[a]	30**
	23/15[b]	10**
4. Blackwell et al. (1976)	8/6	7**
(7) *Relaxation response*		
1. Benson et al. (1974)[c]	11/5	14**
(8) *Multiple methods*		
1. Patel (1973)	12/16	20**
2. Patel (1975)[d]	20/14	32***
3. Patel and North (1975)[e]	26/15[f]	34**
	28/15[g]	

*Patients not on medication.

**Patients on hypotensive medication.

***Mixed group: medicated subjects not separately analyzed.

[a] All subjects; reported as "no significant change".

[b] Ten subjects; with highest SBP during baseline period separately analyzed.

[c] Hypnotic relaxation preceded by progressive relaxation.

[d] Yoga, GSR, feedback, progressive relaxation, autogenic exercise, meditation components present.

[e] As above in [d], but with the addition of EMG biofeedback.

[f] Treatment group followed by control period.

[g] Former control group actively treated; treatment group as controls.

designed to demonstrate their nature and origins, their clinical efficacy and potential side effects, and their indications and contraindications in therapy. Accordingly, for each of these 5 methods, material and data reported in the literature have been examined using the clinical pharmacological format developed for the study of other therapeutic agents in man (Fig. 1, Tables I and II).

The results of this analysis indicate that most of the studies have been of the Phase I type, i.e., demonstration of effects in small numbers of subjects in acute (short term) treatment situations. Phase II studies, i.e., controlled clinical trials, with comparison with known effective agents, are sparse. Phase III studies, i.e., the data derived when large scale clinical use of the new therapy, without controls, are undertaken, may be beginning, although Phase II efficacy and safety have not been established.

The information currently available from these Phase I studies indicates effects on blood pressure which are small (e.g., 5—25 mm Hg MBP) with minimal data about the duration of such effects. The relationships of these therapies to the use of pharmacologic agents need considerable clarification. From current data, these methods are adjunctive and not alternative, particularly in patients with moderate to severe hypertension (e.g. those in the > 105 mm Hg range). The problem of compliance with therapy would seem to be similar with the non-pharmacological as with the pharmacological modalities.

At the present time, the major differences between the 5 methods appear to be in the ease with which they can be taught to patients and adapted to their way of life. Accordingly, widespread application of any of the non-pharmacological methods cannot currently be recommended. Their concurrent use with drugs, further study of their long term effects and careful comparison in cooperative studies of non-pharmacological and pharmacological influences are appropriate, while further basic and clinical research into mechanisms and outcomes should be encouraged.

ACKNOWLEDGEMENT

Work supported by the National Heart, Lung and Blood Institute, D.H.E.W. Complete manuscript of review, of which this is an abstract, will be published elsewhere.

REFERENCES

Benson, H., Shapiro, D., Tursky, B. and Schwartz, G.E. (1971) Decreased systolic blood pressure through operant conditioning techniques in patients with essential hypertension. *Science*, 173: 740—742.

Benson, H. and Wallace, R.K. (1972) Decreased blood pressure in hypertension subjects who practice meditation. *Circulation*, 46, Suppl. II: 130.

Benson, H., Rosner, B.A., Marzetta, B.R. and Klemchuk, H.M. (1974a) Decreased blood pressure in borderline hypertensive patients who practice meditation. *J. chron. Dis.*, 27: 163—169.

Benson, H., Marzetta, B.R. and Rosner, B.A. (1974b) Decreased blood pressure associated with the regular elicitation of the relaxation response: a study of hypertensive subjects. In *Contemporary Problems in Cardiology, Vol. 1, Stress and the Heart*, R.S. Eliot and Mt. Kisco (Eds.), Futura, New York, pp. 293—302.

Benson, H., Rosner, B.A., Marzetta, B.R. and Klemchuk, H.M. (1974c) Decreased blood pressure in pharmacologically treated hypertensive patients who regularly elicited the relaxation response. *Lancet*, 1: 289—291.

Blackwell, B., Bloomfield, S. and Gartside, P. (1976) Transcendental meditation in hypertension. *Lancet*, 1: 223—226.

Blanchard, E.B., Young, L.D. and Haynes, M.R. (1975) A simple feedback system for the treatment of elevated blood pressure. *Behav. Ther.*, 6: 241—245.

Brener, J. and Kleinman, R.A. (1970) Learned control of decreases in systolic blood pressure. *Nature (Lond.)*, 226: 1063—1064.

Datey, K.K., Deshmuckh, S.N., Dalvi, C.P. and Vinekar, M.B. (1969) "Shavasan": a yogic exercise in the management of hypertension. *Angiology*, 20: 325—333.

Deabler, H.L., Fidel, E. and Dillenkorfer, R.L. (1973) The use of relaxation and hypnosis in lowering blood pressure. *Amer. J. clin. Hypn.*, 16: 75—83.

Elder, S.T., Ruiz, Z.R., Deabler, H.L. and Dillenkorfer, R.L. (1973) Instrumental conditioning of diastolic blood pressure in essential hypertensive patients. *J. appl. behav. Anal.*, 6: 377—382.

Elder, S.T. and Eustis, N.K. (1975) Instrumental blood pressure conditioning in out-patient essential hypertension. *Behav. Res. Ther.*, 13: 185—188.

Fey, S.G. and Lindholm, E. (1975) Systolic blood pressure and heart rate changes during three sessions involving biofeedback or no feedback. *Psychophysiology*, 12: 513—519.

Goldman, H., Kleinman, K.M., Snow, M.Y., Bidus, D.R. and Korol, B. (1975) Relationship between essential hypertension and cognitive functioning: effects of biofeedback. *Psychophysiology*, 12: 569—573.

Jacobson, E. (1939) Variation of blood pressure with skeletal muscle tension and relaxation. *Ann. intern. Med.*, 12: 1194—1212.

Klumbies, G. and Eberhardt, G. (1966) Results of autogenic training in the treatment of hypertension. In *IV World Congress of Psychiatry, Madrid, September, 1966, International Congress Series, No. 117*, J.J. Ibor (Ed.), Excerpta Medica Foundation, Amsterdam, pp. 46—47.

Kristt, D.A. and Engel, B.T. (1975) Learned control of blood pressure in patients with high blood pressure. *Circulation*, 51: 370—378.

Littler, W.A., Honour, A.J., Carter, R.D. and Sleight, P. (1975) Sleep and blood pressure. *Brit. med. J.*, 3: 346—348.

Luthe, W. (1969) *Autogenic Therapy, Vols. I—VI*, Grune and Stratton, New York.

Patel, C.H. (1973) Yoga and feedback in the management of hypertension. *Lancet*, 2: 1053—1055.

Patel, C.H. (1975) 12-month follow-up of yoga and biofeedback in the management of hypertension. *Lancet*, 1: 62—64.

Patel, C.H. and North, W.R. (1975) Randomized controlled trial of yoga and biofeedback in management of hypertension. *Lancet*, 2: 93—95.

Redmond, D.P., Gaylor, M.S., McDonald, R.H. and Shapiro, A.P. (1974) Blood pressure and heart rate response to verbal instructions and relaxation in hypertension. *Psychosom. Med.*, 36: 285—297.

Schwartz, G.E. (1971) Learned control of cardiovascular integration in man through operant conditioning. *Psychosom. Med.*, 33: 57—62.

Schwartz, G.E. (1972) Voluntary control of human cardiovascular integration and differentation through feedback and reward. *Science*, 175: 90—93.

Schwartz, G.E. (1974) Toward a theory of voluntary control of response patterns in the cardiovascular system. In *Cardiovascular Psychophysiology*, P.A. Obrist, A.H. Black, J. Brener and L.V. Di Cara (Eds.), Aldine, Chicago, pp. 406—441.

Shapiro, D., Tursky, B., Gershon, E. and Stern, M. (1969) Effect of feedback and reinforcement on the control of human systolic blood pressure. *Science*, 163: 588—589.

Shapiro, D., Tursky, B. and Schwartz, G.E. (1970) Control of blood pressure in man by operant conditioning. *Circulat. Res.*, 26, Suppl. 1: I-27—I-32.

Shapiro, D., Schwartz, G.E. and Tursky, B. (1972) Control of diastolic blood pressure in man by feedback and reinforcement. *Psychophysiology*, 9: 296—304.

Shoemaker, J.E. and Tsato, D.L. (1975) The effects of muscle relaxation on blood pressure of essential hypertensives. *Behav. Res. Ther.*, 13: 29—43.

Stone, R.A. and DeLeo, J. (1976) Psychotherapeutic control of hypertension. *New Engl. J. Med.*, 294: 80—84.

Biofeedback and Cardiovascular Self-regulation: Neurophysiological Mechanisms

GARY E. SCHWARTZ

Department of Psychology, Yale University and Department of Psychiatry, Yale University School of Medicine, New Haven, Conn. 06520 (U.S.A.)

INTRODUCTION

In one way or another, almost everything man does involves corrective feedback, both external and internal (Weiner, 1948). The concept of feedback in its simplest form is so obvious that it is often overlooked by health professionals and patients alike. It is common knowledge that it is essential to have external visual feedback and internal kinesthetic and proprioceptive feedback to learn to tie a knot or to serve a tennis ball. Placed in a more neurophysiological perspective, it becomes clear that the brain requires feedback of what it is doing and of its surroundings in order to appropriately regulate itself and its body (Schwartz, in press a).

The recent product of biomedical technology, biofeedback is a special form of information. With the aid of electronics it is possible to accurately monitor a variety of internal physiological responses and to convert these signals into visual or auditory signals that can be consciously perceived and processed by the brain, and consequently self-regulated by the brain (within the limits of specific central and peripheral constraints). From an evolutionary perspective this is an important event in human history; man has provided the brain with a dynamic form of bioinformation not part of its original neurophysiological structure (Schwartz, 1976).

This capacity for new perception and regulation of the brain has stimulated extensive research on the voluntary control of visceral and skeletal responses (reviewed in Schwartz and Beatty, 1977) and the application of biofeedback to the behavioral treatment of psychophysiological disorders (Birk, 1973), such as hypertension (e.g. Schwartz and Shapiro, 1973). Although a neurophysiological interpretation of biofeedback and its applications to the treatment of functional (Whatmore and Kohli, 1974) or disregulation (Schwartz, in press a, b) disorders is emphasized, this approach is recent in origin and does not reflect the historical development of biofeedback (Kimmel, 1974).

Much of the early research was derived from learning theory, emphasizing the application of instrumental or operant conditioning procedures (Miller, 1969). As noted by numerous authors, investigators taking a feedback approach emphasize the role of *information* in self-regulation, whereas researchers taking a learning approach tend to emphasize *incentives* or motivation in the development of self-control. It turns out that information and incentives are *both* important to learned self-regulation, and their integration is emphasized in current neurophysiological theory (Schwartz, in press a, b).

SPECIFICITY AND PATTERNING OF CARDIOVASCULAR SELF-REGULATION

One of the most important and intriguing discoveries involving biofeedback procedures has been the development of rapidly learned self-regulation of specific autonomic responses. The discovery of the capacity for learned specificity of visceral self-regulation has revised the classic, over simplistic conception of the autonomic nervous system as being totally automatic, diffuse and tightly coupled (Miller, 1969). For example, we now know that the cardiovascular system is finely toned to both anticipate and respond to specific behavioral demands in a differentiated, patterned manner (Cohen and Obrist, 1975). The patterning of cardiovascular responses, under normal conditions, represents an adaptive CNS reaction designed to maintain the bodily organs. This capacity for patterned regulation of cardiovascular responses by the brain in its dynamic commerce with the external environment, reflects, in Cannon's words, a "wisdom of the body" that markedly extends his original statement of homeostatic processes (Cannon, 1939).

It is now well established that normotensive subjects can learn to regulate their systolic and diastolic blood pressure depending upon the precise combination of biofeedback and instructions used (comprehensively reviewed in Schwartz, in press c). If subjects are given simple binary (yes—no) feedback for relative increases or decreases in systolic pressure at each beat of the heart, and are given *minimal* instructions about what they are to do (they are not told what specific response they are to control, nor are they told in what direction their physiology is to change), subjects rapidly learn within twenty-five 1 min trials to increase or decrease voluntarily their systolic blood pressure without producing similar changes in heart rate (Shapiro et al., 1969, 1970a). Conversely, if the feedback is provided for increases or decreases in heart rate, and minimal instructions are again used, subjects rapidly learn to increase or decrease their heart rate without similarly changing their systolic blood pressure (Shapiro et al., 1970b).

These data illustrate how biofeedback procedures can enable subjects to learn to control *specific* responses associated with the feedback. The data suggest that under these conditions of feedback and instructions, subjects are regulating parameters other than heart rate (e.g. stroke volume and/or peripheral resistance) to regulate their systolic pressure. In more neurophysiological terms, if the brain is required to process the external feedback without any "preconceived notions", it readily learns to regulate only those specific neural processes required to activate the periphery and thereby control the biofeedback.

However, subjects can learn to regulate two or more responses simultaneously if the feedback and reward is systemically given for the desired *pattern* of responses. For example, if subjects are given feedback only when their systolic blood pressure (BP) and heart rate (HR) simultaneously increase ($BP^{up}HR^{up}$) or simultaneously decrease ($BP_{down}HR_{down}$) subjects now learn to regulate *both* responses (Schwartz et al., 1971, 1972). Interestingly, teaching subjects to control *patterns* of responses uncovers biological linkages and constraints between systems not readily observed when controlling the individual functions alone (Schwartz, 1974, 1975, 1976). For example, when subjects are taught to lower both their systolic pressure and heart rate simultaneously ($BP_{down}HR_{down}$) they tend to show more rapid learning, produce somewhat larger changes, and experience more of the subjective concomitants of relaxation than when they are given feedback for either function alone (Schwartz, 1972). When subjects are given pattern biofeedback for making these responses go in opposite directions ($BP^{up}HR_{down}$ or $BP_{down}HR^{up}$), regulation of the two responses is attenuated. These observations highlight the concept of physiological patterning in both basic research and clinical treatment, and emphasize the inherent central and peripheral constraints that must limit the degree of neural control possible.

Since binary biofeedback for systolic blood pressure does not lead to corresponding changes in heart rate, and vice versa, this implies that the phasic relationship between systolic BP and HR must be so arranged that consistent feedback for one results in *random* reinforcement of the other simultaneously. Supporting this interpretation, when the frequency of the four possible BP—HR patterns is measured, each is found to occur about 25% of the time (Schwartz, 1972).

However, this is not the case for diastolic blood pressure and heart rate. Shapiro et al. (1972) noted that when subjects were given simple binary feedback for diastolic as opposed to systolic pressure, some corresponding change in heart rate was observed. Since the magnitude of the observed heart rate change was *less* than that for direct heart rate feedback (Shapiro et al., 1970b), it was predicted that diastolic blood pressure and heart rate must be partially, but not completely coupled. Consistent with this prediction, measurement of the 4 possible diastolic BP—HR patterns reveals that these responses tend to covary phasically in the same direction two-thirds of the time.

Based on this observation, it was further predicted that subjects given pattern biofeedback for diastolic $BP^{up}HR^{up}$ or $BP_{down}HR_{down}$ would acquire rapid control of *both* responses, whereas feedback for $BP^{up}HR_{down}$ or $BP_{down}HR^{up}$ would result in minimal learned dissociation (Schwartz et al., 1972). These predictions were confirmed (see Schwartz, 1974). Altogether, it appears that the nature and extent of learned specificity or patterning of cardiovascular responses depends initially on (1) the precise nature of the relationships between various responses over time, and (2) the exact manner in which the biofeedback is administered (e.g., for single responses, or more explicitly for patterns of responses).

In all of the above mentioned studies, subjects were given *minimal* instructions about the task. Interestingly, when subjects are *specifically instructed* to control their heart rate, the subjects *may* demonstrate immediate cardiovascular self-regulation, even in the absence of any feedback (Brener,

1974; Bell and Schwartz, 1975). However, it is a mistake to conclude that instructional control is identical to regulation gained through biofeedback. Whereas single system biofeedback leads to learned specificity (particularly with extensive training) instructions often result in more complex patterns of responses. Hence, the *verbal* instruction to control systolic blood pressure can lead to the *immediate* and simultaneous control of heart rate as well, whereas single system biofeedback for systolic blood pressure with *minimal instructions* can lead to the *development* of learned blood pressure regulation in the absence of heart rate control.

It follows that the precise nature of the biofeedback and the specific instructions used *both* contribute to the final *pattern* of responses that the subject will learn to regulate. It should not be surprising to recognize that instructions can differentially influence peripheral cardiovascular effectors in a biofeedback setting, since the average adult brain can draw on a variety of neural strategies in its conscious repertoire to regulate the feedback. Depending upon the specific nature of the instructions, the biocognitive strategies will vary.

PATTERNING OF EEG AND CARDIOVASCULAR SELF-REGULATION

One of the most challenging frontiers facing researchers in biofeedback and the self-regulation of cardiovascular responses concerns the specification of *patterns* of CNS processes involved in the regulation of complex variables such as blood pressure. Describing mechanisms underlying blood pressure regulation is complicated by a host of definitional and structural considerations that have been frequently confused in the literature. As illustrated in Table I, mechanisms of blood pressure regulation can be meaningfully discussed at five different levels — no single level is a "complete" description of blood pressure, since all levels interact at all times (from Schwartz, 1977). Blood pressure (level 1) is a composite of patterns of hemodynamic factors (level 2) which are created by patterns of effector organs (level 3) innervated by patterns of peripheral neural and humoral mechanisms (level 4) which are expressions of (regulated by) patterns of central neurogenic processes (level 5). Describing the system in this fashion is important because it clarifies how (a) changes at any level are determined by *patterns* of changes at the next lowest level, and (b) each level *directly* interacts *only* with its adjacent level.

Biofeedback for "blood pressure" (level 1) is ultimately feedback for *patterns of central neurogenic processes* (level 5), the system responsible for active learning in the human organism. However, the brain does not "directly" control blood pressure. Rather, the brain (level 5) regulates patterns of peripheral neural and humoral processes (level 4) which control the patterned activity of the peripheral organs (level 3) that produce patterns of hemodynamic changes (level 2) which are integrated and expressed as "blood pressure" (level 1).

Since it is presently impossible to accurately and continuously monitor relevant processes at all of these levels in the normal, intact person, it is not surprising that cardiovascular researchers have not been encouraged to develop

TABLE I

A CONCEPTUAL AND GENERAL DESCRIPTION OF LEVELS OF
ANALYSIS OF MECHANISMS UNDERLYING THE REGULATION
OF BLOOD PRESSURE
See text for details. (From Schwartz, 1977.)

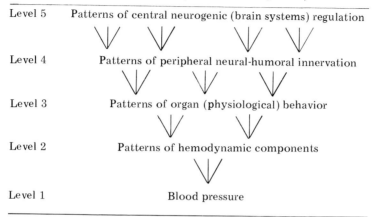

Level 5 — Patterns of central neurogenic (brain systems) regulation

Level 4 — Patterns of peripheral neural-humoral innervation

Level 3 — Patterns of organ (physiological) behavior

Level 2 — Patterns of hemodynamic components

Level 1 — Blood pressure

this line of reasoning. Although neurophysiological theory, physiological techniques and behavioral paradigms each have their own limitations at this time, it is possible to make initial inroads by integrating current neuropsychology, recent cerebral psychophysiology of localization of function, and advances in specifying behavioral tasks that reflect more focused and definable patterns of underlying psychobiological processes.

For example, it is now feasible to examine EEG processes (level 5) involved in the differential regulation of cardiovascular effector organs (level 3). Hassett and Schwartz (1975) have found that it is possible to teach subjects using biofeedback procedures to control the *relationship* between EEG alpha (8—13 Hz activity) recorded from the occipital region, and heart rate. Subjects can be readily trained to generate all 8 possible combinations of occipital alpha (OA) and heart rate (HR): OA^{off} or OA_{on}; HR_{up} or HR_{down}; $OA^{off}HR^{up}$ or $OA_{on}HR_{down}$; $OA^{off}HR_{down}$ or $OA_{on}HR^{up}$. Interestingly, the findings for the pattern regulation conditions indicate that heart rate control is somewhat enhanced over HR^{up} control when occipital EEG is simultaneously self-regulated in an arousal pattern ($OA^{off}HR^{up}$). Conversely, differentiation of heart rate and occipital alpha ($OA_{on}HR^{up}$) leads to an impairment of heart rate regulation, compared to single system heart rate control (HR^{up}). These data suggest that when subjects are required via biofeedback to regulate neural processes in the occipital region, cardiovascular adjustment *may* be brought into play. However, since subjects can utilize a variety of neural mechanisms other than their occipital cortex for regulating heart rate, biofeedback for heart rate per se will not *necessarily* require the regulation of occipital processes.

It has been noted that cardiac and skeletal motor processes are often, but not always, coupled (Obrist, 1976), since one of the primary functions of the cardiovascular system is to meet the dynamic needs of the skeletal tissues. As reviewed in Cohen and Obrist (1975), skeletal activity does not simply initiate brain regulation of cardiovascular processes via peripheral feedback from the musculature itself. There are also cortical/subcortical feedback loops between the motor cortex and the limbic system and brain stem that can integrate these processes as well. Based on current neuropsychological theory (reviewed in Davidson and Schwartz, 1976), if a subject regulated his or her heart rate by means of skeletal motor strategies, the subject would typically be regulating left hemisphere activity of the sensorimotor cortex. On the other hand, if the subject were regulating his or her heart rate using a more "cognitive" strategy, such as thinking arousing thoughts, he or she would likely be regulating right hemisphere activity in the mode specific sensory regions.

We have conducted a series of experiments to document differential EEG patterning during heart rate regulation. In one experiment, Neyer and Schwartz (in preparation) recorded monopolar EEG activity using surface electrodes over the left sensorimotor cortex and left occipital regions. Subjects were *instructed* either (1) to control their heart rate with HR biofeedback by increasing and decreasing their muscle activity, or (2) to regulate their heart rate with HR biofeedback by sitting still and thinking arousing and relaxing thoughts. It was predicted that subjects instructed to regulate their heart rate by controlling their skeletal muscle activity would show corresponding changes in EEG activation over the left sensorimotor region and *not* over the left occipital region. It was further predicted that to the extent that affective imagery involves right hemisphere processes (Schwartz et al., 1975; Davidson and Schwartz, 1976), subjects instructed to regulate heart rate by thinking arousing thoughts would show little differential EEG activity over *either* left hemisphere site recorded in this experiment. Both predictions were supported by the data.

The separation of sensorimotor and occipital EEG activity with biofeedback *and* instructions is one of the simplest of EEG differentiations, yet the questions stimulated by this observation are numerous and deserving of further research. For example, it might be useful to train subjects using *EEG* biofeedback to regulate *patterns* of these EEG processes and look for corresponding patterns in cardiovascular activity. Or, it might be interesting to extend the Hassett and Schwartz (1975) study to train patterns of sensorimotor EEG and heart rate versus patterns of occipital EEG and heart rate. To the extent that sensorimotor EEG reflects neural processes that are more tightly linked to the regulation of heart rate, voluntary dissociation of sensorimotor EEG and heart rate should be more difficult to achieve than voluntary differentiation of occipital EEG and heart rate.

More sophisticated EEG procedures, including evoked potentials and contingent negative variation measures, can be incorporated within a biofeedback patterning framework to investigate CNS processes in cardiovascular self-regulation. The important considerations are to (1) select recording sites on the basis of current neurophysiological theory, (2) select the instructional and behavioral tasks to match the theory as closely as possible, and (3) analyze the EEG patterning both across sites (parallel process) and over time (serial process). This research should include EEG analyses *within* the hemispheres (e.g., Neyer and Schwartz, in preparation) and *between* the hemispheres (e.g., Davidson and Schwartz, 1976). We believe that programmative research in this direction will, in the long run, increase our understanding of general CNS mechanisms underlying self-regulation in the intact person, and more specific CNS mechanisms involved differentially in the regulation of those specific patterns of cardiovascular responses that are ultimately expressed as changes in blood pressure. The study of CNS mechanisms in different types of hypertension is a logical extension of this approach.

DISREGULATION AND THE NEURAL BASIS OF BEHAVIORAL TREATMENTS IN HYPERTENSION

Basic research on biofeedback and the patterning of cardiovascular processes, especially when viewed within a neurophysiological context, can provide a conceptual framework for viewing the role of central mechanisms in the etiology and behavioral treatment of hypertension. Although links between basic research on feedback mechanisms and applications to clinical disorders are in the formative stage and are therefore speculative, they nonetheless provide the beginnings of a foundation for integrating CNS processes in the normal and pathologic regulation of blood pressure. The concept of feedback is central to an understanding of health and disease. As originally posited by the French physiologist Claude Bernard in the last century and elaborated by Walter Cannon in his classic volume (1939), there is a biological necessity to maintain physiological variables within adaptive limits for the purpose of survival. This is accomplished by homeostasis, a feedback mechanism requiring an intact nervous system. The feedback is negative in the sense that the peripheral signal acts to dampen overresponding by the brain in a corrective and stabilizing manner.

However, what happens if the negative feedback circuitry (at the periphery, or centrally) is altered or made ineffective? It follows that normal self-regulation will not occur, and the system will become unstable. This instability can be called disregulation (Schwartz, in press a,b), a concept similar to Miller and Dworkin's (1977) concept of anti-homeostasis. The basic components comprising the feedback self-regulatory system are shown in Fig. 1 (From Schwartz, in press a).

Space precludes a comprehensive discussion of the model (see Schwartz, in press a,b). However, the general theory can be briefly described as follows: When the environment (stage 1) places demands on a person, the brain (stage 2) performs the necessary peripheral organ regulation (stage 3) to meet the specific demands. Depending upon the nature of environmental stresses, certain bodily systems will be activated by the brain, while others may be simultaneously inhibited. However, if this process continues to the point where the organ (stage 3) becomes damaged, the negative feedback loop of the homeostatic mechanism (stage 4) will normally be accentuated, forcing the brain to change its course of action. In most stress related disorders this negative feedback loop results in the experience of pain.

For example, if a person is very active and eating on the run, the stomach may fail to function properly. Consequently, the stomach may generate sufficient negative feedback to the brain, which is experienced consciously as

324

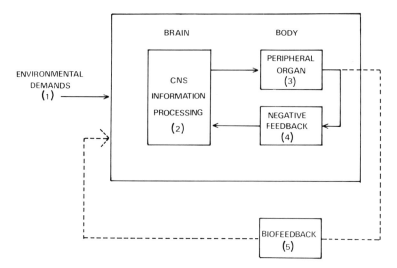

Fig. 1. Block diagram depicting (1) environmental demands influencing (2) the brain's regulation of its (3) peripheral organs, and (4) negative feedback from the peripheral organ back to the brain. Disregulation can be initiated at each of these stages. Diagram also shows how biofeedback (5) is a parallel feedback loop to (4), detecting the activity of the peripheral organ (3), and converting it into environmental stimulation (1) that can be used by the brain (2) to increase self-regulation. (From Schwartz, in press a.)

pain. This corrective signal from the periphery should serve the important function of causing the brain to change its regulation in specific ways, such as leading the person to slow down and to allow digestion to occur more normally. The pain serves a second function in that it "teaches" the brain what it can and cannot do if the stomach is to work properly. The adaptive brain is one that can learn through its mistakes, and learn to anticipate the needs of its organs for the sake of their health.

However, the brain may fail to regulate itself effectively to meet the stomach's need. The reasons for this can be quite varied, and highlight the multiplicity of etiologic factors involved in disregulation and the interactive role of environmental, behavioral and medical factors in treatment.

Stage 1: environmental demands. The stimuli from the external environment may be so demanding that the brain (stage 2) is *forced* to *ignore* the negative feedback (stage 4) generated by the stomach (stage 3). This is the classic case of the person placed in unavoidable stress who must continue to act in certain ways despite negative feedback to the contrary. Many previous theories of psychosomatic disorders have emphasized this factor.

To the extent that environmental demands act as pressor stimuli in a hypertensive patient, it becomes clear that the therapeutic *manipulation* of the external environment may lead to a corresponding decrease in pressure. Manipulations such as hospitalization or vacations act in part through a change in stage 1.

Stage 2: CNS information processing. The brain may be so programmed, initially through genetics and/or subsequently modified through learning, to respond inappropriately to the stimuli in the external environment. This is what in psychological or behavioral terms is referred to as personality or life style. Thus, although feedback from the abused organ may be present, the person's brain may fail to deal with it appropriately.

To the extent that CNS factors are acting as pressor stimuli in a given hypertensive patient, it becomes clear that the therapeutic manipulation of the patient's perceptions, cognitions and actions may lead to a corresponding decrease in pressure. Manipulations such as psychotherapy, behavior therapy, relaxation and meditation procedures, as well as biofeedback, act by changing processes in stage 2.

Stage 3: peripheral organ. The organ in question may itself be hyper- or hyporeactive to the neural or hormonal stimulation regulated by the brain. This is the literal translation of what has sometimes been called the "weak organ" or target organ theory of psychosomatic disorders. It can explain why, in response to similar environmental stresses (stage 1), people differ in the organ that ultimately becomes dysfunctional. When problems are initiated specifically at stage 3, it is possible that the brain *cannot* regulate itself to compensate for the altered feedback it is receiving from the organ in question, or in the case of a diseased organ, finds itself no longer capable of modifying the functioning of the organ.

To the extent that peripheral organ factors are themselves acting as pressor stimuli in a hypertensive patient, it becomes clear that direct medical manipulation of organ functioning will be indicated. Manipulations of a pharmacologic and/or surgical variety may be the treatment of choice in this instance.

Stage 4: negative feedback. Finally, the negative feedback derived from the organ in question may itself be inappropriate. In other words, it is possible for the protective negative feedback system to become less effective, and, in extreme cases, be inactivated. An extreme example of this condition can be seen in persons born without the normal pain response system. These individuals are constantly in danger of severely injuring themselves, because they lack the protective mechanisms for detecting and coping with injury.

To the extent that peripheral negative feedback factors are themselves failing to act as depressor stimuli in a given hypertensive patient, then direct medical manipulation of the controlling mechanisms such as the baroreceptors may be called for (e.g., Schwartz et al., 1967). This analysis also illustrates the unfortunate similarity between the hypertensive patient and the example of persons born without the normal pain response system. Since hypertensive patients are for the most part deprived of the conscious stimulus from the feedback system, they are usually unaware of their condition, lack symptoms of discomfort, and are correspondingly unmotivated to seek and sustain treatment.

Although the etiology of disregulation can occur at any of these four stages, the general consequence is the same in each case. By not responding appropriately to the negative feedback (stage 4), the brain (stage 2) fails to maintain stable regulation of the organs in question (stage 3), and disregulation (with its accompanying instability) emerges.

It is important to recognize that not only can disregulation occur at each of the four stages in the system, but also, it is possible for problems to occur *simultaneously at multiple stages.* In an extreme case, if a person was (1) exposed to demanding stimulation in his environment, requiring continued adaptation (stage 1), *and* (2) his brain processed the sensory information and reacted inappropriately due to genetic and/or learning factors (stage 2), *and* (3) the peripheral organs themselves reacted inappropriately due to genetic and/or maturational factors (stage 3), *and* (4) the baroreceptors were also ineffective (stage 4), this *pattern* would combine so as to increase the likelihood that the person would develop hypertension. Since the brain and cardiovascular system are composed of multiple effector organs that must be coordinated in an integrated fashion, it becomes necessary to examine *each* component, and then consider how they *combine* so as to produce the final outcome or disease.

This holistic perspective to hypertension illustrates how the functioning of the *system as a whole* requires the adaptive coordination by the brain of all of its components. By emphasizing the concept of feedback, the disregulation model provides a framework for understanding how biofeedback can be viewed as the addition of a new corrective feedback loop (stage 5) that augments the negative feedback (stage 4) inherent in man's biological structure (see Fig. 1). From this perspective the *use* of "biofeedback" can be quite broad, since the feedback can be used to (1) help the person determine which aspects of the environment (stage 1) are acting as pressor stimuli for him, and (2) help the person change his perceptions, cognitions and actions (stage 2) so as to decrease the biofeedback and hence the blood pressure.

Traditional medical intervention is also based on a feedback model, although medical treatment is typically not conceptualized in these terms. For example, the selection of combinations of drugs and dosages to lower pressure requires that the physician has (and correctly responds to) feedback of the patient's pressure. Similarly, the use of electrical stimulation of the baroreceptors requires that the surgeon utilizes feedback of the patient's pressure. By emphasizing the concept of *self-regulation*, however, the goal is to place more of the responsibility for health care in the hands (or more precisely, in the brains) of the patients by directing them to more actively participate in the processing and regulation of the feedback. The hope is that by increasing patient awareness and responsibility for health and sickness, it is possible to develop preventive approaches in medicine by manipulating stages 1 and 2 before organ pathology in stages 3 and 4 has a chance to develop.

The purpose of describing disregulation in simple terms is not meant to ignore the complexity of central and peripheral mechanisms underlying hypertension. Rather, the goal is to provide a *general* framework that can stimulate the recognition of the complex interaction of environmental, central and peripheral factors (including organ pathology and peripheral feedback) in the etiology, and hence the treatment, of hypertension. The central organizing system, or final common pathway for the regulation of pressure is the brain. This realization provides the necessary link between the environment and behavior on one hand and the peripheral nervous system and organs on the other. Research that documents the role of the brain in the regulation of blood pressure provides the best foundation for developing environmental (stage 1) and behavioral (stage 2) strategies in the comprehensive biobehavioral treatment of selected hypertensive disorders.

SUMMARY

This paper reviews research on biofeedback and the self-regulation of cardiovascular processes, emphasizing the control of human blood pressure. The importance of examining *patterns* of central and peripheral neural mechanisms in the self-regulation of blood pressure is emphasized. First, research is presented demonstrating (1) specificity of control of heart rate, systolic pressure and diastolic pressure, and (2) patterning of heart rate, systolic pressure and diastolic pressure. Then, research is presented applying pattern biofeedback procedures to the regulation of combinations of EEG and cardiovascular responses. This research provides a new paradigm for studying neurophysiological mechanisms underlying cardiovascular self-regulation in the intact person. Finally, research examining both inter- and intrahemispheric EEG patterning is presented as a means of illustrating some of the central mechanisms involved in learned cardiovascular self-regulation. Implications for the study of hypertension are described, including a neurophysiological model of disregulation in psychosomatic disorders. It is argued that these *neurophysiological* considerations provide a necessary foundation for the *behavioral* treatment of certain types of hypertension.

REFERENCES

Bell, I.R. and Schwartz, G.E. (1975) Voluntary control and reactivity of human heart rate. *Psychophysiology*, 12: 339—348.

Birk, L. (Ed.) (1973) *Biofeedback: Behavioral Medicine*, Grune and Stratton, New York.

Brener, J. (1974) A general model of voluntary control applied to the phenomena of learned cardiovascular change. In *Cardiovascular Psychophysiology*, P.A. Obrist, A.H. Black, J. Brener and L.V. DiCara (Eds.), Aldine, Chicago, Ill., pp. 365—391.

Cannon, W.B. (1939) *The Wisdom of the Body*, Norton, New York.

Cohen, D.H. and Obrist, P.A. (1975) Interactions between behavior and the cardiovascular system. *Circulat. Res.*, 37: 693—706.

Davidson, R.J. and Schwartz, G.E. (1976) Patterns of cerebral lateralization during cardiac biofeedback versus the self-regulation of emotion: sex differences. *Psychophysiology*, 13: 62—68.

Hassett, J. and Schwartz, G.E. (1975) Relationships between heart rate and occipital alpha: a biofeedback approach. *Psychophysiology*, 12: 228 (abstract).

Kimmel, H.D. (1974) Instrumental conditioning of autonomically mediated responses in human beings. *Amer. Psychol.*, 29: 325—335.

Miller, N.E. (1969) Learning of visceral and glandular responses. *Science*, 169: 434—445.

Miller, N.E. and Dworkin, B.R. (1977) Critical issues in therapeutic applications of biofeedback. In *Biofeedback: Theory and Research*, G.E. Schwartz and J. Beatty (Eds.), Academic Press, New York, pp. 129—162.

Obrist, P.A. (1976) The cardiovascular-behavioral interaction: as it appears today. *Psychophysiology*, 13: 95—107.

Schwartz, G.E. (1972) Voluntary control of human cardiovascular integration and differentiation through feedback and reward. *Science*, 175: 90—93.

Schwartz, G.E. (1974) Toward a theory of voluntary control of response patterns in the cardiovascular system. In *Cardiovascular Psychophysiology*, P.A. Obrist, A.H. Black, J. Brener and L.V. DiCara (Eds.), Aldine, Chicago, Ill., pp. 406—440.

Schwartz, G.E. (1975) Biofeedback, self-regulation, and the patterning of physiological processes. *Amer. Sci.*, 63: 314—324.

328

Schwartz, G.E. (1976) Self-regulation of response patterning: implications for psychophysiological research and therapy. *Biofeedback and Self-Regulation*, 1: 7—30.

Schwartz, G.E. (In press a) Psychosomatic disorders and biofeedback: a psychobiological model of disregulation. In *Psychopathology: Experimental Models*, J.D. Maser and M.E.P. Seligman (Eds.), W.H. Freeman, San Francisco.

Schwartz, G.E. (In press b) Biofeedback and the treatment of disregulation disorders. In *Ways of Health*, D.S. Sobel (Ed.), Viking Press, New York.

Schwartz, G.E. (1977) Biofeedback and patterning of autonomic and central processes: CNS-cardiovascular interactions. In *Biofeedback: Therapy and Research*, G.E. Schwartz and J. Beatty (Eds.), Academic Press, New York, pp. 183—220.

Schwartz, G.E. and Shapiro, D. (1973) Biofeedback and essential hypertension: Current findings and theoretical concerns. In *Biofeedback: Behavioral Medicine*, L. Birk (Ed.), Grune and Stratton, New York, pp. 133—144.

Schwartz, G.E. and Beatty, J. (Ed.) (1977) *Biofeedback: Theory and Research*, Academic Press, New York.

Schwartz, G.E., Shapiro, D. and Tursky, B. (1971) Learned control of cardiovascular integration in man through operant conditioning. *Psychosom. Med.*, 33: 57—62.

Schwartz, G.E., Shapiro, D. and Tursky, B. (1972) Self-control of patterns of human diastolic blood pressure and heart rate through feedback and reward. *Psychophysiology*, 9: 270 (abstract).

Schwartz, G.E., Davidson, R.J. and Maer, F. (1975) Right hemisphere lateralization for emotion in the human brain: interactions with cognition. *Science*, 190: 286—288.

Schwartz, S.I., Griffith, L.S.C., Neistadt, A. and Hagfors, N. (1967) Chronic carotid sinus nerve stimulation in the treatment of essential hypertension. *Amer. J. Surg.*, 144: 5—15.

Shapiro, D., Tursky, B., Gershon, E. and Stern, M. (1969) Effects of feedback and reinforcement on the control of human systolic blood pressure. *Science*, 163: 588—589.

Shapiro, D., Tursky, B. and Schwartz, G.E. (1970a) Control of blood pressure in man by operant conditioning. *Circulat. Res.*, 26, Suppl. 1: I-27—I-32.

Shapiro, D., Tursky, B. and Schwartz, G.E. (1970b) Differentiation of heart rate and blood pressure in man by operant conditioning. *Psychosom. Med.*, 32: 417—423.

Shapiro, D., Schwartz, G.E. and Tursky, B. (1972) Control of diastolic blood pressure in man by feedback and reinforcement. *Psychophysiology*, 9: 296—304.

Weiner, N. (1948) *Cybernetics or Control and Communication in the Animal and Machine*, M.I.T. Press, Cambridge, Mass.

Whatmore, G.E. and Kohli, D.R. (1974) *The Physiopathology and Treatment of Functional Disorders*, Grune and Stratton, New York.

PHARMACOLOGICAL ASPECTS OF CENTRAL ACTING ANTIHYPERTENSIVE DRUGS AND INFLUENCE ON PERIPHERAL EFFECTOR MECHANISMS

Chairmen: A. Sjoerdsma (Strasbourg)
P. Van Zwieten (Amsterdam)

L-DOPA Effect on Blood Pressure in Man

D.B. CALNE and P.F. TEYCHENNE

National Institute of Neurological and Communicative Disorders and Stroke, National Institutes of Health, Department of Health, Education and Welfare, Bethesda, Md. 20014 (U.S.A.)

INTRODUCTION

Oral levodopa commonly induces a reduction of the blood pressure in man. This hypotensive effect is seldom severe, usually clears spontaneously, and has not posed a serious problem in the treatment of Parkinsonian patients. Nevertheless, the hypotensive action of levodopa is of some interest, since administration of the precursor of norepinephrine might reasonably have been predicted to induce a rise, rather than a fall in the blood pressure. Evidence bearing on the mechanism of the hypotensive action of levodopa will be reviewed, considering first the problem of whether the disease for which levodopa is being given, idiopathic Parkinsonism, itself contributes to any abnormality of blood pressure control. Where possible, a distinction will be made between the set of the blood pressure (represented by values obtained when the patient is lying supine) and the baroreflexes (represented by values obtained in the standing position, or from measurements of the responses to Valsalva's maneuver).

THE BLOOD PRESSURE IN PARKINSON PATIENTS NOT RECEIVING LEVODOPA

The set of the blood pressure in idiopathic Parkinsonism

It is widely thought that Parkinsonism patients have a lower blood pressure than normal, but there are no adequate published observations to confirm or refute this claim. The largest study (Aminoff et al., 1975), in which blood pressures were compared when patients and normal subjects were first seen by a physician (termed the "casual" blood pressure), indicated that there were no significant differences between the 411 Parkinsonian subjects and controls matched for age and sex.

The baroceptor reflexes in Parkinsonism

Reid et al. (1971) have quantified the response to Valsalva's maneuver and found that baroceptor reflex responses were reduced in Parkinsonian patients when compared to healthy young adults, but when age was taken into account, no significant difference could be detected.

THE SITE OF THE HYPOTENSIVE ACTION OF LEVODOPA

From the above studies it appears that the set of the blood pressure and its control in response to postural changes are not altered by the presence of idiopathic Parkinsonism. Such patients are, therefore, a suitable group in which to study the action of levodopa on the blood pressure.

The next problem approached, in analyzing the effects of levodopa, was whether the hypotension was induced by pharmacological actions operating inside or outside the central nervous system. Carbidopa, an extracerebral decarboxylase inhibitor, was employed as a tool to answer this question.

The site of actions on the set of the blood pressure

Reid et al. (1972a) recorded the blood pressure in patients lying supine, during treatment with levodopa alone, and in the same patients receiving levodopa plus carbidopa. The dose of levodopa was reduced from 3.5 to 0.8 g/day (means) when taking carbidopa, and it was confirmed that this reduction did not lead to a fall in the plasma concentrations of levodopa (Reid et al., 1972b). The supine blood pressure was 98 ± 2.8 mm Hg ($\pm$ S.E.M.) on levodopa alone and 99 ± 2.6 mm Hg on levodopa plus carbidopa. Since administration of carbidopa did not modify the hypotensive action of levodopa in supine patients, it may be concluded that the inhibition of peripheral formation of catecholamines did not influence the set of the blood pressure and hence this hypotensive action must be mediated inside the central nervous system.

The site of action on the baroceptor reflexes

In contrast to the observations on the supine blood pressure, Reid et al. (1972b) reported, in the same patients, that administration of carbidopa virtually reversed the impairment of the baroceptor reflexes induced by levodopa. They inferred from this finding that the orthostatic hypotension induced by levodopa was dependent upon extracerebral formation of catecholamines and thus mediated at the periphery.

IDENTIFICATION OF THE TRANSMITTERS INVOLVED

Levodopa itself is pharmacologically inert in the tissue concentrations encountered in treating Parkinsonism. Its action stems from active metabolites, the catecholamines dopamine and noradrenaline, which are capable of modulating other transmitters such as serotonin, acetylcholine and gamma-aminobutyric acid. It is also possible that levodopa may influence some

TABLE I

MEAN RESULTS OF RECORDING THE BLOOD PRESSURE SUPINE AND AFTER 1
MIN STANDING IN 18 PATIENTS WITH IDIOPATHIC PARKINSONISM

Values in mm Hg ± S.E.M. (From Greenacre et al., 1976.)

	Placebo		Bromocriptine	
	Systolic	Diastolic	Systolic	Diastolic
Supine	145.3 ± 5.4	88.0 ± 2.7	143.9 ± 5.3	86.6 ± 2.7
Erect	142.0 ± 6.3	93.9 ± 3.8	135.9 ± 5.5	89.4 ± 3.1

of the transmitters by competing with other precursors, such as L-tryptophan, for transport systems or enzymic transformations.

Biochemical evidence (Calne et al., 1969) indicates that most of the levodopa administered to Parkinsonian patients is converted to dopamine, so we have investigated the actions of certain artificial dopaminergic agonists on the blood pressure. We have studied two ergoline derivatives, bromocriptine and lergotrile, both of which are potent dopaminergic agents with considerably less effect than levodopa on other transmitter systems. Bromocriptine was found to induce a significant impairment of baroceptor reflexes, and slight

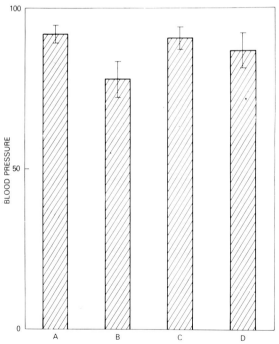

Fig. 1. Mean blood pressure (mm Hg) recorded lying supine. Bars represent S.E.M. Averaged values derived from 4 patients. A: before lergotrile. B: 8 days after starting lergotrile (mean dose 9 mg/day). C: 29 days after starting lergotrile (mean dose 50 mg/day). D: on placebo. The 8 day value is significantly less than before lergotrile ($P < 0.005$) and placebo ($P < 0.01$) phases (paired t test).

334

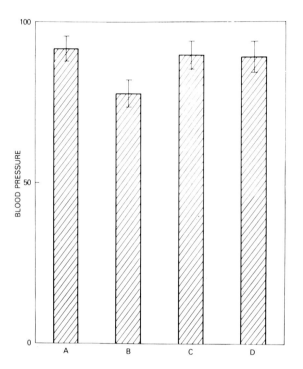

Fig. 2. Mean blood pressure (mm Hg) recorded standing erect. Bars represent S.E.M. Averaged values derived from 4 patients. A: before lergotrile. B: 8 days after starting lergotrile (mean dose 9 mg/day). C: 29 days after starting lergotrile (mean dose 50 mg/day). D. on placebo. The 8 day value is significantly less than before lergotrile ($P < 0.005$) and placebo ($P < 0.005$) phases (paired t test).

reduction of the supine blood pressure (which was not statistically significant). These findings are summarized in Table I from Greenacre et al. (1976). Our studies with lergotrile are not completed, but we have observed definite supine and orthostatic hypotension (Figs. 1 and 2); in one patient this was sufficiently severe to prevent the drug's use for continued treatment of her Parkinsonism. We conclude that augmented dopaminergic function, in both the central nervous system and at the periphery, is likely to be an important factor contributing to the hypotensive action of levodopa in man.

DISCUSSION

This interpretation of the hypotensive effects of levodopa in man is consonant with the studies of Dhasmana and Spilker (1973). These workers found that in the cat levodopa induced a central reduction in the set of the blood pressure, and a peripheral impairment of baroceptor reflexes.

While it is not possible, from current evidence, to offer any precise identification of the peripheral site or mechanism of action of levodopa it is tempting to speculate that the hypotension may be by "functional blockade" of sympathetic ganglia. Evidence in support of this view derives from experiments on dogs and cats by Antonaccio and Robson (1974). Furthermore, Greengard (1976) has recently demonstrated that there is an inhibitory interneuron in the superior cervical ganglion of the cat, and if any homologue exists in man, activation of this neuron would provide a ready explanation for the impairment of baroceptor reflexes induced by levodopa. The attraction of this simple conclusion is marred by the presence of other, equally plausible hypotheses, such as dopaminergic partial agonism leading to inhibition of α-noradrenergic receptors; activation of noradrenergic receptors on presynaptic sympathetic nerve endings resulting in decreased release of norepinephrine; or direct dopaminergic vasodilatation in the renal and mesenteric vascular beds. There is also the possibility that levodopa may induce changes in aldosterone, renin or angiotensin.

Analysis of the central mechanisms of action of levodopa is equally difficult. There are few dopaminergic pathways that would be expected to reduce the blood pressure, though modulation of dopamine in the brain stem might alter cardiac output by modifying the pulse rate; we are currently investigating this possibility. Changes in dopaminergic transmission in the median eminence might also lead to alterations in pituitary function that could upset blood pressure control. Alternatively, or in addition, the partial agonist properties of dopamine at central noradrenergic receptors might play a role. Augmented presynaptic receptor activity could lead to reduced postsynaptic effects or, if the inhibitory features of a partial agonist prevail, there could be direct blockade of the postsynaptic noradrenergic receptor.

It is quite possible that several of these mechanisms are contributing to the central and peripheral hypotensive actions of levodopa. The pharmacology is, unfortunately, still not sufficiently well defined for any compelling single hypothesis to emerge.

SUMMARY

The hypotensive action of levodopa has two components, one central, involving the set of the blood pressure, and the other peripheral, leading to impairment of baroceptor reflexes. Dopamine receptor agonists, such as bromocriptine and lergotrile, also impair the set and baroreflex control of the blood pressure. The complexity of transmitter interactions which are currently considered possible are such that no simple explanation can yet be formulated to account for the hypotensive action of levodopa in terms of a firmly based, unified hypothesis.

ACKNOWLEDGEMENTS

We wish to thank Miss V. Bergmeyer for typing the manuscript.

336

REFERENCES

Aminoff, M.J., Gross, M., Laatz, B., Vakil, S.D., Petrie, A. and Calne, D.B. (1975) Arterial blood pressure in patients with Parkinson's disease. *J. Neurol. Neurosurg. Psychiat.*, 1: 73—77.

Antonaccio, M.J. and Robson, R.D. (1974) An analysis of the peripheral effects of L-DOPA on autonomic nerve function. *Brit. J. Pharmacol.*, 52: 41—50.

Calne, D.B., Karoum, F., Ruthven, C.R.J. and Sandler, M. (1969) The metabolism of orally administered L-dopa in Parkinsonism. *Brit. J. Pharmacol.*, 37: 57—68.

Dhasmana, K.M. and Spilker, B.A. (1973) On the mechanism of L-dopa induced postural hypotension in the cat. *Brit. J. Pharmacol.*, 47: 437—451.

Greenacre, J.K., Teychenne, P.F., Petrie, A., Calne, D.B., Leigh, P.N. and Reid, J.L. (1976) The cardiovascular effects of bromocriptine in Parkinsonism. *Brit. J. clin. Pharmacol.*, 3: 571—574.

Greengard, P. (1976) Possible role for cyclic nucleotides and phosphorylated membrane proteins in postsynaptic actions of neurotransmitters. *Nature (Lond.)*, 260: 101—108.

Reid, J.L., Calne, D.B., George, C.F., Pallis, C. and Vakil, S.D. (1971) Cardiovascular reflexes in Parkinsonism. *Clin. Sci.*, 41: 63—67.

Reid, J.L., Calne, D.B., Vakil, S.D., Allen, J.G. and Davies, C.A. (1972a) Plasma concentration of levodopa in Parkinsonism before and after inhibition of peripheral decarboxylase. *J. neurol. Sci.*, 17: 45—51.

Reid, J.L., Calne, D.B., George, C.F. and Vakil, S.D. (1972b) The action of L(—)-dopa on baroreflexes in Parkinsonism. *Clin. Sci.*, 43: 851—859.

Sites of Action of Clonidine: Centrally Mediated Increase in Vagal Tone, Centrally Mediated Hypotensive and Sympatho-inhibitory Effects

MICHEL LAUBIE and HENRI SCHMITT

Département de Pharmacologie, Faculté de Médecine, Broussais-Hôtel-Dieu, 75270 Paris Cedex 06 and Département de Pharmacologie, IRS, Suresnes (France)

It is now well established that clonidine decreases blood pressure, heart rate and sympathetic discharges by acting on the central nervous system. Clonidine slows heart rate by decreasing the sympathetic tone and increasing the vagal tone (Hoefke and Kobinger, 1966; Laubie and Schmitt, 1974). Transection experiments localize the main site of action into the medulla oblongata (Hukuhara et al., 1968; Schmitt and Schmitt, 1969). The spinal cord is shown to be a less sensitive site of action (Neumayr et al., 1972; Sinha et al., 1973; De Groat et al., 1975; Franz et al., 1975) and some experiments suggest that clonidine can act upon hypothalamic cardiovascular structures (Struyker-Boudier and Van Rossum, 1974). However, in the medulla oblongata two structures are proposed as the sites of action of clonidine: (a) the nucleus tractus solitarii (NTS) (Schmitt et al., 1971; Haeusler, 1974); (b) the S zone located on the ventral surface of the medulla oblongata (Bousquet and Guertzenstein, 1973).

The present work proposes that the NTS is the probable site of action of clonidine for increasing vagal tone; however, other sites of action are responsible for the hypotensive and sympatho-inhibitory effects of the drug.

(1) SITE OF ACTION OF THE VAGALLY MEDIATED BRADYCARDIA

Kobinger and Walland (1971, 1972a,b) reported that clonidine increased the vagal cardiodepressor reflex elicited by a rise in blood pressure through a central effect. However, the site of action of this effect is as yet uncertain and furthermore, it is not known if peripheral mechanisms also participate in this potentiation.

(a) Peripheral mechanism

Dogs of either sex weighing 18—25 kg were anaesthetized with pentobarbital (30 mg/kg i.v.). Blood pressure was recorded at the femoral artery by means of a Statham P 23 Db pressure transducer on a Brush recorder and on one beam of the 5031 Tektronix oscilloscope using the DC channel. The trachea was intubated and dogs were ventilated with a Bird Mark VII pump. The sino-carotid nerve was isolated, stripped free from its sheath and placed on a

338

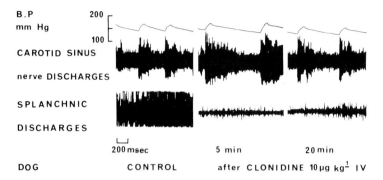

B.P
mm Hg
200
100

CAROTID SINUS

nerve DISCHARGES

SPLANCHNIC

DISCHARGES

200 msec

DOG   CONTROL   after CLONIDINE 10μg kg^{1} IV

5 min   20 min

Fig. 1. Increased baroreceptor discharges induced by clonidine. The figure shows blood pressure, carotid sinus nerve discharges and splanchnic discharges. Clonidine (10 μg/kg i.v.) induced a hypertension followed by a hypotension (20 min). The drug increased baroreceptor discharges during both phases of changes in blood pressure and markedly reduced splanchnic discharges. The figure shows the increased discharges of sino-carotid nerve for the same level of blood pressure (control and at 5 min). (From Laubie et al., 1976.)

pair of Ag-AgCl electrodes. The discharges were amplified with a 122 Tektronix preamplifier and exposed on the second beam of the 5034 Tektronix oscilloscope.

The discharges of the carotid sinus nerve were pulse synchronous; usually two bursts were observed: an initial one at the beginning of the systole and a smaller and later one during the dicrotic wave. Clonidine (10 μg/kg) was injected intravenously. During the hypertensive phase the discharges of the carotid sinus nerve were continuous and strongly increased; during the hypotensive phase they were more pronounced than before the administration of clonidine. For a similar level of blood pressure, the discharges were higher following the administration of the drug than before (Fig. 1).

These experiments indicate that clonidine sensitized the baroreceptors of the carotid sinus to their natural stimuli.

(b) Central component

Dogs of either sex weighing 17—24 kg were anaesthetized with chloralose (90 mg/kg i.v.). Blood pressure was recorded as in the preceding experiments. The right vertebral artery was isolated and a polyethylene catheter was inserted. The animals were given the potent β-adrenoceptor blocking agent S2395 [DL-(hydroxy-2′-butylamino-3′-propoxy)8-thiochromane, 50 μg/kg i.v.] (Laubie et al., 1973). Two other groups of dogs were used. In one group, guanethidine (3 mg/kg) was administered intravenously and the experiments were performed 30 min later. In the other group, a large dose of guanethidine (15 mg/kg) was injected intravenously in order to deplete the peripheral stores of noradrenaline and the dogs were used 24 hr later.

In these dogs clonidine (2 μg/kg) was injected into the vertebral artery. In dogs pretreated with the β-adrenoceptor blocking agent, clonidine induced a bradycardia and a fall in blood pressure. In the group of dogs treated with the small dose of guanethidine, clonidine induced a bradycardia and a small

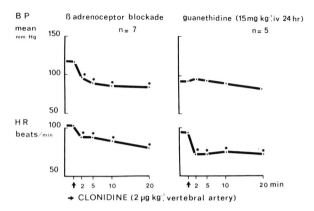

Fig. 2. Effect of clonidine on heart rate and blood pressure after administration of a
β-adrenoceptor blocking agent or guanethidine. After β-adrenoceptor blockade (S2395,
50 μg/kg), clonidine (2 μg/kg) injected into the vertebral artery decreased blood pressure and
heart rate, 24 hr after the administration of guanethidine (15 mg/kg), clonidine (2 μg/kg)
injected into the vertebral artery reduced heart rate but did not change blood pressure.
These experiments demonstrate a centrally mediated increase in vagal tone.

decrease in blood pressure, but in the dogs treated with the high dose of
guanethidine, only a bradycardia appeared (Fig. 2). As the pretreatment
prevented the appearance of any effect mediated by the sympathetic system, it
is clear that clonidine induced heart slowing by centrally increasing the vagal
tone.

Clonidine (10 μg/kg) injected intravenously to dogs having the spinal cord
transected at C_2-C_3 induced a decrease in heart rate confirming the preceding
results but increased blood pressure.

(c) Central sensitization to baroreceptor impulses by clonidine

In a group of chloralose anaesthetized dogs deafferentation was performed
according to the technique described by Edis and Shepherd (1971). Both
carotid sinus nerves were cut and in addition both aortic nerves were isolated at
the level of the laryngeal nerves and then cut. The success of the
deafferentation was ascertained by a marked increase in blood pressure and the
failure of occlusion of both carotid arteries to increase blood pressure. The
integrity of the afferent and efferent vagal pathways was demonstrated by the
bradycardia and hypotension elicited by veratridine (2 μg/kg i.v.), a drug known
to activate cardiopulmonary receptors.

The β-adrenoceptor blocking agent S2395 (50 μg/kg) was injected
intravenously and induced a fall in blood pressure (from 238± 11 to 163±
10 mm Hg) and reduced heart rate. Subsequent administration of clonidine
(2 μg/kg) into the vertebral artery reduced blood pressure but had no effect on
heart rate (Fig. 3). Therefore these experiments indicate that the baroreceptor
pathways mediated the vagal bradycardia induced by clonidine at central sites.

Another series of experiments shows that clonidine sensitized centrally to
baroreceptor impulses. In dogs anaesthetized with pentobarbital and treated

340

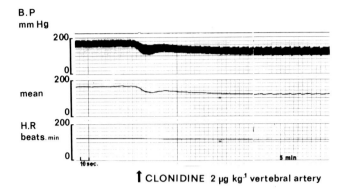

↑ CLONIDINE 2 μg kg⁻¹ vertebral artery

Fig. 3. Effect of clonidine in baroreceptor denervated dogs. Baroreceptor pathways were cut according to the Edis and Shepherd technique. After β-adrenoceptor blockade with S2395 (50 μg/kg i.v.), clonidine (2 μg/kg into the vertebral artery) reduced blood pressure but did not change heart rate.

with the β-adrenoceptor blocking agent S2395 the left carotid sinus nerve was isolated, cut and the central end was placed in a pair of platinum electrodes and stimulated at increasing frequencies. A frequency bradycardiac response curve was drawn before and after the injection of clonidine (1 μg/kg) into the vertebral artery. Clonidine increased the bradycardia induced by the electrical stimulation of the carotid sinus nerve and this effect was more marked at high frequencies of stimulation (Fig. 4).

These observations duplicate, but more directly confirm, the results published by Kobinger and Walland (1971, 1972a,b) by showing an increased bradycardia in response to a rise in blood pressure after clonidine.

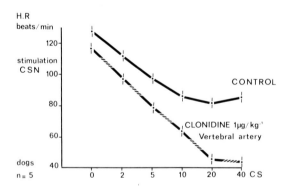

Fig. 4. Influence of clonidine on the bradycardia elicited by carotid sinus nerve stimulation. The figure shows the frequency-bradycardiac response curve produced by stimulations of the carotid sinus nerve in dogs with β-adrenoceptor blockade. Clonidine injected into the vertebral artery (1 μg/kg) potentiated the bradycardia especially at high frequencies of stimulation (20—40 Hz) (Laubie et al., 1976).

(d) The NTS as the site of the vagally mediated bradycardia induced by clonidine

Chloralose anaesthetized dogs weighing 9—11 kg, treated with the β-adrenoceptor blocking agent S2395 (50 μg/kg), were placed into a stereotaxic apparatus (La Précision Cinématographique Française), the muscles of the neck were incised and reclined in order to expose the occipito-atlantoid membrane. The membrane was incised and a portion of the occipital bone was removed. A fine stainless steel teflon coated electrode was inserted into the NTS. The stimulations were performed at weak intensity (1—2 V), with increasing frequencies (10—40 Hz) at a pulse width of 1 msec. These stimulations induced a bradycardia increasing with the frequency of stimulation. Since the displacement of the electrode by 0.5 mm in anterior regions eliminated the bradycardia, the stimulation of efferent parasympathetic pathways found in more anterior regions was ruled out as the cause of the bradycardia. Clonidine injected into the vertebral artery (1 μg/kg) did not significantly change the frequency bradycardiac response curve of these stimulations (Fig. 5).

In other experiments the nucleus ambiguus was stimulated and vertebral artery administration of clonidine (1 μg/kg) did not significantly alter the frequency bradycardiac response curve of these stimulations.

In another group of dogs weighing 9—11 kg anaesthetized with chloralose (90 mg/kg) the NTS was bilaterally destroyed. The procedure was similar to the preceding experiments but electrolytical lesions were performed bilaterally in both nuclei by passing a direct current (5 mA) through the electrode. Two lesions were performed in each side 1 and 2 mm rostrally to the obex, 3 mm laterally and 2 mm in depth.

These lesions induced a fulminating hypertension and a tachycardia. Blood pressure of these dogs did not significantly differ from blood pressure of deafferented dogs; in addition section of both carotid sinus nerves and of both aortic nerves did not further increase blood pressure and heart rate. Therefore the baroreceptor pathways would appear to have been interrupted into the NTS. Histological examination revealed large lesions in the NTS and in the dorsal motor nucleus of the vagus (Fig. 6).

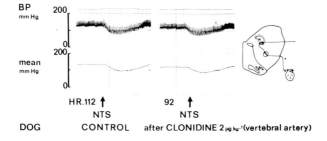

Fig. 5. Influence of clonidine on the bradycardia induced by stimulation of the nucleus tractus solitarii (NTS). Stimulation of the NTS (2 V, 40 Hz, 1 msec) induced bradycardia and a hypotension in a dog with β-adrenoceptor blockade. The injection of clonidine (2 μg/kg) into the vertebral artery did not change these effects.

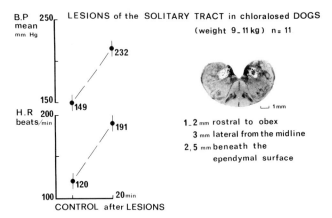

Fig. 6. Effects of bilateral destruction of the nuclei tractus solitarii on blood pressure and heart rate. The figure shows the increase in mean blood pressure and heart rate induced by bilateral destruction of both nuclei tractus solitarii. The upper corner shows the extent of the lesions. In these dogs clonidine did not change heart rate after β-adrenoceptor blockade.

The injection of the β-adrenoceptor blocking agent S2395 (50 μg/kg) significantly reduced blood pressure and heart rate. Clonidine injected into the vertebral artery (1 μg/kg) induced a long-lasting decrease in blood pressure but did not change heart rate.

These experiments indicate therefore that clonidine facilitates the transmission of baroreceptor impulses at the level of the NTS which is thought to be the site of the first synapse of the baroreceptor pathway (Crill and Reis, 1968; Seller and Illert, 1969) and that this effect is entirely responsible for the vagal part of the bradycardia induced by the drug. These results are in marked contrast with those obtained with the narcotic analgesic agents. In recent experiments fentanyl is shown to facilitate the transmission in the NTS, but other sites of action appear to be involved. In fact fentanyl reduces blood pressure and heart rate after deafferentation or bilateral destruction of the NTS in dogs with β-adrenoceptor blockade. As second order neurones are assumed to be stimulated by the electrode inserted into the NTS (Thomas and Calaresu, 1974), the present experiments would seem to indicate that clonidine either increases the release of the unknown neurotransmitter from the endings of the afferent baroreceptor nerves or facilitate the effect of this neurotransmitter on postsynaptic receptors. Previous experiments (Kobinger and Walland, 1971, 1972a,b) show that this effect is an α-sympathomimetic one and suggest that noradrenaline might regulate the transmission of baroreceptor impulses at their level. In fact noradrenaline containing neurones have been found in these nuclei (Dahlström and Fuxe, 1964).

(2) SITES OF ACTION FOR THE HYPOTENSIVE AND SYMPATHO-INHIBITORY EFFECTS OF CLONIDINE

Since clonidine decreased blood pressure in dogs with bilateral NTS lesions, other sites of action may be indicated for this effect. Similarly the sympatho-inhibitory component of the bradycardia seems to be localized in other structures.

Experiments were also performed in pentobarbital anaesthetized cats (30 mg/kg i.p.). The femoral blood pressure was recorded. The muscles of the neck were incised and retracted and a portion of the occipital bone was removed in order to expose the floor of the IVth ventricle. A stainless steel teflon coated electrode was positioned into the NTS and a direct current (5 mA) was passed through the electrode. Four lesions at 1 mm interval were performed on each side. These lesions did not induce hypertension in pentobarbital anaesthetized cats in contrast to their effects in chloralose anaesthetized dogs. In these cats clonidine (10 μg/kg) induced changes in blood pressure not significantly different from the effects of the drug in intact cats: a rise in blood pressure followed by a long-lasting hypotension and a reduction in heart rate (Fig. 7).

Bousquet and Guertzenstein (1973) reported that clonidine applied on the S zone of the ventral surface of the medulla oblongata induced a marked fall in blood pressure. Later Bousquet et al. (1975) reported that after bilateral destruction of this zone clonidine failed to cause the secondary fall in blood pressure. In a group of pentobarbitalized cats the ventral surface of the medulla oblongata was exposed. Bilateral lesions were performed on a region situated 1—2 mm caudal to the trapezoid bodies, 4 mm lateral to the midline, on 1.5 mm length by passing a direct current (5 mA) for 20 sec through the electrode. These coordinates agree with those published by Bousquet et al. (1975). A transient rise or fall in blood pressure occurred at the lesions, after 30 min blood pressure and heart rate were not significantly different from the initial values. Clonidine (10 μg/kg i.v.) induced changes in blood pressure and heart rate in these lesioned cats which were not significantly different from the changes induced in intact cats. It is difficult to account for the discrepancy between these results and those published by Bousquet et al. (1975). Possibly, there was a difference in the extent of the lesions.

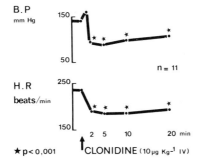

Fig. 7. Effects of clonidine on blood pressure and heart rate in cats with both nuclei tractus solitarii destroyed. In cats with both nuclei tractus solitarii destroyed, clonidine (10 μg/kg i.v.) induced a transient rise in blood pressure followed by a long-lasting hypotension; heart rate was reduced. These effects were not significantly different from those induced in intact cats (n = 11).

Therefore in another group of pentobarbitalized cats more extensive lesions were performed. A direct current (5 mA) was passed for 20 sec through the stainless steel teflon coated electrode. Five bilateral lesions were placed 3 mm lateral to the midline, 1 mm in depth, at 1 mm intervals from the trapezoid bodies to 5 mm caudally (approximately until the level of the obex). Thirty minutes later blood pressure has recovered its initial value, but heart rate was reduced. Clonidine (10 µg/kg) injected intravenously induced a transient rise in blood pressure but the secondary hypotension did not appear. Heart rate was further reduced (Fig. 8). The short duration of the hypertension suggests that clonidine was still able to inhibit the central pressor structures although to a smaller extent than in intact cats. Otherwise the pressor effect would have been much longer as it was reported for spinal or pithed preparations.

Similar experiments were performed in dogs. In a group of pentobarbitalized dogs lesions were performed on the ventral surface of the medulla oblongata from the trapezoid bodies to the level of the obex. In addition discharges of the splanchnic nerve, of the renal nerve or of the sympathetic lumbar chain were recorded. Thirty minutes after the lesions blood pressure and heart rate did not differ significantly from the control values, but sympathetic discharges were reduced. Clonidine (10 and 30 µg/kg) injected intravenously induced an initial hypertension followed by a long-lasting hypotension. Heart rate was reduced (Fig. 9). However, in these lesioned dogs, clonidine did not reduce sympathetic discharges (Figs. 10 and 11). In contrast, the narcotic analgesic agent fentanyl (20 µg/kg i.v.) was still able to reduce splanchnic discharges and this effect was antagonized by nalorphine (2 mg/kg) (Fig. 11). These experiments indicate therefore the existence of different sites and mechanisms of action for the

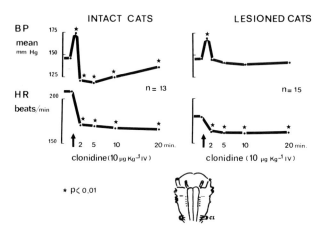

Fig. 8. Effects of clonidine on blood pressure and heart rate in control cats and in cats with extensive lesions in the ventral reticular formation. In intact cats (13 animals), clonidine (10 µg/kg i.v.) induced a rise in blood pressure followed by hypotension and reduced heart rate. Bilateral lesions were placed into the ventral reticular formation between the lateral reticular nucleus and the olivary complex. Thirty minutes later blood pressure was at a similar level to the control period but heart rate was reduced. Clonidine (10 µg/kg i.v.) induced only a transient hypertension but did not have a depressor effect. The drug reduced heart rate.

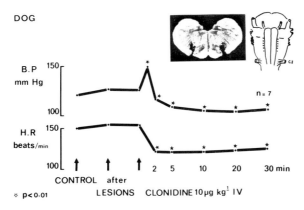

Fig. 9. Effects of clonidine on blood pressure and heart rate in dogs with a large lesion in the ventral reticular formation. In these dogs a large lesion was made into the ventral reticular formation (between the olivary complex and the lateral reticular nucleus). Blood pressure and heart rate did not differ from the control values. Clonidine (10 μg/kg) induced a transient hypertension followed by an hypotension and reduced heart rate. In the right upper corner the extent of the lesions was shown on an anatomical slice and on a drawing of the ventral surface of the medulla oblongata.

sympatho-inhibitory effects of clonidine and fentanyl. The unexpected finding that clonidine reduced blood pressure and heart rate in these dogs without markedly changing sympathetic discharges is difficult to account for. There are several possible explanations. The sympathetic tone might have been reduced in vascular beds innervated by sympathetic fibres from which the activity was not recorded. There is evidence that cooling of the spinal cord (Walther et al., 1970) or asphyxia (Iriki et al., 1971) induced opposite changes in the discharges of visceral and cutaneous sympathetic fibres of rabbits and cats. The periodic components of the sympathetic discharges are composed of 3 Hz and 10 Hz periodicities representing respectively the fundamental organization of brain stem and spinal vasomotor elements. Clonidine as baroreceptor stimulant has

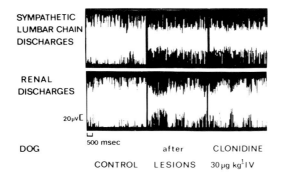

Fig. 10. Effects of clonidine on discharges of the renal nerve and of the lumbar sympathetic chain in a dog with a large lesion into the ventral reticular formation. The lesions were similar to those performed in dogs used for Fig. 9. The lesions reduced discharges in both nerves and clonidine even in large dose (30 μg/kg) did not reduce the discharges.

346

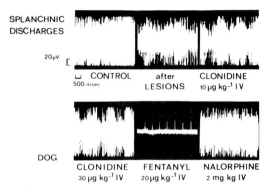

Fig. 11. Effects of clonidine and fentanyl on the splanchnic discharges in a dog with a large lesion into the ventral reticular formation. The lesions were similar to those performed in animals used for Fig. 9. The lesions reduced splanchnic discharges but clonidine (10 and 30 μg/kg i.v.) did not reduce these discharges. However fentanyl (20 μg/kg i.v.) eliminated the discharges and nalorphine (2 mg/kg i.v.) induced a recovery. This experiment indicates that the sites of action of clonidine and fentanyl are different and in addition that classical opiate receptors are involved in the sympatho-inhibitory effect of fentanyl.

recently demonstrated to be more effective in reducing the 10 Hz than the 3 Hz periodicity (McCall and Gebber, 1976). There is therefore a possibility that a shift in the ratio of these periodicities occurred in these dogs. The increased vagal tone induced by clonidine may have reduced heart rate and consequently cardiac output leading to a fall in blood pressure. Clonidine by stimulating presynaptic α-adrenoceptors (Starke et al., 1975) may have reduced noradrenaline release and decreased the sympathetic tone at peripheral sites. Finally clonidine may have stimulated an active vasodilator mechanism as postulated by Beck (1961) and Sakuma and Beck (1961). Further work is needed to examine these different possibilities.

Nevertheless these results show that it is necessary to perform extensive lesions in the medulla oblongata in order to eliminate the secondary fall in blood pressure induced by clonidine in cats or the sympatho-inhibitory effect of the drug in dogs. Histological examination revealed that the destruction involved the ventral reticular formation from the lateral reticular nucleus to the olivary complex. In rats noradrenaline (Dahlström and Fuxe, 1964) and adrenaline (Hökfelt et al., 1974) containing neurones have been found in these regions.

In conclusion, the NTS has been shown to be the site of action for the vagally mediated bradycardia induced by clonidine. This is in contrast to the action of narcotic analgesic agents for which additional sites of action are involved. The ventral reticular formation seems, at least in part, to be involved in the sympatho-inhibitory effect of clonidine.

SUMMARY

Intravenous administration of clonidine increased the discharges in carotid sinus nerve, indicating a sensitization of baroreceptors to their natural stimuli.

A central site of action was detected for the vagally mediated bradycardia, since clonidine induced bradycardia after being administered into the vertebral artery of dogs previously treated with a β-adrenoceptor blocking agent or with guanethidine, and in dogs with spinal transection. Clonidine potentiated the decrease in heart rate induced by carotid sinus nerve stimulation but did not change the effects of the stimulation of the NTS or of the nucleus ambiguus. Clonidine did not decrease heart rate in dogs treated with a β-adrenoceptor blocking agent after bilateral destruction of the NTS or deafferentation.

These experiments indicate that clonidine sensitizes the baroreceptor impulses at the level of the NTS. However, other experiments indicate that the hypotensive effect of clonidine localized at different sites. Lesions in various parts of the medulla oblongata indicate that clonidine could act mainly in different parts of the medulla oblongata depending on the animal species.

REFERENCES

Beck, L. (1961) Active reflex vasodilatation in the innervated hind limb of the dog. *Amer. J. Physiol.*, 201: 123—128.

Bousquet, P., Feldman, J., Velly, J. and Bloch, R. (1975) Role of the ventral surface of the brain stem in the hypotensive action of clonidine. *Europ. J. Pharmacol.*, 34: 151—156.

Bousquet, P. and Guertzenstein, P.G. (1973) Localization of the central cardiovascular action of clonidine. *Brit. J. Pharmacol.*, 49: 573—579.

Crill, W.E. and Reis, D.J. (1968) Distribution of carotid sinus and depressor nerves in the cat brain stem. *Amer. J. Physiol.*, 214: 269—276.

Dahlström, A. and Fuxe, K. (1964) Evidence for the existence of monoamine containing neurones in the central nervous system. *Acta physiol. scand.*, 62, Suppl. 232: 1—55.

De Groat, W., Douglas, J. and Lalley, P. (1975) Effects of clonidine, L-dopa and 5HTP on spinal and supraspinal sympathetic reflexes elicited by visceral and somatic afferent stimulation. *Sixth International Congress of Pharmacology, Helsinki*, Abstract No. 262, p. 520.

Edis, A.J. and Shepherd, J.T. (1971) Selective denervation of aortic arch baroreceptors and chemoreceptors in dogs. *J. appl. Physiol.*, 30: 294—296.

Franz, D.N., Hare, B.D. and Neumayr, R.J. (1975) Reciprocal control of sympathetic preganglionic neurons by monoaminergic, bulbospinal pathways and a selective effect of clonidine. In *Recent Advances in Hypertension, Vol. I*, P. Milliez and M. Safar (Eds.), Société Aliéna, Reims, pp. 85—96.

Haeusler, G. (1974) Further similarities between the action of clonidine and a central activation of the depressor baroreceptor reflex. *Naunyn-Schmiedeberg's Arch. exp. Path. Pharmak.*, 285: 1—14.

Hoefke, W. und Kobinger, W. (1966) Pharmakologische Wirkungen des 2-(2,6-Dichlorophenylamino)-2-Imidazolin Hydrochlorid: einer neuen antihypertensiven Substanz. *Arzneimittel-Forsch.*, 16: 1038—1050.

Hökfelt, T., Fuxe, K., Goldstein, M. and Johansson, O. (1974) Immunohistochemical evidence for the existence of adrenaline neurons in the rat brain. *Brain Res.*, 66: 235—251.

Hukuhara, T.J., Otsuka, R., Tadeka, K. und Sakai, P. (1968) Die zentrale Wirkungen des 2-(2,6-Dichlorophenylamino)-2-Imidazolin Hydrochlorids. *Arzneimittel-Forsch.*, 18: 1147—1153.

Iriki, M., Walther, O.E., Pleschka, K. and Simon, E. (1971) Regional cutaneous and visceral sympathetic activity during asphyxia in the anesthetized rabbit. *Pflügers Arch. ges. Physiol.*, 322: 167—182.

348

Kobinger, W. and Walland, A. (1971) Involvement of adrenergic receptors in central vagus activity. *Europ. J. Pharmacol.*, 16: 120—122.

Kobinger, W. and Walland, A. (1972a) Evidence for a central activation of a vagal cardiovascular reflex by clonidine. *Europ. J. Pharmacol.*, 19: 203—209.

Kobinger, W. and Walland, A. (1972b) Facilitation of vagal reflex bradycardia by an activation of clonidine on central α receptors. *Europ. J. Pharmacol.*, 19: 210—217.

Laubie, M. and Schmitt, H. (1974) Influence of autonomic blockade on the reduction in myocardial performance produced by clonidine. *Europ J. Pharmacol.*, 25: 56—65.

Laubie, M., Schmitt, H., Mouillé, P., Cheymol, G. et Gilbert, J.-C. (1973) Effets adrénolytiques bêta et hémodynamiques du d-1-(hydroxy-2't-butylamino-3'-propyloxy) 8-thiochromane. *Arch. int. Pharmacodyn.*, 201: 334—346.

Laubie, M., Schmitt, H. and Drouillat, M. (1976) Action of clonidine on the baroreceptor pathway and medullary sites mediating vagal bradycardia. *Europ. J. Pharmacol.*, 38: 293—303.

McCall, R.B. and Gebber, G.L. (1976) Differential effect of baroreceptor reflexes and clonidine on frequency components of sympathetic discharges. *Europ. J. Pharmacol.*, 36: 69—78.

Neumayr, R.J., Hare, B.D. and Franz, D.N. (1972) Depression of spinal vasomotor pathways by L-dopa and clonidine. *Abstracts Vth International Congress on Pharmacology (Volunteer Papers), San Francisco*, p. 167, No. 497.

Sakuma, A. and Beck, L. (1961) Pharmacological evidence for active reflex vasodilatation. *Amer. J. Physiol.*, 201: 129—133.

Schmitt, H. and Schmitt, H. (1969) Localization of the site of the central sympatho-inhibitory effects of 2-(2, 6-dichlorophenylamino)-2-imidazoline hydrochlorid (St 155, Catapresan). *Europ J. Pharmacol.*, 6: 8—12.

Schmitt, H., Schmitt, H. and Fénard, S. (1971) Evidence for an α sympathomimetic component in the effects of Catapresan on vasomotor centres; antagonism by piperoxan. *Europ. J. Pharmacol.*, 14: 98—100.

Seller, H. and Illert, M. (1969) The localization of the first synapse in the carotid baroreceptor reflex pathway and its alteration by the afferent input. *Pflügers Arch. ges. Physiol.*, 306: 1—19.

Sinha, J.N., Atkinson, J. and Schmitt, H. (1973) Effect of clonidine and L-dopa on spontaneous and evoked splanchnic nerve discharges. *Europ. J. Pharmacol.*, 24: 113—119.

Starke, K., Montel, H., Endo, T. and Taube, H.D. (1975) Pharmacological consequences of the presynaptic control of noradrenaline release. In *Recent Advances in Hypertension, Vol. I*, P. Milliez and M. Safar (Eds.), Société Aliéna, Reims, pp. 75—84.

Struyker-Boudier, H.A.J. and Van Rossum, J.M. (1974) Clonidine induced cardiovascular effects following stereotaxic application in the hypothalamus of rats. *J. Pharm. Pharmacol.*, 49: 573—579.

Thomas, M. and Calaresu, F. (1974) Localization and function of the medullary sites mediated vagal bradycardia in the cat. *Amer. J. Physiol.*, 226: 1344—1348.

Walther, O.E., Iriki, M. and Simon, E. (1970) Antagonistic changes of blood flow and sympathetic activity in different vascular beds following central thermal stimulation. II. Cutaneous and visceral sympathetic activity during spinal cord heating and cooling in anesthetized rabbits and cats. *Pflügers Arch. ges. Physiol.*, 319: 162—184.

Centrally Induced Hypotension by α-Methyldopa and α-Methylnoradrenaline in Normotensive and Renal Hypertensive Rats

FRANS P. NIJKAMP and WYBREN DE JONG

Rudolf Magnus Institute for Pharmacology, University of Utrecht, Medical Faculty, Utrecht (The Netherlands)

In 1960 Sjoerdsma and associates showed, for the first time, the blood pressure lowering effect of α-methyldopa in hypertensive patients (Oates et al., 1960). The mechanism by which α-methyldopa lowers blood pressure subsequently became the subject of much controversy (Gillespie et al., 1962; Sourkes, 1965; Muscholl, 1966; Haefely et al., 1967; Holtz and Palm, 1967; Stone and Porter, 1967; Henning, 1969). The discovery by Carlsson and Linqvist (1962) that α-methyldopa was converted in vivo to α-methyldopamine led Day and Rand (1963, 1964) to the postulation of the "false-transmitter" theory. According to this idea the α-methylnoradrenaline formed in vivo from α-methyldopa could replace the endogenous transmitter noradrenaline in the nerve terminals. α-Methylnoradrenaline should act as a less effective neuro-transmitter peripherally and thereby decrease sympathetic activity and lead to a reduction in blood pressure and heart rate. Many controversial data on impairment of sympathetic function in different tissues were reported however (for references see articles above). Moreover, many authors did not find a difference between the pressor potencies of noradrenaline and α-methyl-noradrenaline (Maître and Staehelin, 1963; Muscholl and Maître, 1963; Conradi et al., 1965; Trinker, 1971; Heise and Kroneberg, 1973).

The first indication for a site of action of α-methyldopa in the central nervous system came from the observations of Sjoerdsma and associates (Gillespie et al., 1962; Sjoerdsma et al., 1963). These authors demonstrated sedation as well as a hypotensive effect after α-methyldopa administration in man and these effects were not blocked by the peripheral dopa-decarboxylase inhibitor MK-485. Considerable weight was accordingly given to a central site of action of α-methyldopa by an action of its metabolite α-methyl-noradrenaline (for references see Day and Roach, 1975; Henning, 1975; Nijkamp et al., 1975; Van Zwieten, 1975).

We have investigated the mechanism and site of action of α-methyldopa in normotensive and renal hypertensive rats. A permanent indwelling iliac cannula was used to enable continuous recording of blood pressure and heart rate in unanaesthetised rats (Nijkamp et al., 1975). Basal values of the different hypertensive groups ranged from 153 ± 10 mm Hg to 195 ± 8 mm Hg and 374 ± 10 bpm to 439 ± 15 bpm respectively. In the normotensive groups basal

350

values ranged from 99 ± 3 mm Hg to 130 ± 5 mm Hg and 379 ± 22 bpm to 462 ± 11 bpm respectively.

In renal hypertensive animals 200 mg/kg of α-methyldopa administered i.p. causes a profound and long lasting decrease in blood pressure. Heart rate shows an initial increase followed by a decrease (Fig. 1). These decreases are dose-dependent up to 400—800 mg/kg (Fig. 2). Although the fall in blood pressure in the normotensive animals is less, no difference from the hypertensive rats exists if the decrease is calculated as a percentage of the initial value.

Several authors explained the bradycardia after α-methyldopa administration as a consequence of diminished pacemaker sensitivity for noradrenaline and α-methylnoradrenaline (Gillis et al., 1966; Haefely et al., 1967; Doxey and Scutt, 1974). However, we found that in the rat, the bradycardia parallels a drop in body temperature and both effects do not occur at a higher (30°C) environmental temperature (Nijkamp et al., 1975).

Not much agreement exists about the haemodynamic effects of α-methyldopa. In man, a clear reduction in cardiac output is observed after acute oral administration to hypertensive patients (Wilson et al., 1962; Onesti et al., 1964; Sannerstedt et al., 1970). After chronic use, however, both a decrease in

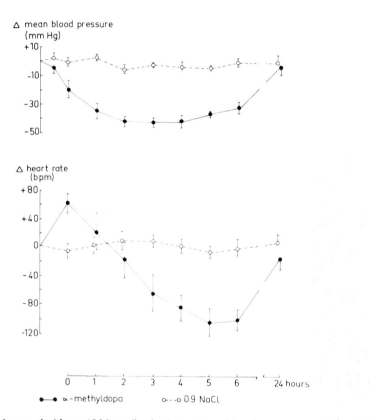

Fig. 1. Effect of α-methyldopa (200 mg/kg i.p.) on mean blood pressure and heart rate of unanaesthetised renal hypertensive rats. Data shown are means ± S.E.M. of 7—9 animals.

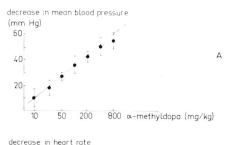

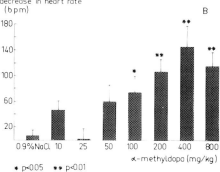

Fig. 2. Dose-response effect of intraperitoneal α-methyldopa on mean blood pressure (A) and heart rate (B) of unanaesthetised renal hypertensive rats. Data shown are means ± S.E.M. of 6—9 animals.

cardiac output with a lesser effect on the peripheral resistance is observed (Lund-Johansen, 1972), as well as a decrease of peripheral resistance without a decrease of cardiac output (Chamberlain and Howard, 1964). We measured the changes in cardiac output after acute i.p. administration of α-methyldopa to unanaesthetised renal hypertensive rats. Measurements were performed according to a modified thermodilution method by Richardson et al. (1962) and Van der Werf (1965) (see Nijkamp, 1975). α-Methyldopa (400 mg/kg) causes a decrease in cardiac output, with a maximum decrease of 31% (18 ± 5 ml/min/100 g) after 4 hr (basal value: 48 ± 3 ml/min/100 g) (Fig. 3). The decrease in cardiac output completely explains the fall in blood pressure, since only minor changes were observed in the calculated peripheral resistance. A decrease in stroke volume seems to be mainly responsible for the fall in cardiac output during the whole period of measurement. After 2—3 hr, stroke volume decreases by about 25% while after 4 and 6 hr decreases of 28% and 18% respectively are observed. A partial explanation for this fall in stroke volume could be provided by the false transmitter theory, since in the isolated heart of the rat, positive inotropic action of α-methylnoradrenaline is only 1/3 of that of noradrenaline (Brunner et al., 1967).

In our experiments a clear indication for a central site of action of α-methyldopa came from the observation that infusion of a peripherally ineffective dose of α-methyldopa (10 mg/kg) into the lateral brain ventricle of unanaesthetised renal hypertensive rats caused a large decrease in blood pressure and heart rate (Fig. 4). A 20-fold higher dose was required to produce

352

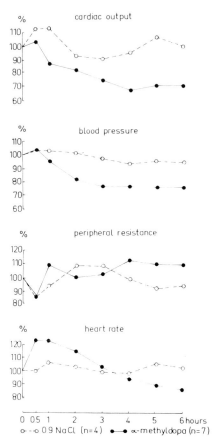

Fig. 3. Effect of α-methyldopa (400 mg/kg i.p.) on cardiac output, mean blood pressure, heart rate and peripheral resistance of unanaesthetised renal hypertensive rats.

the inhibiting effects when the drug was given systemically (Fig. 2). Day et al. (1973) and Heise and Kroneberg (1972, 1973) could also evoke hypotension after intraventricular administration of low doses of α-methyldopa in anaesthetised and non-anaesthetised rats and cats. This action of α-methyldopa seems to be dependent on the existence of central receptors, resembling peripheral α-adrenoceptors, since Heise and Kroneberg could prevent the hypotension by previous central administration of the α-adrenoceptor antagonists yohimbine and phentolamine. The inhibition of the antihypertensive action by some tricyclic antidepressants presumably could also be explained by blockade of central α-adrenoceptors (Van Spanning and Van Zwieten, 1975; Van Zwieten, 1975).

In order to elucidate the central site of action the rostral part of the brain was separated from the lower parts of the brain stem by midcollicular decerebration. In these animals the blood pressure lowering effect of systemically administered α-methyldopa was unchanged (Nijkamp and De Jong, 1974). A site of action therefore, appears to be localised in the lower part of the brain stem or in the spinal cord. A site of action in this part of the central nervous system is also suggested on the basis of transection experiments for the antihypertensive agents clonidine and L-DOPA (Schmitt and Schmitt, 1969; Henning et al., 1972). The importance of the medulla oblongata for the hypotensive action of α-methyldopa was shown in the elegant study of Henning and Van Zwieten (1968) in anaesthetised cats. These authors demonstrated a significant decrease in blood pressure after intravertebral infusion of a peripherally ineffective dose of α-methyldopa. We infused small doses of α-methyldopa into the vertebral artery of unanaesthetised renal hypertensive rats. The technique for injection of drugs into the vertebral artery according to Henning and Van Zwieten (1968) was modified to prevent disturbances of respiration in conscious rats (Wellens et al., 1976). After infusion into the vertebral artery of 25 mg/kg α-methyldopa, blood pressure decreased gradually reaching a minimum 5 hr after starting the infusion (Fig. 5). The decrease in blood pressure observed after infusion of the same dose of α-methyldopa into

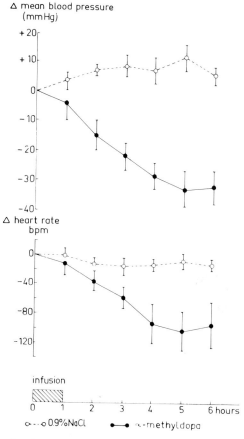

Fig. 4. Effect of α-methyldopa (10 mg/kg) on mean blood pressure and heart rate of unanaesthetised renal hypertensive rats after central administration into the lateral ventricle via an hour infusion to unanaesthetised renal hypertensive rats. Data shown are means ± S.E.M. of 7—10 animals.

354

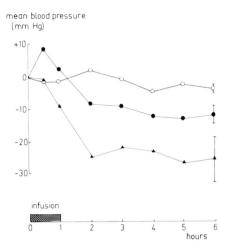

Fig. 5. Effect of α-methyldopa on mean blood pressure of unanaesthetised renal hypertensive rats after an hour infusion into the vertebral artery and jugular vein. Data shown are means ± S.E.M. of 3—7 animals. ○-○, 10 mg/kg i.v.; ▲-▲, 25 mg/kg i.v.; ●-●, 25 mg/kg i. vert.

the jugular vein, however, was more pronounced. Consequently these results are not in accord with those of Henning and Van Zwieten (1968). An explanation for this difference was provided, since radioactive microspheres injected into the vertebral artery of the rat are mainly found in the neck muscles on the injected side and not in the brain. In addition, cerebrovascular methylmetacrylate casts of the rat brain vasculature showed that the sidebranches of the basilar artery providing the pontomedullary structures are mainly filled by material injected via the common carotid artery (Wellens et al., 1976). In contrast, the major proportion of vertebral artery blood in cats and (to a lesser degree) dogs, goes to the pontomedullary structures of the brain (Reneman et al., 1974; Wellens et al., 1975).

In series of experiments we investigated whether α-methyldopa itself, or one of its metabolites, accounted for the inhibitory cardiovascular effects observed in our model. After inhibition of the peripheral conversion of α-methyldopa into α-methyldopamine by means of the dopa-decarboxylase inhibitor Ro 4-4602 (± seryl2,3,4-trihydroxybenzyl-hydrazine hydrochloride, 4 x 50 mg/kg, i.p.) the decrease in blood pressure was not prevented (Nijkamp et al., 1975). The initial increase in heart rate, however, was blocked while the secondary decrease was diminished. Accordingly, only the initial increase in heart rate seems to be mediated by a peripheral effect of α-methyldopa metabolites. Release of endogenous dopamine through replacement of the stores by α-methyldopamine might explain this initial increase in heart rate (Robson, 1971). Inhibition of central dopa-decarboxylase activity with Ro 4-4602 (3 x 0.15 mg/kg i.c.v.) completely prevented the decrease in heart rate and blood pressure (Nijkamp et al., 1975). The initial increase in heart rate, however, was not affected. Heart rate was even still slightly elevated 7 hr after injection of α-methyldopa. Interestingly, the fall in body temperature was also prevented after inhibition of central dopa-decarboxylase activity.

Obviously central conversion of α-methyldopa at least to α-methyldopamine is necessary for the inhibitory effects on the cardiovascular system. These data are consistent with those of Davis et al. (1963) and of Henning (1967, 1969). After simultaneous inhibition of peripheral as well as central dopamine-β-hydroxylase activity with FLA-63 (bis(4-methyl-1-homo-piperazinyl-thiocarbonyl) disulphide) in a dose of 25 mg/kg i.p., virtually no decrease in blood pressure and heart rate was observed after i.p. α-methyldopa administration (Fig. 6). The initial increase in heart rate was still present. These data are in agreement with those of Henning and Rubenson (1971) and Day et al. (1973), who used different inhibitors of dopamine-β-hydroylase activity and prevented the blood pressure lowering effect of α-methyldopa in normotensive and metacorticoid hypertensive rats. That α-methyldopamine is not the direct active metabolite is supported by the observations of Heise and Kroneberg (1972, 1973) and Finch et al. (1975). Although these authors observed a decrease in blood pressure after intraventricular injection of α-methyldopamine to anaesthetised cats and unanaesthetised hypertensive rats, the depressor effect was absent after pretreatment with a dopamine-β-hydroxylase inhibitor (Finch et al., 1975). Uptake of α-methyldopa into adrenergic nerve terminals seems necessary since no decrease in blood pressure is observed after destruction of central adrenergic neurones with 6-hydroxydopamine (Finch and Haeusler, 1973); data which also point to the necessity of conversion to α-methylnoradrenaline.

It is of interest that the previously mentioned centrally acting hypotensive agents, L-DOPA and clonidine also caused a centrally mediated decrease in heart rate (Schmitt and Schmitt, 1969; Osborne et al., 1971) and body temperature (Tsoucaris-Kupfer and Schmitt, 1972; Maj and Pawlowski, 1973). Central administration of α-adrenoceptor blocking agents prevents the hypothermic actions of clonidine and α-methylnoradrenaline (Marley and Stephenson, 1970; Tsoucaris-Kupfer and Schmitt, 1972) as well as the hypotensive action of clonidine and α-methyldopa (Finch and Haeusler, 1973; Schmitt et al., 1973a,b). These findings may indicate that the central effects of

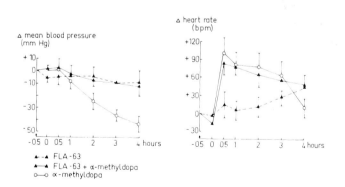

Fig. 6. Effect of α-methyldopa (400 mg/kg i.p.) on mean blood pressure and heart rate after inhibition of peripheral and central dopamine-β-hydroxylase activity with FLA-63 (25 mg/kg i.p.) of unanaesthetised renal hypertensive rats. Data shown are means ± S.E.M. of 6—7 animals.

α-methyldopa, L-DOPA and clonidine on blood pressure, body temperature and indirectly on heart rate are mediated through a common pathway in the brain.

The results presented so far demonstrate that α-methyldopa exerts its blood pressure lowering effect through an action of its metabolite α-methylnoradrenaline in the lower parts of the brain stem, presumably the medulla oblongata. The medulla oblongata of the brain stem is important for the overall cardiovascular control as demonstrated by employing brain stem transections or electrical stimulation (for references see De Jong et al., 1975b). An important role is played by the nucleus tractus solitarii (NTS) of the medulla oblongata, a primary site of termination of afferent carotid sinus baroreceptor fibres (Seller and Illert, 1969; Miura and Reis, 1969, 1972; Doba and Reis, 1973; De Jong et al., 1975a,b). Ablation of this area elicits an immediate and severe hypertension (Doba and Reis, 1973; De Jong et al., 1975a, b) while electrical stimulation of this site decreases blood pressure (Scherrer, 1967; De Jong et al., 1975a,b). Because of the above mentioned importance of this nucleus together with the data that α-methyldopa causes a clear reduction of the carotid occlusion reflex in the anaesthetised cat and dog (Stone et al., 1962; Dhasmana and Spilker, 1973; Antonaccio et al., 1974), we studied the influence on blood pressure and heart rate of microinjections of α-methylnoradrenaline in the area of the NTS. The experiments were performed on normotensive rats anaesthetised with urethane. Bilateral micro-injections of α-methylnoradrenaline were given through a stereotaxically inserted cannula (φ 0.2 mm) 0.5 mm lateral to the obex (De Jong, 1974; Nijkamp and De Jong, 1975). The obex corresponding with the rostral part of the area postrema was used as a stereotaxic zero. The effect of 23 nM α-methylnoradrenaline is shown in Fig. 7. Blood pressure and heart rate started to fall immediately after completion of the injections and reached a maximum after 5 resp. 10 min. A non-specific vasoconstriction was ruled out since pressor doses of angiotensin as well as of vasopressin applied into the NTS failed to elicit hypotension (Nijkamp and De Jong, 1975). The cardiovascular inhibitory action of α-methylnoradrenaline is dose-related as shown in Fig. 8. In order to determine the most effective localisation in the NTS, the dose of 23 nM α-methylnoradrenaline was applied in 16 different sites of the medulla oblongata. The maximal blood pressure lowering effect occurred just caudal of the obex level (De Jong and Nijkamp, 1976). However, a similar but less pronounced effect on blood pressure was observed up to 0.5 mm rostral and 1.0 mm caudal of the obex. The blood pressure lowering effect was associated with decreases in heart rate. The effective sites for the inhibiting cardiovascular effects are located inside an area which has a high density of catecholaminergic terminals (Fuxe, 1965). Noradrenaline also causes a blood pressure lowering effect after local application into the NTS (De Jong, 1974; De Jong et al., 1975a,b). Accordingly mimicking of the effects of the endogenous neuro-transmitter by α-methylnoradrenaline in this part of the brain seems a possibility. The effects on cardiovascular functions exerted by noradrenaline and α-methylnoradrenaline in the NTS are stereospecific since (+)-noradrenaline and (+)-α-methylnoradrenaline in doses up to 200 nmoles failed to induce changes in blood pressure and heart rate (De Jong and Nijkamp, 1975; Zandberg and De Jong, 1977).

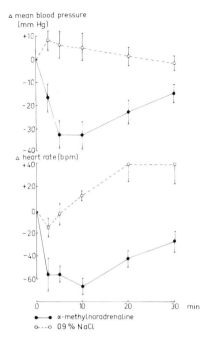

Fig. 7. Effect of bilateral microinjection of α-methylnoradrenaline (23 nmoles) on mean blood pressure and heart rate after local administration into the area of the nucleus tractus solitarii of anaesthetised normotensive rats. Data shown are means ± S.E.M. of 6—9 animals.

In order to compare the potencies of noradrenaline and α-methylnoradrenaline, we injected three different doses of these catecholamines, as well as adrenaline, into the area of the NTS (5.8, 23, 96 nmoles). The maximal decrease in blood pressure after administration of the respective doses of

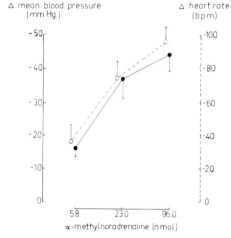

Fig. 8. Effect of graded doses of α-methylnoradrenaline on mean blood pressure and heart rate after local administration into the area of the nucleus tractus solitarii of anaesthetised normotensive rats. Data shown are means ± S.E.M. of 6—7 animals.

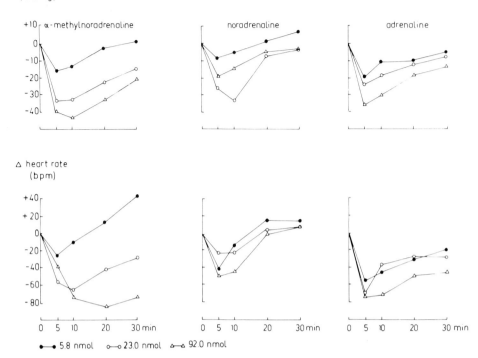

Fig. 9. Effect of different doses of α-methylnoradrenaline, noradrenaline and adrenaline on mean blood pressure and heart rate of anaesthetised normotensive rats (n = 4—9). (Data from De Jong and Nijkamp, 1976, reproduced with permission of *Brit. J. Pharmacol.*)

adrenaline and noradrenaline was reached 2.5—5 min before that of α-methyl-noradrenaline (Fig. 9). The effect of α-methylnoradrenaline was also most pronounced. Calculated from the dose-response curves it appeared to be three times more potent than noradrenaline. A similar pattern was observed for the effects on heart rate. Because of the more prolonged effect of α-methyl-noradrenaline than noradrenaline, it is tempting to speculate that α-methyldopa produces its inhibitory effects on the cardiovascular system through α-methyl-noradrenaline which in the central nervous system (NTS) may be a more effective neurotransmitter on noradrenergic receptor sites. Also after intra-ventricular administration to conscious cats of α-methylnoradrenaline and noradrenaline the response to α-methylnoradrenaline was much more prolonged than that to noradrenaline (Day and Roach, 1974).

Prior administration of the α-adrenoceptor blocking agent phentolamine into the area of the NTS transformed the decrease of blood pressure and heart rate induced by α-methylnoradrenaline into an increase (Fig. 10). Phentolamine followed by 0.9% NaCl had no significant effect. This finding is in agreement with the blocking effect of intraventricularly injected phentolamine in rats on the blood pressure lowering effect of α-methyldopa (Finch and Haeusler, 1973). The increase in blood pressure and heart rate after α-adrenoceptor blockade might be caused by an effect on β-adrenoceptors, since α-methylnoradrenaline possesses β-agonistic activity (Satchell et al., 1971) and intraventricular injection of β-mimetics, like isoprenaline, sometimes causes pressor responses and tachycardia (Toda et al., 1969; Bhargava et al., 1972; Day and Roach, 1974). After pretreatment with systemically administered atropine and vagotomy, the decrease in blood pressure after local injection of α-methylnoradrenaline into the area of the NTS is augmented (Fig. 11). So, although the central inhibitory noradrenergic cardiovascular effects might be mediated by a decrease in central sympathetic activity (Baum and Shropshire, 1973; Sinha and Schmitt, 1974), the cholinergic system seems to be involved as well. In addition, the hypotensive effect of systemic administered α-methyldopa presumably is mediated by a decrease in central sympathetic outflow (Ingenito et al., 1970; Tauberger and Kuhn, 1971; Baum et al., 1972; Finch and Haeusler, 1973). An opposite effect of the parasympathetic system could be present since systemic atropine causes a small potentiation of the hypotensive effect of α-methyldopa (Nijkamp, 1975).

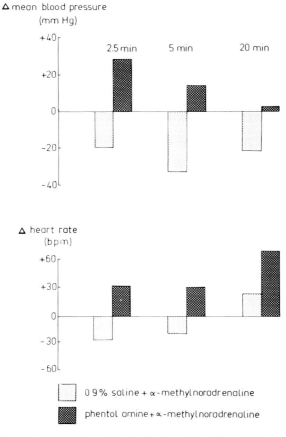

Fig. 10. Effect of bilateral injection of α-methylnoradrenaline (23 nmoles) into the area of the nucleus tractus solitarii on mean blood pressure and heart rate after local bilateral pretreatment with phentolamine (23 nmoles) of anaesthetised normotensive rats. Data shown are means ± S.E.M. of 8—10 animals.

360

In unanaesthetised dogs, atropine antagonises the blood pressure increase following intraventricular injection of acetylcholine into the brain (Lang and Rush, 1973; Laubie, 1975), while the hypertensive response is potentiated by physostigmine. We found a dose-dependent increase in blood pressure after local injection of 1 and 5 μg physostigmine into the area of the NTS (unpublished results). Thus the more pronounced decrease in blood pressure might

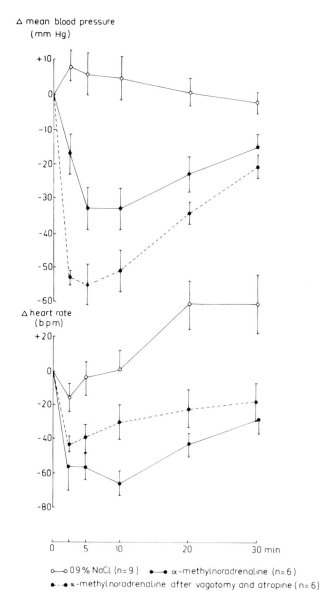

Fig. 11. Effect of bilateral injection of α-methylnoradrenaline (23 nmoles) into the area of the nucleus tractus solitarii on mean blood pressure and heart rate of anaesthetised normotensive rats and of vagotomized rats treated with atropine-sulphate (5 mg/kg i.p.). (Data from De Jong and Nijkamp, 1976, reproduced with permission of *Brit. J. Pharmacol.*)

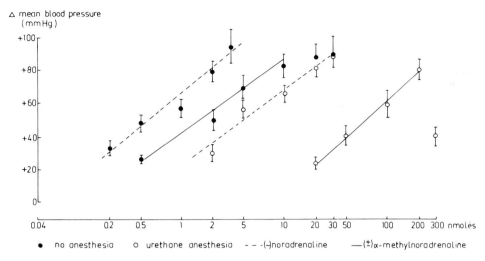

Fig. 12. Dose-response effect of α-methylnoradrenaline and noradrenaline on mean blood pressure after intravenous administration to anaesthetised and non-anaesthetised normotensive rats. Data shown are means ± S.E.M. of 6—10 animals.

be explained by an inhibition of the activation of muscarinic receptors. A neurotransmitter function for acetylcholine mediating the stimulating properties of α-methyldopa seems possible since Palkovits and Jacobowitz (1974) showed that a reasonable amount of acetylcholinesterase is present just under the NTS. An inhibitory role of the cholinergic system has also been suggested in the action of the antihypertensive drug clonidine (Laubie, 1975; Schmitt, 1975).

In anaesthetised and conscious normotensive rats i.v. injection of (—)-noradrenaline as well as (±)-α-methylnoradrenaline causes dose-dependent increases in blood pressure (Fig. 12). The (+)-isomer of α-methylnoradrenaline has a several hundred times weaker pressor action than the (—)-isomer (Muscholl, 1972) and causes in the doses used no increase in blood pressure. Calculated on base of the (—)-isomers there is a difference in pressor activity in between the two catecholamines of 6.5 times in the anaesthetised rats and 1.8 times in the conscious rats. These results might partly explain the controversial results reported in literature about relative pressor potencies between noradrenaline and α-methylnoradrenaline (Brunner et al., 1967; Holtz and Palm, 1967; Schmitt and Pétillot, 1970; Kelly and Burks, 1974; Heise and Kroneberg, 1973). On basis of our results, however, we cannot exclude an additional peripheral effect of α-methyldopa, by an action of α-methylnoradrenaline as a less effective neurotransmitter.

In the central nervous system the hypothalamus also was examined in conscious rats for a potential site of action of α-methyldopa and α-methylnoradrenaline. Unanaesthetised renal hypertensive rats were used with permanently implanted cannulas (φ 0.4 mm) into the hypothalamus (Hulst and De Wied, 1967; Nijkamp, 1975). After local application of 5—10 μg α-methyldopa (substance) into different sites of the hypothalamus, small increases in blood

362

pressure were observed in the ventral part (Fig. 13A). Maximal responses occurred after about 90 min. After local injection of 5—160 μg α-methylnoradrenaline (solution) a direct increase in blood pressure was also observed, with a maximum response occurring within 3 min. This hypertensive effect appeared not to be restricted to a certain area of the hypothalamus. The initial increase accordingly was followed by a decrease of blood pressure below basal levels, with a maximum after about 40 min. The decrease seems to be restricted to the borderline of the hypothalamus posterior and anterior (Fig. 13B). The pressor effect was dose-dependent, in contrast with the depressor response. We therefore do not exclude the possibility that the hypotensive effects of

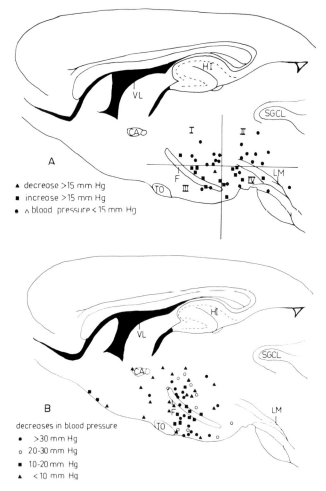

Fig. 13. Effect of implantation of α-methyldopa (5—10 μg) (A) and microinjection of α-methylnoradrenaline (5—160 μg) (B) into the area of the hypothalamus on mean blood pressure and heart rate of unanaesthetised renal hypertensive rats. The localisations (0.2—1.5 mm of the midline) are projected on a diagram of the L 950 μm transection according to König and Klippel (1963). Abbreviations: CA = commissura anterior; F = columna fornicis; HI = hippocampus; LM = lemniscus medialis; SGCL = substantia grisea centralis lateralis; VL = ventriculus lateralis; TO = tractus opticus.

α-methylnoradrenaline are caused by leakage to surrounding structures or the third ventricle. Hypotensive responses are not only found after injection of α-methylnoradrenaline into the hypothalamus but after noradrenaline and adrenaline injections also (Struyker Boudier et al., 1974; Toivolo and Gale, 1970).

CONCLUSION

α-Methyldopa exerts its antihypertensive effect by a central action of its metabolite α-methylnoradrenaline. Our results point to the nucleus tractus solitarii of the medulla oblongata as a main site of action. The blockade of the inhibitory cardiovascular effects by phentolamine suggests a role for an α-adrenoceptor. The greater effectiveness of α-methylnoradrenaline than noradrenaline to induce hypotension after central administration together with the smaller peripheral pressor action most likely explains the hypotensive mechanism of action of α-methyldopa.

SUMMARY

After acute i.p. administration to conscious renal hypertensive rats α-methyl-dopa caused a dose-dependent decrease in blood pressure and heart rate. These inhibitory cardiovascular effects were mediated by a decrease in cardiac output. Intraventricular administration of α-methyldopa in a peripherally ineffective dose caused a profound decrease of blood pressure and heart rate. Inhibition of peripheral dopa-decarboxylase activity with Ro 4-4602 did not prevent the inhibitory cardiovascular effect of α-methyldopa. After inhibition of central dopa-decarboxylase and central and peripheral dopamine-β-hydroxylase activity, however, no decreases in blood pressure and heart rate were observed, thus the central formation of α-methylnoradrenaline is an essential requirement for the mechanism of the hypotensive action of α-methyldopa. Since midcollicular transection of the brain did not influence the hypotensive effect of α-methyldopa, the effect seems to be mediated by a site in the lower part of the brain stem. In anaesthetised rats, bilateral injections of α-methylnor-adrenaline, noradrenaline and adrenaline into the area of the nucleus tractus solitarii (NTS) of the brain stem caused dose-dependent decreases of blood pressure and heart rate. The effects of α-methylnoradrenaline were most pronounced and lasted longest. A preceding injection of the α-adrenoceptor blocking agent phentolamine reversed the decrease of blood pressure and heart rate to an increase. Systemic administration of atropine combined with vagotomy potentiated the inhibitory effects of α-methylnoradrenaline on the cardiovascular system.

The pressor potency of α-methylnoradrenaline after intravenous injection was 1.8 times less than that of noradrenaline in the conscious rat, and 6.5 times less in the anaesthetised rat.

Local application of α-methyldopa into the ventral part of the hypothalamus

364

caused small increases in blood pressure. Local injection of α-methylnoradrenaline also caused increases in blood pressure, but these increases were followed by a decrease. In contrast to the increase, the decrease was mainly restricted to the midhypothalamic structures.

REFERENCES

Antonaccio, M.J., Robson, R.D. and Burrell, R. (1974) The effects of L-dopa and α-methyldopa on reflexes and sympathetic nerve function. *Europ. J. Pharmacol.*, 25: 9—18.

Baum, T. and Shropshire, A.T. (1973) Reduction of sympathetic outflow by central administration of L-dopa, dopamine and norepinephrine. *Neuropharmacology*, 12: 49—56.

Baum, T., Shropshire, A.T. and Varner, L.L. (1972) Contribution of the central nervous system to the action of several antihypertensive agents (methyldopa, hydralazine and guanethidine). *J. Pharmacol. exp. Ther.*, 182: 135—144.

Bhargava, K.P., Mishra, N. and Tangri, K.K. (1972) An analysis of central adrenoceptors for control of cardiovascular function. *Brit. J. Pharmacol.*, 45: 596—602.

Brunner, H., Hedwall, P.R., Maître, L. and Meier, M. (1967) Antihypertensive effects of alpha-methylated catecholamine analogues in the rat. *Brit. J. Pharmacol.*, 30: 123—133.

Carlsson, A. and Lindqvist, M. (1962) In vivo decarboxylation of α-methyldopa and α-methylmetatyrosine. *Acta physiol. scand.*, 54: 87—94.

Chamberlain, D.A. and Howard, J. (1964) Guanethidine and methyldopa: a haemodynamic study. *Brit. Heart J.*, 26: 528—536.

Conradi, E.C., Gaffney, T.E., Fink, D.A. and Vangrow, J.S. (1965) Reversal of sympathetic nerve blockade: a comparison of dopa, dopamine and norepinephrine with their α-methylated analogues. *J. Pharmacol. exp. Ther.*, 150: 26—33.

Davis, R.A., Drain, D.J., Horlington, M., Lazare, R. and Urbanska, A. (1963) The effect of α-methyldopa and N-2-hydroxy-benzyl-N-methylhydrazine (NSD 1039) on the blood pressure of renal hypertensive rats. *Life Sci.*, 3: 193—197.

Day, M.D. and Rand, M.J. (1963) A hypothesis for the mode of action of α-methyldopa in relieving hypertension. *J. Pharm. Pharmacol.*, 15: 221—224.

Day, M.D. and Rand, M.J. (1964) A possible mechanism of action for α-methyldopa (Aldomet). *Neuropharmacology*, 3: 173—175.

Day, M.D. and Roach, A.G. (1974) Central α- and β-adrenoceptors modifying arterial blood pressure and heart rate in conscious cats. *Brit. J. Pharmacol.*, 51: 325—333.

Day, M.D., Roach, A.G. and Whiting, R.L. (1973) The mechanism of the anti-hypertensive action of α-methyldopa in hypertensive rats. *Europ. J. Pharmacol.*, 21: 271—280.

De Jong, W. (1974) Noradrenaline: central inhibitory control of blood pressure and heart rate. *Europ. J. Pharmacol.*, 29: 179—181.

De Jong, W. and Nijkamp, F.P. (1975) Hypotensive action of noradrenaline and α-methylnoradrenaline in the area of the nucleus tractus solitarii in the rat brainstem. In *Central Action of Drugs in Blood Pressure Regulation*, D.S. Davies and J.L. Reid (Eds.), Pitman, London, pp. 179—180.

De Jong, W. and Nijkamp, F.P. (1976) Centrally induced hypotension and bradycardia after administration of α-methylnoradrenaline into the area of the nucleus tractus solitarii of the rat. *Brit. J. Pharmacol.*, 58: 593—598.

De Jong, W., Nijkamp, F.P. and Bohus, B. (1975a) Role of noradrenaline and serotonin in the central control of blood pressure in normotensive and spontaneously hypertensive rats. *Arch. int. Pharmacodyn.*, 213: 272—284.

De Jong, W., Zandberg, P. and Bohus, B. (1975b) Central inhibitory noradrenergic cardiovascular control. In *Hormones, Homeostasis and the Brain, Progr. Brain Res., Vol. 42*, W.H. Gispen, Tj. B. Van Wimersma Greidanus, B. Bohus and D.De Wied (Eds.), Elsevier, Amsterdam, pp. 285—298.

Dhasmana, K.M. and Spilker, B.A. (1973) On the mechanism of L-dopa-induced postural hypotension in the cat. *Brit. J. Pharmacol.*, 47: 437–451.

Doba, N. and Reis, D.J. (1973) Acute fulminating neurogenic hypertension produced by brainstem lesions in the rat. *Circulat. Res.*, 32: 584–593.

Doxey, J.C. and Scutt, A. (1974) Effect of α-methyldopa on sympathetic nerve function in the pithed rat. *Europ. J. Pharmacol.*, 29: 320–323.

Finch, L. and Haeusler, G. (1973) Further evidence for a central hypotensive action of α-methyldopa in both the rat and the cat. *Brit. J. Pharmacol.*, 47: 217–228.

Finch, L., Hersom, A. and Hicks, P. (1975) Studies on the hypotensive action of α-methyldopamine. *Brit. J. Pharmacol.*, 54: 445–451.

Fuxe, K. (1965) Evidence for the existence of monoamine neurons in the central nervous system. IV. The distributions of monoamine nerve terminals in the central nervous system. *Acta physiol. scand.*, 247, Suppl. 64: 39–85.

Gillespie, L., Oates, J.A., Crout, J.R. and Sjoerdsma, A. (1962) Clinical and chemical studies with α-methyldopa in patients with hypertension. *Circulation*, 25: 281–291.

Gillis, R.A., Shister, H.E. and Melville, K.I. (1966) Effects of methyldopa (Aldomet) on cardiovascular responses to adrenaline, noradrenaline and tyramine in rabbits. *Arch. int. Pharmacodyn.*, 159: 219–233.

Haefely, W., Hurlimann, A. and Thoenen, H. (1967) Adrenergic transmitter changes and response to sympathetic nerve stimulation after differing pretreatment with α-methyldopa. *Brit. J. Pharmacol.*, 31: 105–119.

Heise, A. and Kroneberg, G. (1972) α-Sympathetic receptor stimulation in the brain and hypotensive activity of α-methyldopa. *Europ. J. Pharmacol.*, 17: 315–317.

Heise, A. and Kroneberg, G. (1973) Central nervous α-adrenergic receptors and the mode of action of α-methyldopa. *Naunyn-Schmiedeberg's Arch. exp. Path. Pharmak.*, 279: 285–300.

Henning, M. (1967) Blood pressure and noradrenaline levels after treatment with α-methyldopa, α-methyldopamine and α-methyl-*m*-tyrosine. *J. Pharm. Pharmacol.*, 19: 775–779.

Henning, M. (1969) Interaction of dopa decarboxylase inhibitors with the effect of α-methyldopa on blood pressure and tissue monoamines in rats. *Acta pharmacol. (Kbh.)*, 27: 135–148.

Henning, M. (1975) Central sympathetic transmitters and hypertension. *Clin. Sci. molec. Med.*, 48: 195s–203s.

Henning, M. and Rubenson, A. (1971) Evidence that the hypotensive action of methyldopa is mediated by central action of methylnoradrenaline. *J. Pharm. Pharmacol.*, 23: 407–411.

Henning, M. and Van Zwieten, P.A. (1968) Central hypotensive effect of α-methyldopa. *J. Pharm. Pharmacol.*, 20: 409–417.

Henning, M., Rubenson, A. and Trolin, G. (1972) On the localization of the hypotensive effect of L-dopa. *J. Pharm. Pharmacol.*, 24: 447–451.

Holtz, P. and Palm, D. (1967) On the pharmacology of α-methylated catecholamines and the mechanism of the antihypertensive action of α-methyldopa. *Life Sci.*, 6: 1847–1857.

Hulst, S.G. Th. and De Wied, D. (1967) Changes in body temperature and water intake following intracerebral implantation of carbachol in rats. *Physiol. Behav.*, 2: 367–371.

Ingenito, A.J., Barrett, J.P. and Procita, L. (1970) A centrally mediated peripheral hypotensive effect of α-methyldopa. *J. Pharmacol. exp. Ther.*, 175: 593–599.

Kelly, R.J. and Burks, T.F. (1974) Relative vasoconstrictor potencies of norepinephrine, alpha-methylnorepinephrine and octopamine. *Arch. int. Pharmacodyn.*, 208: 306–316.

König, J.F.R. and Klippel, R.A. (1963) *The Rat Brain: a Stereotaxic Atlas of the Forebrain and Lower Parts of the Brainstem*, Williams and Wilkins, Baltimore, Md.

Lang, W.J. and Rush, M.L. (1973) Cardiovascular responses to injections of cholinergic drugs into the cerebral ventricles of unanaesthetised dogs. *Brit. J. Pharmacol.*, 47: 196–205.

Laubie, M. (1975) Pharmacological evidence for interactions of cholinergic and noradrenergic mechanisms in central cardiovascular control. In *Proceedings of the Sixth Int. Congr. of Pharmacol. (Helsinki)*, Vol. 4, I. Tuomisto and M.K. Paasonen (Eds.), Pergamon, London, pp. 79–85.

Lund-Johansen, P. (1972) Hemodynamic changes in long-term α-methyldopa therapy of essential hypertension. *Acta med. scand.*, 192: 221—226.

Maître, L. and Staehelin, M. (1963) Effect of α-methyldopa on myocardial catecholamines. *Experientia (Basel)*, 19: 573—575.

Maj. J. and Pawlowski, L. (1973) The hypothermic effect of L-dopa in the rat. *Life Sci.*, 13: 141—149

Marley, E. and Stephenson, J.D. (1970) Effects of catecholamines infused into the brain of young chickens. *Brit. J. Pharmacol.*, 40: 639—658.

Miura, M. and Reis, D.J. (1969) Termination and secondary projections of carotid sinus nerve in the cat brain stem. *Amer. J. Physiol.*, 217: 142—153.

Miura, M. and Reis, D.J. (1972) The role of the solitary and paramedian reticular nuclei in mediating cardiovascular reflex response from carotid baro- and chemoreceptors. *J. Physiol. (Lond.)*, 223: 525—548.

Muscholl, E. (1966) Autonomic nervous system: newer mechanisms of adrenergic blockade. *Ann. Rev. Pharmacol.*, 6: 107—128.

Muscholl, E. (1972) Adrenergic false transmitters. In *Catecholamines*, H. Blaschko and E. Muscholl (Eds.), Springer, Berlin, p. 618.

Muscholl, E. and Maître, L. (1963) Release by sympathetic stimulation of α-methylnoradrenaline stored in the heart after administration of α-methyldopa. *Experientia (Basel)*, 19: 658—659.

Nijkamp, F.P. (1975) *Over de Bloeddrukverlagende Werking van α-Methyldopa. Experimenteel Bewijs voor een Centraal Aangrijpingspunt*, Thesis, University of Utrecht, Utrecht.

Nijkamp, F.P. and De Jong, W. (1974) Conversion of α-methyldopa to α-methylnoradrenaline; an explanation for the central inhibitory effect of α-methyldopa on blood pressure and heart rate of rats. *Ned. T. Geneesk.*, 17: 304—305.

Nijkamp, F.P. and De Jong, W. (1975) α-Methylnoradrenaline induced hypotension and bradycardia after administration into the area of the nucleus tractus solitarri. *Europ. J. Pharmacol.*, 32: 361—364.

Nijkamp, F.P., Ezcr, J. and De Jong, W. (1975) Central inhibitory effects of α-methyldopa on blood pressure, heart rate and body temperature of renal hypertensive rats. *Europ. J. Pharmacol.*, 31: 242—249.

Oates, J.A., Gillespie, L., Udenfriend, S. and Sjoerdsma, A. (1960) Decarboxylase inhibition and blood pressure reduction by α-methyl-3,4-di-hydroxy-D,L-phenyl-alanine. *Science*, 131: 1890—1891.

Onesti, G., Brest, A.N., Novack, P., Kasparian, I. and Moyer, J.H. (1964) Pharmacodynamic effects of alpha-methyldopa in hypertensive subjects. *Amer. Heart J.*, 67: 32—38.

Osborne, M.W., Wenger, J.J. and Willems, W. (1971) The cardiovascular pharmacology of L(-)dopa; peripheral and central effects. *J. Pharmacol. exp. Ther.*, 178: 517—528.

Palkovits, M. and Jacobowitz, D.M. (1974) Topographic atlas of catecholamine and acetylcholinesterase-containing neurons in the rat brain. II. Hindbrain (mesencephalon, rhombencephalon). *J. comp. Neurol.*, 157: 29—42.

Reneman, R.S., Wellens, D., Jageneau, A.H.M. and Stynen, L. (1974) Vertebral and carotid blood distribution in the brain of the dog and the cat. *Cardiovasc. Res.*, 8: 65—72.

Richardson, A.W., Cooper, T. and Pinakatt, T. (1962) Thermodilution method for measuring cardiac output of rats by using a transistor bridge. *Science*, 135: 317—318.

Robson, R.D. (1971) Modification of the cardiovascular effects of L-dopa in anaesthetized dogs by inhibitors of enzymes involved in catecholamine metabolism. *Circulat. Res.*, 28: 662—670.

Sannerstedt, R., Conway, J. and Arbor, A. (1970) Hemodynamic and vascular responses to antihypertensive treatment with adrenergic blocking agents: a review. *Amer. Heart J.*, 79: 122—127.

Satchell, D.G., Freeman, S.E. and Hopkins, S.V. (1971) Effects of α-methylnoradrenaline on cardiac metabolism. *Biochem. Pharmacol.*, 20: 1691—1694.

Scherrer, H. (1967) Inhibition of sympathetic discharge by stimulation of the medulla oblongata in the rat. *Acta neuroveg. (Wien)*, 29: 56—74.

Schmitt, H. (1975) On some unexplained effects of clonidine. In *Recent Advances in*

Hypertension, Vol. II, P. Milliez and M. Safer (Eds.), Boehringer, Ingelheim, pp. 63—74.

Schmitt, H. et Pétillot, N. (1970) Influence du remplacement de la noradrenaline par des faux mediateures et de l'inhibition de la synthése sur l'excitabilité sympathique. *J. Pharmacol. (Paris),* 1: 183—189.

Schmitt, H. and Schmitt, H. (1969) Localization of the hypotensive effect of 2-(2-6-dichlo-rophenyl-amino)-2-imidazoline hydrochloride (St 155, catapresan). *Europ. J. Pharmacol.,* 6: 8—12.

Schmitt, H., Schmitt, H. and Fenard, S. (1973a) Action of α-adrenergic blocking drugs on the sympathetic centres and their interactions with the central sympatho-inhibitory effect of clonidine. *Arzneimittel. Forsch.,* 23: 40—45.

Schmitt, H., Schmitt, H., Fenard, S. and Laubie, M. (1973b) Evidence for a sympatho-mimetic component inhibiting the sympathetic centres: nature of the receptor. In *Symposium on Pharmacological Agents and Biogenic Amines in the Central Nervous System,* J. Knoll and K. Magyar (Eds.), Akademiai Kiadó, Budapest, pp. 177—194.

Seller, H. and Illert, M. (1969) The localization of the first synapse in the carotid sinus baroreceptor reflex pathway and its alteration of the afferent input. *Pflügers Arch. Ges. Physiol.,* 306: 1—19.

Sinha, J.N. and Schmitt, H. (1974) Central sympatho-inhibitory effects of intracisternal and intravenous administrations of noradrenaline in high doses. *Europ. J. Pharmacol.,* 28: 217—221.

Sjoerdsma, A., Vendsalu, A. and Engelman, K. (1963) Studies on the metabolism and mechanism of action of methyldopa. *Circulation,* 28: 492—502.

Sourkes, T.L. (1965) The action of α-methyldopa in the brain. *Brit. med. Bull.,* 21: 66—69.

Stone, C.A. and Porter, C.C. (1967) Biochemistry and pharmacology of methyldopa and some related structures. *Advanc. Drug Res.,* 4: 71—93.

Stone, C.A., Ross, C.A., Wenger, H.C., Ludden, C.T., Blessing, J.A., Totaro, J.A. and Porter, C.C. (1962) Effect of α-methyl-3,4-dihydroxyphenylalanine (methyldopa), reserpine and related agents on some vascular responses in the dog. *J. Pharmacol. exp. Ther.,* 136: 80—88.

Struyker Boudier, H.A.J., Smeets, G.W.M., Brouwer, G.M. and Van Rossum, J.M. (1974) Hypothalamic alpha adrenergic receptors in cardiovascular regulation. *Neuropharmacology,* 13: 837—846.

Struyker Boudier, H.A.J., Smeets, G.W.M., Brouwer, G.M. and Van Rossum, J.M. (1975) Central nervous system α-adrenergic mechanisms and cardiovascular regulation in rats *Arch. int. Pharmacodyn.,* 213: 285—293.

Tauberger, G. und Kuhn, P. (1971) Untersuchungen der zentralnervosen sympathicus dampfenden Wirkungen von α-Methyldopa. *Naunyn-Schmiedeberg's Arch. exp. Path. Pharmak.,* 268: 33—43.

Toda, N., Matsuda, Y. and Shimamoto, K. (1969) Cardiovascular effects of sympatho-mimetic amines injected into the cerebral ventricles of rabbits. *Int. J. Neuropharmacol.,* 8: 451—461.

Toivola, P. and Gale, C.C. (1970) Effect on temperature of biogenic amine infusion into hypothalamus of baboon. *Neuroendocrinology,* 6: 210—219.

Trinker, F.R. (1971) The significance of the relative potencies of noradrenaline and α-methylnoradrenaline for the mode of action of α-methyldopa. *J. Pharm. Pharmacol.,* 23: 306—308.

Tsoucaris-Kupfer, D. and Schmitt, H. (1972) Hypothermic effect of α-sympathomimetic agents and their antagonism by adrenergic and cholinergic drugs. *Neuropharmacology,* 11: 625—635.

Van der Werf, T. (1965) *Directe en Indirecte Stroommeeting in het Hart en de Grote Bloedvaten,* Thesis, University of Groningen, Groningen.

Van Spanning, H.W. and Van Zwieten, P.A. (1975) The interaction between α-methyldopa and tricyclic antidepressants. *Int. J. clin. Pharmacol.,* 11: 65—69.

Van Zwieten, P.A. (1975) Antihypertensive drugs with a central action. *Progr. Pharmacol.,* 1: 1—63.

Wellens, D.L.F., Wouters, L.J.N.R., De Reese, R.J.J., Beirnaert, P. and Reneman, R.S.

(1975) The cerebral blood distribution in dogs and cats. An anatomical and functional study. *Brain Res.*, 86: 429—438.

Wellens, D., Wouters, L., Nijkamp, F.P. and De Jong, W. (1976) Distribution of the blood flow supplied by the vertebral artery in rats: anatomical, functional and pharmacological aspects. *Experientia, (Basel)* 32: 85—87.

Wilson, W.R., Fisher, F.D. and Kirkendall, W.M. (1962) The acute hemodynamic effects of α-methyldopa in man. *J. chron. Dis.*, 15: 907—913.

Zandberg, P. and De Jong, W. (1977) Localization of catecholaminergic receptor sites in the nucleus tractus solitarii involved in the regulation of arterial blood pressure. In *Hypertension and Brain Mechanisms, Progr. Brain Res.*, Vol. 47, W. De Jong, A.P. Provoost and A.P. Shapiro (Eds.), Elsevier, Amsterdam, pp. 117—122.

The Central Hypotensive Action of Clonidine and Propranolol in Animals and Man

J.L. REID, K.K. TANGRI and L.M.H. WING

Department of Clinical Pharmacology, Royal Postgraduate Medical School, London W12 0HS (Great Britain)

There is a considerable amount of evidence from experimental studies that certain drugs can lower blood pressure in animals by a direct action on the central nervous system. Several techniques have been used, including administration into brain tissue or cerebrospinal fluid (Schmitt and Schmitt, 1969), vertebral artery infusion (Henning and Van Zwieten, 1968), cross-circulation experiments or studies using pharmacological manoeuvres, including antagonism of specific receptors (Schmitt et al., 1973) or metabolism of drugs (Henning, 1969). Such studies have clearly established that methyldopa, clonidine and several beta receptor blockers including propranolol can lower blood pressure after central administration in animals by central mechanisms (Van Zwieten, 1973), probably by reducing sympathetic outflow. The central effects of these drugs are modified by pithing (Autret et al., 1971), acute spinal cord transections or ganglionic blockade (Autret et al., 1971; Day and Roach, 1973) and associated with the reduction in activity recorded from splanchnic preganglionic nerves in cats, dogs or rabbits (Schmitt et al., 1974; Lewis and Haeusler, 1975). Similar effects on sympathetic nerve activity have been reported following intravenous injection of clonidine and propranolol suggesting that the central site of action may participate in the hypotensive effect of intravenous or even oral dosing (Lewis and Haeusler, 1975).

In man, the evidence for a quantitatively important central site of action after oral administration of these drugs is largely circumstantial. Clonidine and methyldopa frequently cause side effects of drowsiness and sedation (Prichard and Gillam, 1969; Conolly et al., 1972) and propranolol may provoke hallucinations or vivid dreams which are clearly central in origin (Greenblatt and Shader, 1972; Zacharias et al., 1972). Further, these agents lower both supine and erect blood pressure and do not usually result in side effects of ganglionic blockade or impairment of peripheral adrenergic transmission such as impaired ejaculation in males (Prichard and Gillam, 1969).

The confirmation of a central site of action may be important in establishing a rational basis for treating essential hypertension in man. The development of sensitive assay techniques for catecholamines suggests that in a proportion of hypertensive patients, sympathetic activity as reflected by plasma noradrenaline concentration is increased (Engelman et al., 1970; De Quattro and Chan, 1972; Louis et al., 1973) and this increase in sympathetic activity may be centrally mediated. If agents like clonidine, methyldopa and even propranolol do indeed lower blood pressure by reducing sympathetic activity, then they may be useful, not only in controlling blood pressure, but in reversing an underlying central abnormality which results in the increase in sympathetic activity.

This presentation reviews studies undertaken in animals and man in our laboratory in recent years to obtain more direct evidence for a central component to the cardiovascular effects or oral and intravenous clonidine and propranolol. Clonidine was chosen in these studies because it is believed to act directly in its own right and not like methyldopa through an active metabolite. Further, we have developed a specific mass fragmentographic assay for clonidine sufficiently sensitive to detect the very small amounts in plasma after oral dosing in man (Dollery et al., 1976).

EVIDENCE FOR A CENTRAL ACTION OF CLONIDINE IN THE RABBIT

Although a central action of clonidine in the brain stem has been demonstrated in several species (Kobinger and Walland, 1967; Schmitt and Schmitt, 1969; Dollery and Reid, 1973) there are reports of other actions of the drug which might contribute to the blood pressure fall. These include effects on baroreceptor afferent discharges (Aars, 1972; Korner et al., 1974), spinal cord neurons (Sinha et al., 1973), ganglionic transmission and release of neurotransmitter from postganglionic nerve endings (Starke et al., 1972) and finally direct effects on vascular smooth muscle (Zaimis and Hannington, 1969). In addition, the relative importance of sympathetic withdrawal and enhancement of vagal tone have not been clearly defined.

General anaesthesia, with or without respiratory paralysis and artificial ventilation, profoundly alters cardiovascular regulatory mechanisms and the effects of hypotensive drugs (Vatner and Braunwald, 1975). In the present studies we have attempted wherever possible to use unrestrained conscious preparations. Results obtained immediately after gross mutilating surgical procedures may not reflect effects in the conscious preparation after recovery from trauma and haemorrhage.

Autret and colleagues (1971) reported that, after destruction of the spinal cord and thus the sympathetic outflow by pithing, the biphasic pressor and depressor effect of intravenous clonidine was converted to a prolonged pressor action dependent on the unopposed direct alpha agonist action of clonidine on peripheral alpha adrenoceptors (Kobinger and Walland, 1967). Pithing, however, abolishes all sympathetic reflex tone. To determine the relative contribution of central and peripheral mechanisms we have examined the modification of the blood pressure and heart rate effects of clonidine (30 μg/kg) intravenously in conscious rabbits at intervals up to 7 days after a complete transection of the spinal cord above the level of the first thoracic vertebra (Petty et al., 1976), that is above the level of the sympathetic outflow (Truex and Carpenter, 1969). In this model sympathetic outflow is intact and after a recovery period spinal sympathetic activity is present. Similarly baroreceptor input and vagal outflow are intact. After high spinal cord

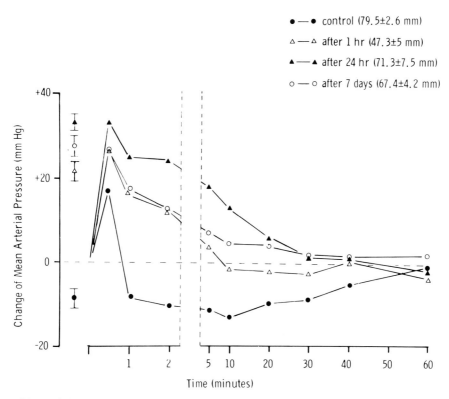

Fig. 1. Mean change in mean arterial pressure in groups (n = 6) of rabbits after clonidine 30 μg/kg i.v. before and 1 hr, 24 hr and 7 days after spinal cord transection at the level of C7. The symbols and bars on the left represent the standard error for a single time interval for each group determined by analysis of variance. Numbers in brackets are the mean ± S.E.M. of predose control mean arterial pressure.

transection, the mean arterial pressure was markedly reduced at 1 hr, but returned to near pre-operated levels at 1 and 7 days. The initial pressor response to i.v. clonidine was potentiated in magnitude and particularly in duration (Fig. 1). The later fall in blood pressure was not seen at any time after transection and was absent at times when resting pressure had returned to near control levels (Fig. 1). The changes in heart rate are shown in Fig. 2 and reveal that the bradycardia persists after transection, although it is of reduced magnitude. These results suggest that the hypotensive action of intravenous clonidine is dependent on an action of the drug above the level of the spinal cord, probably in the brain stem, while the bradycardiac action, expressed through a central increase in vagal tone could still be observed.

The increased magnitude and duration of the pressor effect represented an unopposed peripheral pressor effect, as there was no evidence of marked changes in pressor sensitivity to intravenous phenylephrine at these times (unpublished observations). These studies support the conclusion that withdrawal of sympathetic tone underlies the hypotensive effect of i.v. clonidine. The fall in blood pressure after intracisternal clonidine is also abolished by

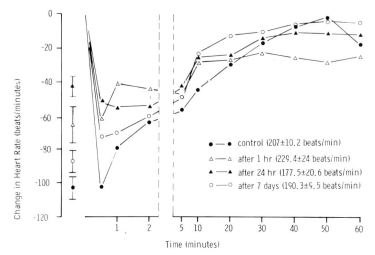

Fig. 2. Mean change in heart rate in groups of rabbit (n = 6) after clonidine 30 μg/kg i.v. before and 1 hr, 24 hr and 7 days after spinal cord transection at the level of C7. The symbols and bars on the left represent the standard error for a single time interval for each group determined by analysis of variance. Numbers in brackets are the mean ± S.E.M. of predose control heart rates.

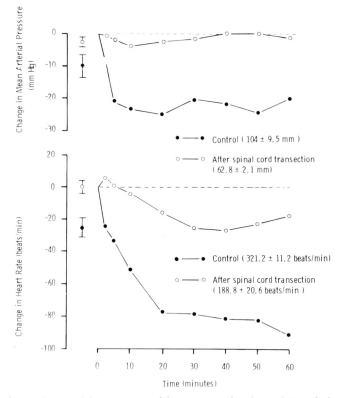

Fig. 3. Mean change in arterial pressure and heart rate after intracisternal clonidine 1 μg/kg in pentobarbitone anaesthetised rabbits before and 7 days after spinal cord transection at the level of C7. The symbols and bars on the left represent the standard error of a single time interval for each group determined by analysis of variance. Mean (± S.E.M.) control values before drug dosing in each group are shown in brackets.

spinal cord transection (Fig. 3) indicating that this direct central action and the effect of i.v. clonidine are both dependent on a similar central mechanism. Peripheral baroreceptor mechanisms are not of primary importance as the depressor action of clonidine is augmented after chronic carotid and aortic baroreceptor denervation (Shaw et al., 1971; Reid et al., 1973). However, this procedure does attenuate the heart rate slowing action and the bradycardia is completely abolished when baroreceptor denervation is combined with spinal cord transection (unpublished observations).

The intravenous dose used in these and similar studies in small mammals (30—100 µg/kg) is much higher than that used orally or intravenously (2—4 µg/kg) in man. In collaboration with E. Neill, M. Petty and P. Tippett, we have recently examined the distribution and elimination of intravenous clonidine in rabbits. A bolus injection of 30 µg/kg has a large volume of distribution and post-distribution plasma levels of 1—2 ng/ml similar to peak plasma concentrations after 4 µg/kg orally to man. However, the elimination half-life (10—20 min) is very much shorter in rabbits than man (5—13 hr) and the duration of drug effect correspondingly shorter, indicating that the doses chosen in animal studies are not disproportionately high in terms of bioavailability of the drug.

EVIDENCE FOR A CENTRAL HYPOTENSIVE ACTION OF CLONIDINE IN MAN

It is well established that clonidine lowers blood pressure in hypertensive man (Conolly et al., 1972). Not so widely recognised is the consistent and significant hypotensive action of single oral doses of 300 µg (4—5 µg/kg) in normotensive individuals (Dollery et al., 1976; Wing et al., 1976) accompanied by a sedative effect and reduction in resting saliva production. The fall in systolic and diastolic blood pressure lasts more than 8 hr and is accompanied by a reduction in plasma noradrenaline and urinary excretion of catechol-amines and metabolites (Hökfelt et al., 1975; Wing et al., 1976). Although this reduction in noradrenaline turnover is compatible with a central action of clonidine in man, it does not exclude an action on the spinal cord or noradrenaline release from peripheral nerve endings.

In an attempt to resolve this problem we have studied the effects of single oral doses of clonidine in normotensive men and compared the results with those in 6 subjects with traumatic transection of the cervical spinal cord under the care of the National Spinal Injuries Unit, Stoke Mandeville Hospital, Aylesbury, England (Reid et al., 1976). All subjects had chronic tetraplegia with complete loss of sensation and voluntary movements below the level of the fifth cervical segment. These individuals had interruption of descending bulbospinal sympathetic pathways but intact baroreceptor afferents and vagal outflow (Truex and Carpenter, 1969). Spinal sympathetic reflex activity was present and could be elicited by manoeuvres such as bladder percussion (Guttman and Witteridge, 1947; Mathias et al., 1975). Although clonidine significantly lowered blood pressure in normotensives between 1 and 8 hr after dosing, oral clonidine did not significantly lower the pressure in the tetraplegics at any time examined (Fig. 4). Peak plasma clonidine concentration measured

374

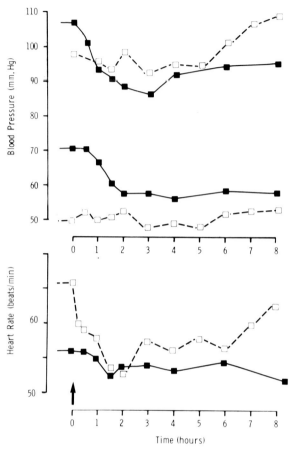

Fig. 4. Mean systolic and diastolic blood pressure and heart rate in 5 normotensive controls (■———■) and 6 tetraplegic subjects (□ — — — □) with chronic cervical spinal cord transection after clonidine 300 μg orally (arrow). Systolic and diastolic pressures after 45 min were significantly reduced in controls ($P < 0.05$) by analysis of variance. At no time did blood pressure fall significantly in the tetraplegics.

by mass fragmentography in controls and tetraplegics was similar (1.39 ± 0.14 and 1.36 ± 0.19 ng/ml) at 90 min and the range of half-life elimination from plasma (plasma $t_{1/2}$) was the same in the two groups (5—13 hr). A pharmacokinetic explanation did not appear likely to underlie the difference in effect on blood pressure as absorption, distribution and elimination of clonidine was similar in the two groups.

A sedative effect and a reduction in saliva production are commonly observed in clinical practice and may limit the dose tolerated (Conolly et al., 1972). Both sedation (Delbarre and Schmitt, 1973) and dry mouth (Rand et al., 1969) are believed to be central nervous effects mediated like the central cardiovascular action by an interaction with alpha adrenoceptors in the CNS. We have assessed the sensitivity of the putative central receptors for clonidine in the two groups by quantifying changes in the level of sedation and resting saliva production after dosing (Dollery et al., 1976). Sedation is measured with a self-assessment 100 mm bipolar visual analogue scale and scored in mm from the wide awake pole. Clonidine 300 µg orally caused a marked increase in sedation maximal between 2 and 4 hr after dosing (100 mm represents deep sleep (Table I)). The effect of clonidine persisted for at least 6—8 hr and was qualitatively similar in the two groups.

Saliva production was measured as the change in weight of pre-weighed dental rolls placed in the mouth opposite the openings of the salivary ducts for exactly 1 min. There was a profound reduction in salivary flow which persisted for 8 hr in both groups (Table I). There was no difference between the magnitude or duration of the effect in the two groups. These results do not indicate any difference in sensitivity of putative central clonidine receptors in the tetraplegics compared to controls. The persistence of the effect on saliva production in tetraplegics shows that sympathetic innervation of the salivary glands does not contribute to this effect of clonidine and would be compatible with a central action on the parasympathetic innervation.

Thus resting supine blood pressure is not significantly lowered by clonidine in tetraplegics while normotensive subjects studied under similar conditions have a consistent fall in blood pressure. In contrast, the fall in heart rate is not only present in tetraplegics but is more marked than in controls. Tetraplegic subjects do not have both sympathetic and vagal components contributing to reflex control of heart rate. The remaining vagal contribution is much more important in regulating heart rate and cardiac output (Frankel et al., 1975). The bradycardia observed represents the central effect of clonidine on the brain stem and further confirms the integrity of vagal mechanisms in these subjects. The absence of a fall in pressure in spite of the exaggerated bradycardia makes it unlikely that cardiac vagal actions contribute to clonidine hypotension. It is more likely that sympathetic withdrawal mediated by a central action of clonidine in the brain rostral to the spinal cord is responsible for the fall in blood pressure. In resting supine tetraplegics and probably also normals, the level of peripheral sympathetic activity is low. Under these conditions we do not observe a quantitatively important peripheral effect on blood pressure through spinal cord, postganglionic neurone release or smooth muscle actions. However, it is possible that when local spinal reflex activity is increased in tetraplegics by urinary tract infection or bladder distension (Mathias et al., 1975), spinal or peripheral effects of clonidine may participate in depressor actions (to be published).

Although changes in discharges in baroreceptor afferents following clonidine have been previously described (Aars, 1972; Korner et al., 1974), peripheral baroreceptor deafferentation in rabbits does not abolish the fall in blood pressure after clonidine (Shaw et al., 1971; Reid et al., 1973). We have been able to study one man who had clinical features of afferent baroreceptor reflex denervation (Sharpey-Schafer, 1956; Love et al., 1971). This syndrome is associated particularly with tabes dorsalis or diabetes mellitus and is characterised by postural hypotension, complete absence of baroreflex responses to tilting or Valsalva's manoeuvre but with normal responses to mental stress or ice-cold water (non-baroreceptor dependent cardiovascular reflexes) and a relatively normal efferent peripheral effector pathway as assessed by pressor sensitivity to intravenous noradrenaline (Love et al., 1971).

TABLE I

MEAN (± S.E.M.) SEDATION SCORE IN MILLIMETRES FROM WIDE AWAKE SCORE ON A BIPOLAR SELF-ASSESSMENT ANALOGUE SCALE AND RESTING SALIVA PRODUCTION (g/min) IN 5 NORMOTENSIVE CONTROLS AND 6 TETRAPLEGICS BEFORE AND UP TO 8 HR AFTER ORAL CLONIDINE 300 µg

	Time (hr) after oral clonidine				
	0	1	2	4	8
Sedation (mm from wide awake)					
Normotensive controls	9.0 ± 2.6	50.4 ± 11.9	76.3 ± 5.0	63.1 ± 6.0	41.6 ± 9.7
Tetraplegics	20.2 ± 10.2	40.3 ± 15.0	54.3 ± 16	62.3 ± 7.3	20.7 ± 11.7
Saliva production (g/min)					
Normotensive controls	1.01 ± 0.34	0.16 ± 0.03	0.12 ± 0.02	0.22 ± 0.06	0.29 ± 0.06
Tetraplegics	0.82 ± 0.10	0.19 ± 0.05	0.14 ± 0.03	0.22 ± 0.04	0.34 ± 0.06

377

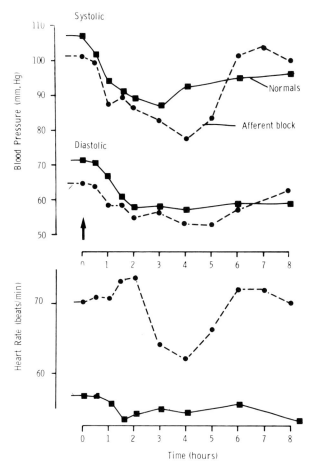

Fig. 5. Mean systolic and diastolic blood pressure and heart rate after oral clonidine 300 μg in 5 normotensive controls (■———■) and one subject with an afferent autonomic neuropathy and clinical evidence of baroreceptor denervation (● — — — ●).

The patient studied had positive syphilitic serology and clinical features of tabes dorsalis in addition to the characteristic cardiovascular reflex pattern. The blood pressure and heart rate response to oral clonidine 300 μg is compared in this subject with afferent autonomic neuropathy and a group of normotensive controls (Fig. 5). The hypotensive effect is present and actually greater in the patient. Bradycardia also occurs due to the central effects of clonidine. Tabes affects sensory fibres and cell bodies and in this case presumably glosso-pharyngeal and vagal sensory afferent involvement underlies the autonomic deficit. Although this is a single clinical observation, without histological evidence, we suggest that these data would indicate that clonidine achieves its central action at a point between the primary sensory afferent and bulbospinal pathways leading to withdrawal of sympathetic tone which is responsible for the fall in blood pressure not only after administration in animals but also after oral dosing in man.

EVIDENCE FOR A CENTRAL ACTION OF PROPRANOLOL IN THE RABBIT

Intracerebroventricular (ICV) propranolol lowers blood pressure in anaesthetized (Srivastava et al., 1973) and conscious animals (Day and Roach, 1973; Reid et al., 1974). The fall in pressure is small in magnitude but relatively long lasting and follows an initial pressor effect. These effects of propranolol have been extensively investigated by several groups including our own (Reid et al., 1974; Myers et al., 1975a,b) and the fall in pressure appears to be a consequence of beta blockade as it only occurs with the beta blocking L-isomer and occurs with some other beta receptor blocking drugs (Srivastava et al., 1973; Sweet et al., 1975). Myers et al. (1975a) also observed a small fall in blood pressure after intravenous infusion of D L-propranolol in conscious rabbits which did not occur after infusion of D-propranolol (Table II). Brain propranolol concentrations after i.v. propranolol were similar to those after ICV dosing suggesting that the observed effects could be centrally mediated. Further evidence of a central contribution to propranolol's hypotensive action in the rabbit is derived from Lewis and Haeusler's report (1975) that sympathetic nerve activity measured from the splanchnic nerve was reduced after intravenous infusion of propranolol. This reduction in nerve activity was much less pronounced than that following clonidine, but occurred in the presence of a fall in systemic blood pressure. Intravenous sodium nitroprusside and haemorrhage which lower blood pressure by peripheral mechanisms increase sympathetic activity (P.J. Lewis, personal communication). The reduction observed after propranolol is compatible with a central action of propranolol. However, the studies described with intravenous propranolol do

TABLE II

EFFECT OF INTRAVENOUS INFUSION OF DL- AND D-PROPRANOLOL ON MEAN ARTERIAL PRESSURE (MAP) IN RABBITS

Myers et al., 1975.

	Change in MAP (mm Hg)		
	Initial	At 60 min	At 120 min
i.v. DL-propranolol infusion (mg/kg/hr)			
1.0 (n = 6)	81 ± 7.3	−9 ± 1.8*	−11 ± 1.8*
2.0 (n = 6)	85 ± 3.6	−8 ± 3.7**	−10 ± 4.4**
i.v. D-propranolol infusion (mg/kg/hr)			
1.0 (n = 6)	84 ± 0.8	−2 ± 3.4	−4 ± 1.9
2.0 (n = 5)	82 ± 5.8	−7 ± 4.1	−6 ± 1.8*
4.0 (n = 6)	84 ± 1.7	−5 ± 3.4	−5 ± 3.4
i.v. saline (ml/kg/hr)			
1.0 (n = 5)	78 ± 3.0	4 ± 1.3	5 ± 2.5

*$P < 0.01$.
**$P < 0.05$.

not conclusively demonstrate a central nervous site of action of the drug. Some or all of propranolol's effect may be mediated by modification of transmitter release from postganglionic neurones by blockade of beta receptors located presynaptically (Langer et al., 1975; Rand et al., 1975). Although the presence and functional significance of presynaptic beta receptors are controversial, there are other serious objections to a hypothesis which attributes an important central effect to propranolol's action. Several other beta blockers which also lower blood pressure are very polar compounds which do not readily enter the central nervous system in animals. Thus, although animal experiments reveal that certain beta blockers can under certain circumstances exhibit a central hypotensive action, it is still uncertain to what extent central mechanisms contribute to the drugs' action after oral or intravenous dosing.

EVIDENCE FOR A CENTRAL ACTION OF PROPRANOLOL IN MAN

If the evidence for a central action is uncertain in animals, it is even more controversial in man. The evidence is mainly circumstantial and derives from clinical reports of hallucination, vivid dreams and other central nervous side effects (Greenblatt and Shader, 1972; Zacharias et al., 1972). Further, other proposed mechanisms of hypotensive action of beta blockers are not entirely satisfactory (Frohlich, 1972).

Propranolol undoubtedly enters the brain in man and a high ratio of brain to plasma concentration develops. We have been able to examine plasma concentration and brain regional concentrations in patients receiving D-propranol who died and had post-mortem examinations (Myers et al., 1975a). Brain concentrations (Table III) were similar to those measured in rabbits after i.v. and ICV dosing. However, although propranolol clearly enters the brain it is unlikely that more polar compounds such as practolol, atenolol or metoprolol can penetrate the blood—brain barrier to the same extent. It is possible that several loci of action, including the CNS in the case of lipophilic beta blockers contribute to the overall effect.

Another possible approach to defining a central component of the hypotensive action of beta blockers is to measure changes in sympathetic activity before and after beta blockers. Beta blockers cause no consistent change in urinary excretion of catecholamines or their metabolites (Hansson and Hökfelt, 1975). Urinary metabolites are usually unchanged even though blood pressure is lowered. Plasma noradrenaline concentration has been used as an index of sympathetic activity. We have found that single oral doses of 200 mg of propranolol cause a small but significant fall in blood pressure. Resting supine plasma noradrenaline is normal or reduced. However, the increase in plasma noradrenaline following exercise is not modified by propranolol and may be potentiated by maximal beta blockade (Maling et al., to be published). Rahn et al. (1976) observed that chronic dosing of beta blockers to hypertensives caused small but significant rises in plasma catecholamines, although urinary excretion was unchanged. Others have observed only small changes in plasma catecholamines (Hansson and Hökfelt, 1975).

TABLE III

REGIONAL BRAIN PROPRANOLOL CONCENTRA-
TION AFTER I.V. INFUSION OF D-PROPANOLOL
0.05—0.40 mg/kg/hr TO MAN FOR 25—264 hr

Myers et al., 1975a.

Brain region	Propranolol content (µg/g)		
	D.H.	E.B.	M.P.
Midbrain	7.74	0.62	3.73
Hypothalamus	8.88	0.68	2.60
Basal ganglia	8.77	0.72	2.28
Internal capsule	7.13.	0.72	2.71
Cerebral cortex (grey matter)	7.52	0.47	2.19
Medulla	7.14	0.50	2.34
Pons	7.31	0.60	1.85
Cerebellum	6.29	0.42	1.57
Plasma	—	1.12	0.69

Thus at present reports of the action of beta blockers on plasma noradrenaline have produced inconsistent results. It appears that marked changes do not occur in plasma or urinary catecholamines in spite of considerable effects on blood pressure. These results do not exclude an action of beta blockers on peripheral sympathetic tone.

Further carefully controlled studies will be essential to determine whether hypotension with beta blockers is accompanied by changes in sympathetic activity. At present it is not at all clear whether central nervous effects or actions on proposed presynaptic receptors participate in the hypotension observed after chronic oral dosing with beta blockers.

SUMMARY

Clonidine and methyldopa lower blood pressure in animals by an action on the central nervous system. The hypotensive action of oral clonidine (300 µg) in man also appears to be centrally mediated as the hypotensive action was abolished in tetraplegic subjects with post-traumatic cervical spinal cord transection.

Similar results in rabbits indicate the importance of the integrity of bulbospinal sympathetic outflow. The integrity of afferent baroreceptor fibres was not essential for the hypotensive action in man or rabbits. Plasma noradrenaline, as an index of sympathetic activity, was reduced after single doses and chronic treatment with clonidine in normotensives and hypertensives.

The beta blocker, propranolol (200 mg orally), lowered blood pressure in normotensive men by a small but significant amount. Plasma noradrenaline changes were much less prominent than following clonidine. Hypertensive patients on chronic oral treatment with propranolol alone did not have significantly different plasma levels of noradrenaline to patients on diuretics or those on no treatment.

Although clonidine appears to exert its hypotensive action via the central nervous system, we have not established that the major site of propranolol's effect is on efferent sympathetic outflow.

ACKNOWLEDGEMENTS

We would like to thank our colleagues who assisted and participated in experiments described and in particular Professor C.T. Dollery, Drs. P. Lewis, M. Myers and T. Maling and Misses M. Petty, E. Neill and P. Tippett.

Ms. C. Hamilton, B. Fraser and J. Daniel gave invaluable technical assistance and Miss B. Edinborough typed the manuscript.

J.L.R. is supported by the Wellcome Trust, K.K.T. is a Fellow of the Commonwealth Universities Association and L.M.H.W. is a Fellow of the National Health and Medical Research Council of Australia.

REFERENCES

Aars, H. (1972) Effects of clonidine on aortic diameter and aortic baroreceptor activity. *Europ. J. Pharmacol.*, 20: 52—59.

Autret, A.M., Schmitt, H. and Fenard, S. (1971) Comparison of haemodynamic effects of alpha sympathomimetic drugs. *Europ. J. Pharmacol.*, 13: 208—217.

Conolly, M.E., Briant, R.H., George, C.F. and Dollery, C.T. (1972) A crossover comparison of clonidine and methyldopa in hypertension. *Europ. J. clin. Pharmacol.*, 4: 222—227.

Day, M.D. and Roach, A.G. (1973) Beta adrenergic receptors in the central nervous system of the cat concerned with control of arterial pressure and heart rate. *Nature New Biol.*, 242: 30—31.

Delbarre, B. and Schmitt, H. (1943) A further attempt to characterize sedative receptors activated by clonidine in chickens and mice. *Europ. J. Pharmacol.*, 22: 355—359.

De Quattro, V. and Chan, S. (1972) Raised plasma catecholamines in some patients with primary hypertension. *Lancet*, i: 806—809.

Dollery, C.T. and Reid, J.L. (1973) Central noradrenergic neurones and the cardiovascular actions of clonidine in the rabbit. *Brit. J. Pharmacol.*, 47: 206—216.

Dollery, C.T., Davies, D.S., Draffan, G.H., Dargie, H.J., Dean, C., Reid, J.L., Clare, R.A. and Murray, S. (1976) Clinical pharmacology and pharmacokinetics of clonidine. *Clin. Pharmacol. Ther.*, 19: 11—18.

Engelman, K., Portnoy, B. and Sjoerdsma, A. (1970) Plasma catecholamine concentration in patients with hypertension. *Circulat. Res.*, 26—27, Suppl. 1: 141—145.

Frankel, H.L., Mathias, C.J. and Spalding, J.M.K. (1975) Mechanisms of reflex cardiac arrest in tetraplegic patients. *Lancet*, ii: 1183—1185.

Frolich, E.D. (1972) Mechanism of beta blockade hypotension. *New Engl. J. Med.*, 287: 1247.

Greenblatt, D.J. and Shader, R.I. (1972) On the psychopharmacology of beta adrenergic blockade. *Curr. Ther. Res.*, 14: 615—625.

Guttman, L. and Witteridge, D. (1947) Effects of bladder distension on automatic mechanisms after spinal cord injuries. *Brain*, 70: 361—404.

Hansson, B.-G. and Hökfelt, T. (1975) Long term treatment of moderate hypertension with penbutolol (Hoe 893 d). Effects on blood pressure, pulse rate, catecholamines in blood and urine, plasma renin activity and urinary aldosterone under basal conditions and following exercise. *Europ. J. clin. Pharmacol.*, 9: 9—19.

Henning, M. (1969) Interactions of dopa decarboxylase inhibitors with the effect of alpha methyldopa on blood pressure and tissue monoamines. *Acta pharmacol. (Kbh.)*, 27: 135—148.

Henning, M. and van Zwieten, P.A. (1968) Central hypotensive effect of alpha methyldopa. *J. Pharm. Pharmacol.*, 20: 409—417.

Hökfelt, B., Hedeland, H. and Hansson, B.-G. (1975) Effect of clonidine and penbutolol respectively on catecholamines in blood and urine, plasma renin activity and urinary aldosterone in hypertensive patients. *Arch. int. Pharmacodyn.*, 213: 307—321.

Kobinger, W. and Walland, A. (1967) Investigation into the mechanism of hypotensive effect of 2-(2,6-dichlorophenylamino)-2-imidazoline HCl. *Europ. J. Pharmacol*, 2: 155—162.

Korner, P.I., Oliver, J.R., Sleight, P., Chalmers, J.P. and Robinson, J.S. (1974) Effects of clonidine on the baroreceptor heart rate reflex and on single aortic baroreceptor fibre discharge. *Europ. J. Pharmacol.*, 28: 189—198.

Langer, S.Z., Enero, M.A., Aaler-Graschinsky, E., Dubocovich, M.L. and Caluchi, S.M. (1975) Presynaptic regulatory mechanisms for noradrenaline release by nerve stimulation. In *Central Actions of Drugs in the Regulation of Blood Pressure*, D.S. Davies and J.L. Reid (Eds.), Pitmans, London, pp. 133—151.

Lewis, P.J. and Haeusler, G. (1975) Reduction of sympathetic nervous activity as a mechanism for hypotensive effect of propranolol. *Nature New Biol.*, 256: 440.

Louis, W.J., Doyle, A.E. and Anavekar, S. (1973) Plasma norepinephrine levels in essential hypertension. *New Engl. J. Med.*, 288: 599—601.

Love, D.R., Brown, J.J., Chinn, R.H., Johnson, R.H., Lever, A.F., Park, D.M. and Robertson, J.I.S. (1971) Plasma renin in idiopathic orthostatic hypotension. Differential response in subjects with probable afferent and efferent autonomic lesion. *Clin. Sci.*, 41: 289—299.

Mathias, C.J., Christensen, N.J., Corbett, J.L., Frankel, H.L., Goodwin, T.J. and Peart, W.S. (1975) Plasma catecholamine, plasma renin activity and plasma aldosterone in tetraplegic man horizontal and tilted. *Clin. Sci. molec. Med.*, 49: 291—299.

Myers, M.G., Lewis, P.J., Reid, J.L. and Dollery, C.T. (1975a) Brain concentration of propranolol in relation to hypotensive effect in the rabbit with observations on brain propranolol levels in man. *J. Pharmacol. exp. Ther.*, 192: 327—335.

Myers, M.G., Lewis, P.J., Reid, J.L. and Dollery, C.T. (1975b) Central noradrenergic mechanisms and the cardiovascular effects of intracerebroventricular (+)- and (−)-propranolol in the conscious rabbit. *Neuropharmacology*, 14: 221—226.

Petty, M., Reid, J.L. and Tangri, K.K. (1976) The cardiovascular effects of clonidine in rabbits after cervical spinal cord transection. *Brit. J. Pharmacol.*, 57: 449—450P.

Prichard, B.N.C. and Gillam, F.M.S. (1969) Treatment of hypertension with propranolol. *Brit. med. J.*, 1: 7—16.

Rahn, K., Gierlicks, H.W., Planz, G., Planz, R. and Stephany, W. (1976) Effect of propranolol on plasma catecholamine in hypertensive patients. *Europ. J. clin. Invest.*, 6: 323.

Rand, M.J., McCulloch, M.W. and Story, D.F. (1975) Pre-junctional modulation of noradrenergic transmission by noradrenaline, dopamine and acetylcholine. In *Central Actions of Drugs in the Regulation of Blood Pressure*, D.S. Davies and J.L. Reid (Eds.), Pitmans, London, pp. 94—132.

Rand, M.J., Rush, M. and Wilson, S. (1969) Some observation in the inhibition of salivation by ST 155. *Europ. J. Pharmacol.*, 5: 168—172.

Reid, J.L., Lewis, P.J. and Dollery, C.T. (1973) Central and peripheral mechanisms in the maintenance of experimental hypertension in the rabbit. *Clin. Sci.*, 45: 701—709.

Reid, J.L., Lewis, P.J., Myers, M.G. and Dollery, C.T. (1974) Cardiovascular effects of intracerebroventricular d-, l, and dl-propranolol in the conscious rabbit. *J. Pharmacol. exp. Ther.*, 188: 294—299.

Reid, J.L., Wing, L.M.H., Mathias, C.J. and Frankel, H.L. (1976) The central hypotensive action of clonidine in man. *Europ. J. clin. Invest.*, 6: 323.

Schmitt, H. and Schmitt, H. (1969) Localization of the hypotensive effect of 2-(2,6-dichlorophenylamino-2-imidazoline hydrochloride (ST 155, Catapresan). *Europ. J. Pharmacol.*, 6: 8—12.

Schmitt, H., Schmitt, H. and Fenard, S. (1973) Action of alpha-adrenergic blocking drugs on the sympathetic centres and their interactions with the central sympatho-inhibitory effect of clonidine. *Arzneimittel-Forsch.*, 23: 40—45.

Schmitt, H., Fenard, S. and Schmitt, H.S. (1974) A technique for recording sympathetic nerve activity in unanaesthetised dogs. *Neuropharmacology*, 13: 347—351.

Sharpey-Schafer, E.P. (1956) Circulatory reflexes in chronic disease of the afferent nervous system. *J. Physiol. (Lond.)*, 134: 1—10.

Shaw, J., Hunyor, S.N. and Korner, P.I. (1971) Sites of central nervous action of clonidine on reflex autonomic function in the unanaesthetised rabbit. *Europ. J. Pharmacol.*, 15: 66—78.

Sinha, J.N., Atkinson, J.M. and Schmitt, H. (1973) Effects of clonidine and L-dopa on spontaneous and evoked splanchnic nerve discharges. *Europ. J. Pharmacol.*, 24: 113—119.

Srivastava, R.K., Kulshrestha, V.K., Singh, N. and Bhargava, K.P. (1973) Central cardiovascular effects of intracerebroventricular propranolol. *Europ. J. Pharmacol.*, 21: 222—229.

Starke, K., Wagner, J. and Schumann, H.J. (1972) Adrenergic neuron blockade by clonidine: comparison with guanethidine and local anaesthetics. *Arch. int. Pharmacodyn.*, 195: 291—308.

Sweet, C.S., Scriabine, A., Wenger, H.C., Ludden, C.T., Vickers, S. and Stone, C.A. (1975) Cardiovascular effects of intracerebroventricular injection versus oral administration of timolol in spontaneously hypertensive rats. In *Central Action of Drugs in Blood Pressure Regulation*, D.S. Davies and J.L. Reid (Eds.), Pitmans, London, pp. 253—255.

Truex, R.C. and Carpenter, M.B. (1969) *Human Neuroanatomy*, 6th ed., Williams and Wilkins, Baltimore, Md., 216 pp.

Van Zwieten, P.A. (1973) The central action of antihypertensive drugs mediated via central alpha receptors. *J. Pharm. Pharmacol.*, 25: 89—95.

Vatner, S.F. and Braunwald, E. (1975) Cardiovascular control mechanisms in the conscious state. *New Engl. J. Med.*, 293: 970—976.

Wing, L.M.H., Reid, J.L., Hamilton, C.A., Davies, D.S. and Dollery, C.T. (1976) The effects of clonidine on biochemical indices of sympathetic activity in normotensive subjects. *Clin. Sci.*, 51: 15—16P.

Zacharias, F.J., Cowen, K.J., Prestt, J., Vickers, J. and Wall, B.G. (1972) Propranolol in hypertension: a study of long term therapy. *Amer. Heart J.*, 83: 755—761.

Zaimis, E. and Hannington, E. (1969) A possible pharmacological approach to migraine. *Lancet*, 3: 298—300.

Interactions Interfering with Central Adrenoreceptor Activity and Hypotension of Centrally Acting Antihypertensive Agents

P.A. VAN ZWIETEN, with the technical assistance of Miss MARION PAUER

Department of Pharmacy, Division of Pharmacotherapy, University of Amsterdam, Amsterdam-C (The Netherlands)

INTRODUCTION

In clinical therapy the simultaneous administration of different drugs occurs very frequently. The average hospitalized patient treated in medical clinics seems to receive 6—8 different drugs simultaneously. It is hardly surprising, therefore, that drug interaction has become an enormous potential problem on which both the physician and the pharmacist should be adequately informed.

Many patients suffering from hypertension simultaneously require treatment for other diseases as well so that in these patients drug interaction problems may be encountered regularly. Most antihypertensive drugs owe their blood pressure lowering properties to a reduction of sympathetic tone. This reduction of peripheral sympathetic activity may be brought about by various mechanisms: blockade of peripheral adrenergic neuron activity (guanethidine, guanoxan, cyclazenine), depletion of noradrenaline (guanethidine, reserpine), ganglionic blockade (trimetaphan), but also through a direct influence of antihypertensive drugs on the brain stem (clonidine, α-methyl-DOPA, and possibly reserpine).

Various possibilities can be imagined, through which other drugs can interfere with these complex antihypertensive mechanisms in such a manner that the antihypertensive effect will usually be diminished or even abolished. Amitriptyline, a tricyclic antidepressant, has been demonstrated to abolish the hypotensive effect of guanethidine (Meyer et al., 1970). Similarly, desipramine is known to block the antihypertensive effect of clonidine in hypertensive patients (Briant et al., 1973) and also in rabbits (Briant and Reid, 1972). The frequently occurring interaction between antihypertensive drugs and tricyclic antidepressants and possibly other psychotropic drugs as well prompted us to study this problem in more detail in animal experiments. Since part of this work has been published in original papers, we shall limit ourselves here to a comprehensive survey.

MATERIALS AND METHODS

The interference of centrally acting antihypertensive drugs and various psychotropic drugs was mainly studied in cats, but two smaller series of experiments were also carried out in the rat. Drugs, dissolved in saline, were slowly infused into the left vertebral artery of mongrel cats of either sex, anesthetized with 60 mg α-glucochloralose/kg. This procedure has been described in full detail elsewhere (Van Zwieten, 1975a). Mean arterial blood pressure was taken from a femoral artery, heart rate was established by means of the pulse wave recorded at high speed of the recording paper. In control experiments drugs were injected into a femoral vein and the same cardio-vascular parameters were determined.

A second series of experiments was carried out in conscious spontaneously hypertensive rats. A catheter was inserted into a common carotid artery under ether anesthesia and subsequently transferred through the skin of the neck and attached in a fixed position. A second catheter was inserted into the vena cava superior and treated likewise as the arterial catheter. The venous catheter was used for drug administration, from the other catheter mean arterial pressure was taken continuously. Recordings were started at least 3—4 hr after recovery from the surgical intervention. Heart rate was established as well when this was thought to be of interest.

RESULTS AND DISCUSSION

(1) Tricyclic antidepressants

An example of the influence of a tricyclic antidepressant is shown in Fig. 1. The potent centrally induced hypotensive effect of clonidine obtained upon infusion of the drug into the left vertebral artery in cats is significantly diminished by pretreatment with desipramine, administered via the same route. The bradycardic effect of clonidine was influenced in a similar although quantitatively less pronounced manner. When injected intravenously much higher doses of the tricyclic antidepressant had to be used in order to obtain the same degree of reduction of the central hypotensive action of clonidine. When injected after infusion of clonidine into the vertebral artery desipramine and also protriptyline readily reversed the already established hypotension. This finding suggests that the interaction may be competitive in nature. This presumption was confirmed by the fact that a parallel shift of the dose-response curve for clonidine was obtained when protriptyline was injected into the vertebral artery prior to the administration of clonidine (see Fig. 2).

The following tricyclic antidepressants have been demonstrated to diminish the central hypotensive effect of clonidine: desipramine; imipramine; amitriptyline; protriptyline; mianserine; iprindole. The phenomenon of interaction is probably not due to the well-known cocaine-like inhibition of reuptake processes, for the following two reasons: (1) cocaine does not diminish the central hypotensive action of clonidine; (2) iprindole is a tricyclic antidepressant which has no cocaine-like properties whatsoever (Ayd, 1969, Berger, 1975), nevertheless iprindole does significantly diminish the central hypotensive effect of clonidine (Van Zwieten, 1976).

We submit the following mechanism for the general principle of interaction between clonidine and tricyclic antidepressants: clonidine as a centrally acting α-adrenergic stimulant excites α-adrenoreceptors in the brain stem and thus

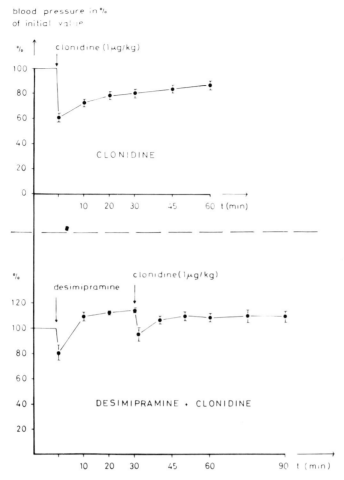

Fig. 1. Hypotensive effect of clonidine (1 μg/kg) alone (top) and that of clonidine after pretreatment with 300 μg desipramine/kg (below). Both clonidine and desipramine were infused into the left vertebral artery of anesthetized cats. Mean values for at least 6 different cats in each series of experiments (± S.E.M.). Note the transient hypotensive effect of desipramine. (From: Van Zwieten (1975b), with permission.)

brings about a reduction in peripheral sympathetic tone and a decrease in arterial pressure and heart rate (Schmitt, 1971; Kobinger, 1973; Van Zwieten, 1975a).

All tricyclic antidepressants employed in the present studies are rather potent α-sympatholytic agents, at least in the periphery. Accordingly we presume that the interaction between clonidine and the antidepressants occurs at the level of the central α-adrenoreceptors in the brain stem, clonidine being the α-agonist and the tricyclic antidepressants the α-antagonists. As already stated the antagonism is probably competitive in nature. An example of interaction at the α-receptor in the brain stem is the blockade of the central hypotensive effect of clonidine by α-sympatholytic agents like piperoxane and yohimbine.

The antagonism is not limited to clonidine and the tricyclic antidepressants.

388

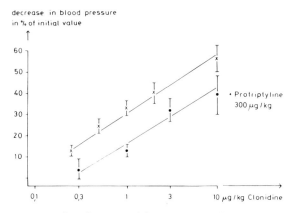

Fig. 2. Dose-response curves for the central hypotensive effect of clonidine; upper curve (x———x): clonidine (vertebral artery); lower curve (●———●): clonidine (vertebral artery) after pretreatment with 300 μg protriptyline/kg, administered via the same route. For details see legend to Fig. 1. (From: Van Zwieten (1975b), with permission.)

In separate studies we have demonstrated that imipramine, desipramine and amitriptyline diminish or abolish the well-known central hypotensive effect of a slow infusion of L-α-methyl-DOPA into the left vertebral artery of chloralose-anesthetized cats (Van Zwieten, 1975b). This interaction can be explained by means of the same mechanism as that described above. α-Methyl-DOPA owes its central hypotensive effect to its metabolite α-methylnoradrenaline, which is formed in the brain. α-Methylnoradrenaline stimulates central α-adreno-receptors and thus induces a decrease in peripheral sympathetic activity and a fall in blood pressure. Again, the tricyclic antidepressants can be expected to block central α-adrenoreceptors and thus reduce the central hypotensive effect of α-methyl-DOPA. The clinical relevance of this phenomenon has not been fully established yet. Some authors described a decrease in antihypertensive efficacy of α-methyl-DOPA when tricyclic antidepressants were administered simultaneously (Simpson, 1973; Boakes, 1974).

Apart from α-methyl-DOPA and clonidine, additional compounds exert some central hypotensive activity when infused into a vertebral artery, through excitation of central α-adrenoreceptors. This mechanism explains the central hypotensive effect of amphetamine and ephedrine as well as its reduction by imipramine (Van Zwieten, 1975b). Again the same type of mechanism may explain the interaction phenomenon.

(2) Neuroleptic agents

The following phenothiazine-type neuroleptic agents, when infused in a dosage of 300 μg/kg into the cat's left vertebral artery, significantly diminish the central hypotensive effect of clonidine: chlorpromazine, thioridazine, promazine, promethazine and thiethylperazine. Similarly, the hypotensive effect of clonidine (i.v.) in conscious, spontaneously hypertensive rats was diminished by chlorpromazine in a dose-dependent manner. The degree of inhibition of clonidine's effect in cats lies within the same order of magnitude as that brought about by the various tricyclic antidepressants. The mechanism is probably the same as the one which we submit for the explanation of the interaction between clonidine and the tricyclic antidepressants. The phenothiazines are potent α-sympatholytic agents as well. Haloperidol, a butyrophenone neuroleptic with weak α-sympatholytic activity in the periphery, slightly reduces the central effect of clonidine. Pimozide, a long-acting neuroleptic agent is not an α-sympatholytic drug and in our experiments it did not significantly influence the central hypotensive effect of clonidine.

The clinical relevance of the interaction between clonidine and phenothiazine neuroleptics remains to be studied. The present animal experiments at least demonstrate the general applicability of the already submitted mechanism of interaction at the level of the central α-adrenoreceptors.

(3) Benzodiazepine tranquillizers

Flurazepam (Dalmadorm®) or chlordiazepoxide (Librium®) when injected into the cat's vertebral artery in appropriate dosage did not significantly diminish the central hypotensive effect of clonidine (1 μg/kg). The lack of blockade of clonidine's hypotensive effect may be explained by the aforementioned mechanism, since benzodiazepines possess none or very little α-sympatholytic activity.

SUMMARY

In chloralose-anesthetized cats the centrally induced hypotensive effect of clonidine, and in some cases α-methyl-DOPA was diminished upon pretreatment with a variety of tricyclic antidepressants and phenothiazine-neuroleptics. This phenomenon could be confirmed by experiments in spontaneously hypertensive rats. Haloperidol was hardly effective, whereas pimozide and benzodiazepine tranquillizers did not diminish the hypotensive response to clonidine. The interaction probably occurs at the level of the central α-adrenoreceptors located in the brain stem. It seems very likely that a competitive antagonism is involved, where clonidine or α-methylnoradrenaline (from α-methyl-DOPA) are the agonists and the tricyclic antidepressants and phenothiazine neuroleptics the antagonists. The lack of interaction with pimozide or the benzodiazepine tranquillizers is explained by the fact that these drugs are not α-blockers.

ACKNOWLEDGEMENT

The generous support of the Dutch Heart Foundation (Nederlandse Hartstichting), the Hague, The Netherlands, is gratefully acknowledged.

REFERENCES

Ayd, F. (1969) Clinical evaluation of a new tricyclic antidepressant: iprindole. *Dis. nerv. Syst.*, 30: 818—824.
Berger, F.M. (1975) Depression and antidepressant drugs. *Clin. Pharmacol. Ther.*, 18: 214—248.

390

Boakes, A.J. (1974) Editorial. *Brit. J. clin. Pharmacol.*, 1: 9—10.

Briant, R.H. and Reid, J.L. (1972) Desmethylimipramine and the hypotensive action of clonidine in the rabbit. *Brit. J. Pharmacol.*, 46: 536P.

Briant, R.H. Reid, J.L. and Dollery, C.T. (1973) Interaction between clonidine and desipramine in man. *Brit. med. J.*, 1: 522—526.

Kobinger, W. (1973) Pharmacological basis of the cardiovascular actions of clonidine. In *Hypertension, Mechanisms and Management*, G. Onesti, K.E. Kim and J.H. Moyer (Eds.), Grune and Stratton, New York, pp. 369—380.

Meyer, J.C., McAllister, K. and Goldberg, L.I. (1970) Insidious and prolonged antagonism of guanethidine by amitriptyline. *J. Amer. med. Ass.*, 213: 1487—1491.

Schmitt, H. (1971) Action des alpha-sympathicomimétiques sur les structures nerveuses. *Actualités Pharmacol.*, 24: 93—131.

Simpson, F.O. (1973) Antihypertensive drug therapy. *Drugs*, 6: 333—363.

Van Zwieten, P.A. (1975a) Antihypertensive drugs with a central action. *Progr. Pharmacol.*, 1: 1—63.

Van Zwieten, P.A. (1975b) The interaction between centrally acting hypotensive drugs and tricyclic antidepressants. *Arch. Int. Pharmacodyn.*, 214: 12—30.

Van Zwieten, P.A. (1977) Reduction of the hypotensive effect of clonidine and alpha-methyl-DOPA by various psychotropic drugs. In *Congress of the International Society for Hypertension, Sydney*, 1976, *Clin. Sci. molec. Med.*, in press.

Clonidine and Related Imidazolidines: Structure–Activity Relationship with Respect to Various Cardiovascular Actions

P.B.M.W.M. TIMMERMANS and P.A. VAN ZWIETEN

Department of Pharmacy, Division of Pharmacotherapy, University of Amsterdam, Amsterdam (The Netherlands)

INTRODUCTION

Clonidine (Catapresan[®], 2-[2,6-dichlorophenylimino]imidazolidine · HCl) probably exerts its hypotensive effect via the excitation of central α-adrenergic receptors, which brings about a peripheral decrease in sympathetic tone (Schmitt, 1971; Kobinger, 1973; Van Zwieten, 1975).

The more or less accidental discovery of clonidine as a potent hypotensive drug has led to the synthesis of a large number of related compounds. The structure-activity relationship (SAR) with respect to the centrally mediated hypotensive action of clonidine and a limited number of structurally related imidazolidines has been considered by Laverty (1969), Walland and Hoefke (1974), Stähle (1974), Hoefke et al. (1975) and Kobinger and Pichler (1975). These investigations indicate that for the central depressor effect lipophilicity is probably a factor of importance in conjunction with the peripheral α-adrenergic stimulating potency of the molecules. However, no quantitative correlations have been presented as yet which do allow any conclusions concerning the SAR at the central α-receptor level. The present study was undertaken in order to obtain a better understanding of the molecular features determining the hypotensive activity of clonidine-like drugs.

For clonidine and 27 structurally related imidazolidines, which differ in substitution in the aromatic moiety, the main cardiovascular effects, i.e. decrease in blood pressure and heart rate, were quantified with the aid of three different animal models. A quantitative comparison between the cardiovascular potencies in these three animal models will be reported. In addition, attempts for a quantitative treatment of the SAR at the level of the central α-receptor will be presented.

METHODS

The hypotensive and bradycardic effects of clonidine and its related derivatives were measured in pentobarbital (75 mg/kg i.p.) anesthetized, normotensive male Wistar rats following intravenous administration. Dose-response curves were used to quantify the hypotensive potency by means of an

ED_{30} and an ED_{25} was calculated for the bradycardic activity. A procedure similar to the one described above was followed for clonidine and a number of its derivatives in order to quantify these cardiovascular effects in the conscious, spontaneously hypertensive rat (SHR-NIH/Cpb, TNO, Zeist, The Netherlands), which yielded an ED_{20} for the antihypertensive activity as well as for the potency in decreasing cardiac frequency. By means of infusions into the left vertebral artery of the chloralose-anesthetized cat, the central mode of action of a number of compounds was investigated. The details of this technique have been reported previously in extenso (Henning and Van Zwieten, 1968; Bock and Van Zwieten, 1971). Studies with piperoxane were carried out in this animal model to establish whether central α-adrenergic receptors are involved in the mechanism of action of these drugs. The central hypotensive activity was quantified by means of an ED_{25}.

As a measure for lipophilic behavior the apparent partition coefficients of the compounds between octanol and a phosphate buffer (pH = 7.4) were obtained (log APC).

For all the equations presented in this paper the technique of the least squares was used and as a basis for the statistical significance of the regressions standard statistical tests were performed which involved the correlation coefficient, r, the standard deviation, S, and the significance of the regression, F.

Drugs used and their sources were: clonidine (Catapresan®; Boehringer Sohn, Ingelheim) and a number of related imidazolidines, the majority of which was synthesized by the authors; ($\pm$)-piperoxane hydrochloride (Janssen Pharmaceutica, Beerse).

RESULTS AND DISCUSSION

In the anesthetized, normotensive rat and in the conscious, spontaneously hypertensive rat all the compounds show the same profile of action as that manifested by clonidine following intravenous administration. The decrease in blood pressure was preceded by a transient hypertensive effect and bradycardia was provoked by all the substances. The derivatives administered via the vertebral artery of the anesthetized cat immediately reduced arterial blood pressure. Systemic injections of the same doses were less effective. In addition, piperoxane significantly diminished the centrally mediated hypotensive response to clonidine and several related imidazolidines after infusion into the cat's vertebral artery. In connection with these results it seems likely that central α-adrenergic receptors play a substantial part in the mode of action of the imidazolidine derivatives in a similar manner as in the mechanism of clonidine.

In the three animal models large differences in hypotensive and bradycardic activity were obtained within this series of structurally very similar molecules (> 4 log units). Clonidine and 2-(2-bromo-6-chlorophenylimino)imidazolidine·HCl were found most potent while the unsubstituted analogue appeared almost devoid of activity.

Equation 1 describes the correlation between the hypotensive activity in the anesthetized, normotensive rat (log ED_{30}) and the centrally induced hypotensive potency in the anesthetized cat (log ED_{25}). The relationship between the hypotensive activity in the anesthetized, normotensive rat (log ED_{30}) and the antihypertensive potency in the conscious, spontaneously hypertensive rat (log ED_{20}) is given by equation 2.

$$\log ED_{30} = 0.891 \log ED_{25} + 0.702 \qquad \text{(eq. 1.)}$$
$$n = 8; r = 0.974; S = 0.284; F = 109 \ (P < 0.001)$$

$$\log ED_{30} = 1.083 \log ED_{20} - 0.340 \qquad \text{(eq. 2.)}$$
$$n = 7; r = 0.978; S = 0.127; F = 111 \ (P < 0.001)$$

These linear correlations strongly indicate that all factors which determine the relative hypotensive potencies are the same in these three animals and that the central α-adrenergic receptors in these species possess a similar character.

In view of the complexity of blood pressure as a parameter, other cardiovascular actions which are provoked by clonidine and its derivatives were examined as well. An excellent correlation was obtained between the blood pressure lowering activity (log ED_{30}) and the heart rate decreasing potency of the molecules (log ED_{25}) in the anesthetized, normotensive rat (Fig. 1). The relationship between the blood pressure decreasing activity, log $ED_{20}(BP)$, and the potency of the drugs in diminishing heart rate, log $ED_{20}(HR)$, in the conscious, spontaneously hypertensive rat is described mathematically by equation 3.

$$\log ED_{20}(BP) = 1.041 \log ED_{20}(HR) - 0.186 \qquad \text{(eq. 3.)}$$
$$n = 7; r = 0.989; S = 0.079; F = 222 \ (P < 0.001)$$

Consequently, the hypotensive potency of the imidazolidines is accompanied by a parallel running decrease in cardiac frequency.

Another important factor consists of the peripheral α-sympathomimetic activity of the title compounds which induces a transient rise in arterial blood pressure following intravenous application. Although this peripheral effect is of a much shorter duration, its influence on the centrally mediated hypotensive response cannot be predicted. Recently, the α-sympathomimetic activity of clonidine and a number of its derivatives was quantified in the pithed rat by Rouot (1974). Thirteen of these compounds correspond with those in our series. The correlation which was obtained between the central hypotensive potency (log $1/ED_{30}$) and the peripheral hypertensive activity (pH_{100}, i.e. the logarithm of the reciprocal concentration connected with an increase in blood pressure of 100%), both calculated for the percentage protonated form, is given by equation 4. This relationship is hardly significant, but was considerably improved by adding a term in lipophilicity (log APC) (equation 5.).

$$\log 1/ED_{30} = 1.150 \, pH_{100} - 0.907 \qquad \text{(eq. 4.)}$$
$$n = 13; r = 0.713; S = 0.854; F = 11.4 \ (P < 0.01)$$

$$\log 1/ED_{30} = 0.641 \log APC + 0.828 \, pH_{100} - 0.276 \qquad \text{(eq. 5.)}$$
$$n = 13; r = 0.920; S = 0.500; F = 27.6 \ (P < 0.001)$$

394

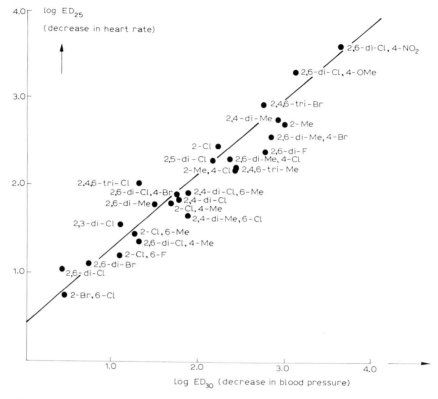

Fig. 1. Relationship between the hypotensive activity (log ED_{30}) and the bradycardic potency (log ED_{25}) for clonidine and its structurally related imidazolidines in the anesthetized, normotensive rat. log ED_{30} = 1.212 log ED_{25} — 0.494 (n = 26; r = 0.960; S = 0.248).

The appearance of log APC points to the importance of the ability of the molecules to penetrate into the brain in determining the central hypotensive activity. The positive correlation indicates that the hypotensive activity is not affected by the peripheral hypertensive effect and furthermore suggests that there are no differences between the peripheral and central α-adrenergic receptors which are excited by these molecules.

The validity of using log APC as a measure for the tendency of the imidazolidines to penetrate into the brain was proved by a highly significant relationship between this parameter and log $(C_{brain}/C_{i.v.})$ in which C_{brain} represents the rat brain concentration reached following intravenous application of a certain dose $(C_{i.v.})$ (equation 6., Fig. 2.).

$$\log (C_{brain}/C_{i.v.}) = -0.133 \ (\log APC)^2 + 0.574 \log APC - 0.094$$

$$(eq. 6.)$$

$$n = 14; \ r = 0.987; \ S = 0.139; \ F = 212 \ (P < 0.001)$$

Equation 6. was used to calculate for all the compounds the brain concentration connected with a decrease in blood pressure of 30%. This ED_{30}

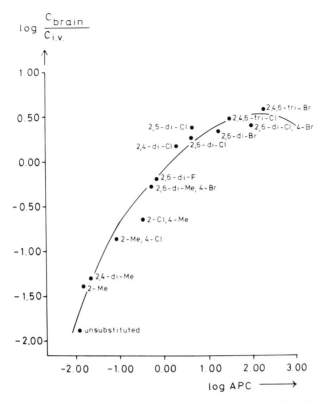

Fig. 2. The dependence of the ability to penetrate across the blood—brain barrier, log $(C_{brain}/C_{i.v.})$, upon lipophilic behavior, log APC, for clonidine and a number of its structurally related derivatives. The relation is expressed mathematically by equation 6 (see text).

can be considered a measure for the concentration of the drugs at the level of the central α-adrenergic receptor and is independent of the transport processes which precede the excitation of these receptors. Therefore, this biological parameter will be more suitable for the considerations concerning structure and activity.

Preliminary multiple regression analysis studies reveal that the SAR at the central α-receptor level is determined by the electronic and the steric features of the molecules. Properties described by quantum chemical parameters (Meerman-Van Benthem et al., 1975; Timmermans et al., submitted for publication) probably play also an additional role.

SUMMARY

Quantitative linear relationships were obtained between the hypotensive and bradycardic potencies of clonidine and a number of its structurally related imidazolidines, as quantified in the anesthetized, normotensive rat, the conscious, spontaneously hypertensive rat, following intravenous administration, and in the anesthetized cat, upon infusion via the vertebral artery.

In the anesthetized, normotensive rat a significant correlation between the hypotensive and the hypertensive activity resulted when the ability of the compounds to penetrate into the brain was taken into account. This finding points to a similarity between peripheral and central α-adrenergic receptors.

Brain disposition could be described extrathermodynamically by a parabolic equation containing the octanol/buffer partition coefficients.

The structure-activity relationship (SAR) with respect to the hypotensive action of the present clonidine-like drugs has been considered at the level of the central α-adrenergic receptor.

REFERENCES

Bock, J.U. and Van Zwieten, P.A. (1971) The central hyperglycaemic action of clonidine. *Europ. J. Pharmacol.*, 16: 303—310.

Henning, M. and Van Zwieten, P.A. (1968) Central hypotensive action of α-methyl-DOPA. *J. Pharm. Pharmacol.*, 20: 409—417.

Hoefke, W., Kobinger, W. and Walland, A. (1975) Relationship between activity and structure in derivatives of clonidine. *Arzneimittel-Forsch.*, 25: 786—793.

Kobinger, W. (1973) Pharmacological basis of the cardiovascular actions of clonidine. In *Hypertension: Mechanisms and Managements*, G. Onesti, K.E. Kim and J.H. Moyer (Eds.), Grune and Stratton, New York, pp. 369—380.

Kobinger, W. and Pichler, L. (1975) Investigations into some imidazoline compounds with respect to peripheral α-adrenoceptor stimulation and depression of cardiovascular centers. *Naunyn-Schmiedeberg's Arch. exp. Path. Pharmak.*, 291: 175—191.

Laverty, R. (1969) A comparison of the behavioural effects of some hypotensive imidazoline derivatives in rats. *Europ. J. Pharmacol.*, 9: 163—169.

Meerman-Van Benthem, C.M., Van der Meer, K., Mulder, J.J.C., Timmermans, P.B.M.W.M. and Van Zwieten, P.A. (1975) Clonidine base: evidence for conjugation of both ring systems. *Molec. Pharmacol.*, 11: 667—670.

Rouot, B. (1974) *Clonidine et Analogues, Relations entre Structure et Activité*, Ph. D. Thesis, University Louis Pasteur, Strasbourg, France.

Schmitt, H. (1971) Actions des alpha-sympathomimétiques sur les structures nerveuses. *Actualités pharmacol.*, 24: 93—131.

Stähle, H. (1974) Medicinal chemistry related to the central regulation of blood pressure. In *Proceedings of the 4th International Symposium on Medicinal Chemistry*, J. Maas (Ed.), Elsevier, Amsterdam, pp. 75—105.

Van Zwieten, P.A. (1975) Antihypertensive drugs with a central action. *Progr. Pharmacol.*, 1: 1—63.

Walland, A. and Hoefke, W. (1974) Relationship between activity and structure in derivatives of clonidine. *Naunyn-Schmiedeberg's Arch. exp. Path. Pharmak.*, 282: R104.

Central and Reflex Control of Renin Release

ALBERTO ZANCHETTI, ANDREA STELLA and ROGER DAMPNEY

Istituto di Ricerche Cardiovascolari, Università di Milano and Centro di Ricerche Cardiovascolari, CNR, Milan (Italy)

Many recent findings indicate that the sympatho-adrenergic system can influence renin release or secretion (Zanchetti and Stella, 1975; Davis and Freeman, 1976). As summarized in Fig. 1, there is evidence in the literature that peripheral plasma renin activity or renin release is affected by (1) intra-arterial or intravenous injection of catecholamines (Vander, 1965; Wathen et al., 1965; Bunag et al., 1966; Johnson et al., 1971; Winer et al., 1971), (2) endogenous norepinephrine released by tyramine (Bunag et al., 1966), (3) electrical stimulation of the renal nerves (Vander, 1965; Johnson et al., 1971; Loeffler et al., 1972; Coote et al., 1972; Lagrange et al., 1973), and (4) electrical stimulation of the brain (Ueda et al., 1967; Passo et al., 1971; Richardson et al., 1974). Furthermore, the renin producing juxtaglomerular cells are richly supplied by adrenergic nerve endings (Barajas, 1964).

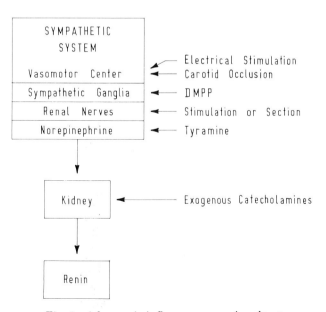

Fig. 1. Adrenergic influences on renin release.

The demonstration of a sympathetic influence on renin release raises several issues, which must be solved in order to understand the actual role of the sympathetic system in regulating the activity of juxtaglomerular cells including the role of sympathetic release of renin in circulatory homeostasis. We will discuss the mechanism of the sympathetic activation of renin release, the central organization of the neural control of renin release, and the reflex modulation of renin release.

MECHANISMS OF SYMPATHETIC INFLUENCE ON RENIN RELEASE

Renal nerves can influence renin release through at least 3 mechanisms: (1) by changing the stretch of the afferent arteriole activating the so-called vascular

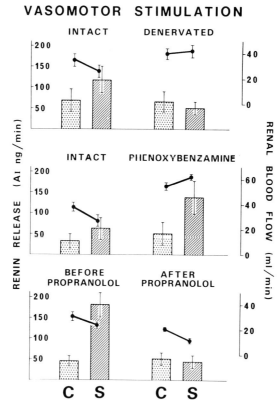

Fig. 2. Effect of electrical stimulation of the brain stem in cats on renin release (ng angiotensin I/min) and renal blood flow. Mean values ± S.E.M. are shown for renin release (histograms and bars, left ordinates) and for renal blood flow (● and bars, right ordinates) measured just before (C) and at the end of a 5 min stimulation period (S). Top row: comparison of innervated kidney and contralateral denervated kidney (12 experiments in 7 cats). Middle row: comparison of an intact kidney and contralateral kidney pretreated with intra-arterial phenoxybenzamine (6 experiments in 4 cats). Bottom row: comparison of effects before and after intravenous administration of propranolol (8 experiments in 8 cats). AI = angiotensin I (Richardson et al., 1974).

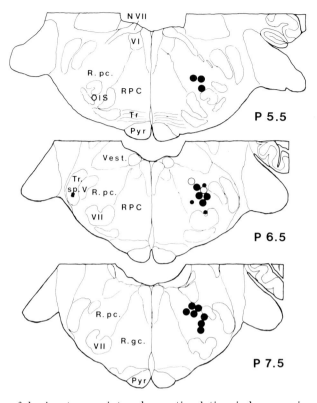

Fig. 3. Location of brain stem points whose stimulation induces renin release from the kidney in cats. Large filled circles indicate sites giving rise to large responses, smaller filled circles smaller responses, hollow circles no response. P5.5, P6.5, and P7.5 represent transverse sections of the brain stem posterior to the transverse interaural plane. N VII, seventh nerve; OIS, superior olive; Pyr, pyramids; R.gc., nucleus reticularis gigantocellularis; R.pc. nucleus reticularis parvocellularis; RPC, nucleus reticularis pontis caudalis; Vest., vestibular nuclei; Tr, trapezoid body; Tr. sp. V, spinal bigeminal tract; VI and VII, nuclei of the sixth and seventh nerves.

receptor, (ii) by changing the glomerular filtration rate with consequent involvement of the macula densa receptor, and (iii) by directly acting on the juxtaglomerular cells.

We have recently performed experiments to prove that sympathetic stimulation does release renin from the kidney independently of local vasomotor changes. Fig. 2 summarizes the results obtained from 3 different groups of cats. In these animals the response of an intact kidney to electrical stimulation of the vasomotor centre (Fig. 3) was compared to the response of the contralateral kidney which had been either previously denervated (Fig. 2, top row) or treated with phenoxybenzamine (Fig. 2, middle row). Electrical stimulation of the brain stem produced a sharp increase in renin release and a fall in renal blood flow to the innervated kidney, while no change in renin release and a slight passive increase in blood flow occur in the contralateral denervated kidney. In these experiments, therefore, vasoconstriction and renin release were associated. Dissociation of vasomotor and renin releasing effects of brain stem stimulation can be obtained by intrarenal infusion of a miniscule amount of the α-adrenergic blocker, phenoxybenzamine. In fact, renin release occurs from both kidneys, though it is greater from the phenoxybenzamine treated kidney, while renal vasoconstriction is present only in the innervated side. A reverse dissociation of the vasomotor and renin releasing effects of sympathetic stimulation is obtained by infusing the β-adrenergic blocker propranolol (Fig. 2, bottom row) which completely inhibits any increase in renin release while leaving renal vasoconstriction unaffected.

Since it had been demonstrated that renal nerves can act directly on juxtaglomerular cells (Johnson et al., 1971; Lagrange et al., 1973), it must then be determined what type of adrenergic receptors mediate renin release. Our data with propranolol confirm that the renin-releasing action of sympathetic fibres may be mediated by intrarenal β-adrenergic receptors (Michelakis et al., 1969; Veyrat and Rosset, 1972; Vandongen et al., 1973; Aoi et al., 1974). Moreover, the greater response in renin release after local injection of phenoxybenzamine may also be due to an inhibitory influence of the α-adrenergic receptors on renin release as recently proposed by the findings of Vandongen and Peart (1974) on the isolated rat kidney, and by Nolly et al. (1974) on kidney slices incubated in vitro.

CENTRAL ORGANIZATION OF THE NEURAL CONTROL OF RENIN RELEASE

There is also evidence that the sympathetic control of renin release is centrally organized, as should be expected of an influence participating in cardiovascular homeostasis. Renin release can be increased by electrical stimulation of structures in the pons and the medulla oblongata (Passo et al., 1971; Richardson et al., 1974) (Fig. 3), and the mesencephalon (Ueda et al., 1967), as well as by stimulation of the hypothalamus (Zanchetti and Stella, 1975). Fig. 4 illustrates an example of our recent experiments in which we stimulated the so-called defence-area of the lateral hypothalamus, commonly assumed to influence defence or emotional behaviour (Folkow et al., 1965; Zanchetti, 1976). Despite the transient nature of the vasoconstriction, the intact kidney markedly increased its output of renin while the denervated one showed no response. Although the lateral hypothalamus has an excitatory action, Zehr and Feigl (1973) have recently shown suppression of plasma renin activity in the conscious dog after stimulation of the so-called sympatho-inhibitory area in the anterior hypothalamus. These findings pose a first example of opposite influences on renin release exerted by areas of the brain known to be differently involved in haemodynamic and behavioural control.

NEURAL AND NON-NEURAL MECHANISMS IN RENIN RELEASE TO VARIOUS STIMULI.

Renin release can be affected by several physiological and pathological conditions such as upright posture, acute and chronic salt depletion, haemorrhage, and reduction of renal perfusion pressure (Davis and Freeman, 1976). But

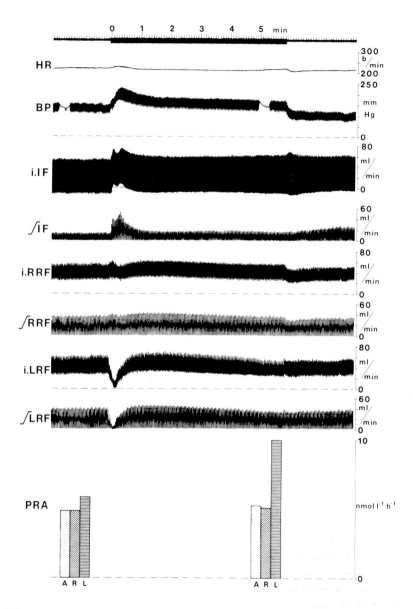

Fig. 4. Effect of electrical stimulation of the hypothalamic defence area on renin release from the kidney in cats. The top tracing records time: the period of stimulation is indicated by its wide portion. From above downwards are shown heart rate (HR), phasic arterial pressure (BP), instantaneous left iliac flow (i.IF), mean left iliac flow (∫IF), instantaneous right renal flow (i.R.R.F.), mean right renal flow (∫RRF), instantaneous left renal flow (i.LRF), mean left renal flow (∫LRF). The bars indicating plasma renin (PRA) (nmol angiotensin I l^{-1} h^{-1}) also denote the time at which blood samples were drawn. A,R and L indicate arterial plasma, and right and left renal venous plasma. The right kidney was denervated (Zanchetti and Stella, 1975).

402

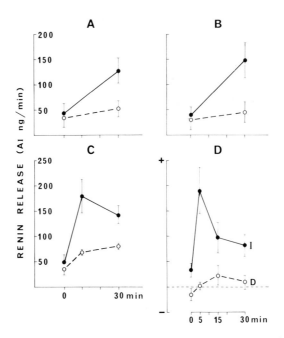

Fig. 5. Renin release from innervated (filled circles continuous line) and denervated kidneys (open circles dashed lines) in cats during (A) head-up tilting $60°$, (B) infusion of low doses of furosemide, (C) infusion of high doses of furosemide, (D) suprarenal aortic stenosis in cats. Values are mean ± S.E.M. AI = angiotensin I.

the response of juxtaglomerular cells to various mechanisms of renin control, particularly of neural factors is still controversial. While comparing the response of an intact kidney with the response of the contralateral denervated one, we studied the role of renal innervation under some of these conditions (Stella and Zanchetti, 1977). Fig. 5, upper left quadrant, shows that head-up tilting of 30 min duration in anaesthetized cats significantly increased renin release from innervated kidneys, in contrast to a small and inconstant increase observed in denervated kidneys. The same results were noted when a small, but definitely diuretic dose of furosemide (0.75 mg/kg in 30 min) was infused (Fig. 5, upper right quadrant). Adrenalectomy completely negated the small increase from the denervated kidney. Different results were, however, obtained when a much larger dose of furosemide (6 mg/kg in 30 min) was infused: although the innervated kidney again released renin in a much greater amount, the denervated kidney also consistently increased its renin output (Fig. 5, lower left quadrant) and this effect was still observed in adrenalectomized cats. Likewise, bilateral reduction in renal perfusion pressure by suprarenal aortic stenosis increased renin release disproportionately more from the innervated than from the denervated kidney, although the denervated organ was still consistently stimulated (Stella et al., 1976).

When the time course of the response was studied, as we did when employing large doses of furosemide and aortic stenosis, it was apparent that the neural and non-neural mechanisms have a different time course: the neural one being very prompt, while the non-neural mechanism becoming evident only at the end of the stimulation period. The early involvement of the neural mechanism suggests that neural influences, however triggered, may be more important for release of renin (i.e., the passage of preformed renin from storage granules into the blood stream) than in production (i.e. the synthesis of new renin within the juxtaglomerular cells). Alternatively, the neural mechanism may be involved in intrarenal activation of an inactive precursor, such as prorenin, recently found in peripheral plasma or in the kidney.

REFLEX REGULATION OF RENIN RELEASE

Several afferent pathways may be involved in reflex release of renin by the various stimuli already discussed.

The conspicuous early component of renin release caused by reducing renal perfusion pressure may involve renal arterial baroreceptors and afferent fibres from the kidney, but this reasonable hypothesis has not been substantiated by our recent experiments (Calaresu et al., 1976). Stimulation of afferent renal fibres (Fig. 6) induced reflex hypertension and vasoconstriction, rather than hypotension and vasodilatation expected from the baroreceptors; and renin release was not affected in either direction. The reflex source of renin stimulation by aortic stenosis may come from outside the kidney; or, alternatively, the neural component may not be reflex in nature, but simply result from sympathetic stimuli facilitating the action of other stimuli in

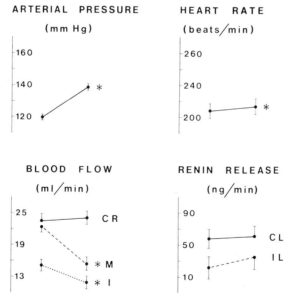

Fig. 6. Effect of electrical stimulation of an afferent renal nerve on mean arterial pressure, heart rate, mesenteric blood flow (M), iliac blood flow (I), contralateral renal blood flow (CR) and on renin release from the ipsilateral denervated (IL) and contralateral innervated (CL) kidneys in cats. Values are mean ± S.E.M. Asterisks indicate statistical significance. (From Calaresu et al., 1976.)

turn influencing the juxtaglomerular cells through the classical intrarenal mechanisms.

It is likely, however, that stimuli such as tilting and small doses of furosemide, which activate the juxtaglomerular cells through entirely neural mechanisms, act reflexively. Identification of the reflex or, possibly, of the reflexes is, however, more difficult and still controversial. It is reasonable to think of volume receptors in the cardiopulmonary area as being the source of a tonic inhibitory discharge reducing the sympathetic drive to the juxta-glomerular cells; when tilting and furosemide reduce central blood volume they may also decrease the tonic reflex inhibition and stimulate renin release. Cardiopulmonary receptors are known to feed mainly into the vagi (Guazzi et al., 1962; Mancia et al., 1973), and indeed there have been reports that interruption of vagal conduction increases plasma angiotensin or renin release (Hodge et al., 1969; Mancia et al., 1975). We have recently investigated this issue by comparing the effects of vagotomy in the innervated and denervated kidney (Zanchetti et al., 1976). Though our experiments are still underway, it appears (Fig. 7) that vagotomy can stimulate renin release from the innervated (not from the denervated) kidney, but this is an early and transient response

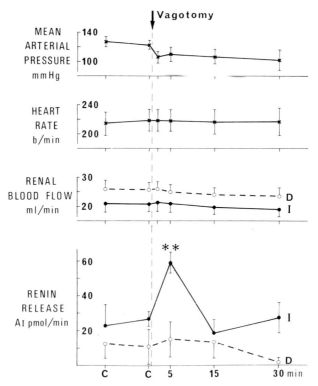

Fig. 7. Effect of vagotomy on mean arterial pressure, heart rate, and on renal blood flow and renin release from innervated (I) and denervated (D) kidneys in cats. Values are mean ± S.E.M. before (C) and after vagotomy. Arrow indicates the time of vagotomy. Asterisks indicate statistical significance (Zanchetti et al., 1976).

that soon disappears, and it is not observed in all experimental conditions. We are now trying to define the experimental conditions in which this tonic vagal restraint of renin release occurs, and to question whether interfering factors are represented by vagal control of vasopressin release, as has been suggested (Schrier and Bert, 1972), or by the coexistence of other reflexes from volume receptors, or by other factors interfering peripherally at the juxtaglomerular level.

In conclusion, evidence to date indicates that the sympathetic system can control renin release by directly influencing the juxtaglomerular cells, without the involvement of the vascular or macula densa receptors.

The time characteristics of this influence make the sympathetic system well adapted to a prompt moment-to-moment control of renin release, and there are many stimuli of physiological and pathological significance that have been shown to influence the juxtaglomerular cells through sympathetic innervation. Whether sympathetic regulation is limited to prompt adjustments, and is mainly concerned with release rather than production, is open to question and, therefore, to further investigation.

That volume receptors in the cardiopulmonary area may represent important sensors in the control of the sympathetic outflow to the juxtaglomerular cells is also likely, but we hope that more information on this crucial point will be forthcoming in current investigations.

SUMMARY

Growing evidence indicates that the sympathetic system can directly influence renin release of juxtaglomerular cells without the involvement of the vascular or macula densa receptors. Central neural mechanisms participate in the adrenergic control of renin release, the medullary vasomotor centre and the hypothalamic defence area playing an excitatory role, the hypothalamic sympatho-inhibitory area a depressor one. Stimuli, such as head-up tilting and the injection of moderate amounts of furosemide, release renin through entirely neural mechanisms, whereas large doses of furosemide and the reduction of renal perfusion pressure mobilize both neural and non-neural mechanisms of release. Among the afferent pathways for reflex control of renin release, renal nerve afferents would appear to play no role, while participation of sino-aortic afferents remains controversial. Volume receptors connected with vagal fibres are, however, likely to be involved, but interaction of reflex control of renin and vasopressin requires further experimental clarification.

REFERENCES

Aoi, W., Wade, M.B., Rosner, D.R. and Weinberger, M.H. (1974) Renin release by rat kidney slices in vitro: effects of cations and catecholamines. Amer. J. Physiol., 227: 630—634.

Barajas, L. (1964) Innervation of the juxtaglomerular apparatus: electron microscopic study of the innervation of the glomerular arterioles. Lab. Invest., 13: 916—930.

Bunag, R.D., Page, I.H. and McCubbin, J.W. (1966) Neural stimulation of renin release. Circulat. Res., 21: 851—858.

406

Calaresu, F.R., Stella, A. and Zanchetti, A. (1976) Haemodynamic responses and renin release during stimulation of afferent renal nerves in the cat. *J. Physiol. (Lond.)*, 255: 687—700.

Coote, J.H., Johns, E.J., Macleod, V.M. and Singer, B. (1972) Effects of renal nerve stimulation, renal blood flow and adrenergic blockade on plasma renin activity in the cat. *J. Physiol. (Lond.)*, 226: 15—36.

Davis, J.O. and Freeman, R.H. (1976) Mechanisms regulating renin release. *Physiol. Rev.*, 56: 1—56.

Folkow, B., Heymans, C. and Neil, E. (1965) Integrated aspects of cardiovascular regulation. In *Handbook of Physiology, Vol. 3, Circulation*, W.F. Hamilton and P. Dow (Eds.), American Physiological Society, Washington, D.C.,pp. 1787—1823.

Guazzi, M., Libretti, A. and Zanchetti, A. (1962) Tonic reflex regulation of the cat's blood pressure through vagal afferents from the cardiopulmonary region. *Circulat. Res.*, 11: 7—16.

Hodge, R.L., Lowe, R.D., Ng, K.K.F. and Vane, J.R. (1969) Role of the vagus nerve in the control of the concentration of angiotensin II in the circulation. *Nature (Lond)*, 221: 177—179.

Johnson, J.A., Davis, J.O. and Witty, R.T. (1971) Effects of catecholamines and renal nerve stimulation on renin release in the nonfiltering kidney. *Circulat. Res.*, 29: 646—653.

Lagrange, R.G., Sloop, C.H. and Schmid, H.E. (1973) Selective stimulation of renal nerves in the anesthetized dog. Effect on renin release during controlled changes in renal hemodynamics. *Circulat. Res.*, 33: 704—712.

Loeffler, J.R., Stockigt, J.R. and Ganong, W.F. (1972) Effect of alpha- and beta-adrenergic blocking agents on the increase in renin secretion produced by stimulation of the renal nerves. *Neuroendocrinology*, 10: 129—138.

Mancia, G., Donald, D.E. and Shepherd, J.T. (1973) Inhibition of adrenergic outflow to peripheral blood vessels by vagal afferents from the cardiopulmonary region in the dog. *Circulat. Res.*, 33: 713—724.

Mancia, G., Romero, J.C. and Shepherd, J.T. (1975) Continuous inhibition of renin release in dogs by vagally innervated receptors in the cardiopulmonary region. *Circulat. Res.*, 36: 529—535.

Michelakis, A.M., Caudle, J. and Liddle, G.W. (1969) In vitro stimulation of renin production by epinephrine, norepinephrine, and cyclic AMP. *Proc. Soc. exp. Biol. (N.Y.)*, 130: 748—753.

Nolly, H.L., Reid, I.A. and Ganong, W.F. (1974) Effect of theophylline and adrenergic blocking drugs on the renin response to norepinephrine in vitro. *Circulat. Res.*, 35: 575—579.

Passo, S.S., Assaykeen, T.A., Otsuka, K., Wise, B.L., Goldfien, A. and Ganong, W.F. (1971) Effect of stimulation of the medulla oblongata on renin secretion in dogs. *Neuroendocrinology*, 7: 1—10.

Richardson, D., Stella, A., Leonetti, G., Bartorelli, A. and Zanchetti, A. (1974) Mechanisms of renal release of renin by electrical stimulation of the brainstem in the cat. *Circulat. Res.*, 34: 425—434.

Schrier, R.W. and Bert, T. (1972) Mechanism of the antidiuretic effect associated with interruption of parasympathetic pathways. *J. clin. Invest.*, 51: 2613—2620.

Stella, A. and Zanchetti, A. (1977) Effects of renal denervation on renin release in response to tilting and furosemide. *Amer. J. Physiol.*, in press.

Stella, A., Calaresu, F. and Zanchetti, A. (1976) Neural factors contributing to renin release during reduction in renal perfusion pressure and blood flow in cats. *Clin Sci. molec. Med.*, 51: 453—461.

Ueda, H., Yasuda, H., Takabatake, Y., Iizuka, M., Iizuka, T., Ihori, M., Yamamoto, M. and Sakamoto, Y. (1967) Increased renin release evoked by mesencephalic stimulation in the dog. *Jap. Heart J.*, 8: 498—506.

Vander, A.J. (1965) Effect of catecholamines and renal nerves on renin secretion in anesthetized dogs. *Amer. J. Physiol.*, 209: 659—662.

Vandongen, R. and Peart, W.S. (1974) The inhibition of renin secretion by alpha-adrenergic stimulation in the isolated rat kidney. *Clin. Sci. molec. Med.*, 47: 471—479.

Vandongen, R., Peart, W.S. and Boyd, G.W. (1973) Adrenergic stimulation of renin secretion in the isolated perfused rat kidney. *Circulat. Res.*, 32: 290—296.

Veyrat, R. and Rosset, E. (1972) In vitro renin release by human kidney slices: effect of norepinephrine, angiotensin II and I, and aldosterone. In *Hypertension '72*, J. Genest and E. Koiw (Eds.), Springer, New York, pp. 37—44.

Wathen, R.L., Kingsbury, W.S., Stouder, D.A., Schneider, E.G. and Rostorfer, H.H. (1965) Effects of infusion of catecholamines and angiotensin II on renin release in anesthetized dogs. *Amer. J. Physiol.*, 209: 1012—1024.

Winer, N., Chokshi, D.S. and Walkenhorst, W.G. (1971) Effects of cyclic AMP, sympatho-mimetic amines, and adrenergic receptor antagonists on renin secretion. *Circulat. Res.*, 29: 239—248.

Zanchetti, A. (1976) Hypothalamic control of circulation. In *The Nervous System in Arterial Hypertension*, S. Julius and M.O. Esler (Eds.), Thomas, Springfield, Ill., pp. 397—429.

Zanchetti, A. and Stella, A. (1975) Neural control of renin release. *Clin. Sci. molec. Med.*, 48, Suppl 2: 215—223.

Zanchetti, A., Dampney, R.A., Ludbrook, J., Mancia, G. and Stella, A. (1976) Baroreceptor reflexes from different vascular areas in animals and man. *Clin. Sci. molec. Med.*, In press.

Zehr, J.E. and Feigl, E.O. (1973) Suppression of renin activity by hypothalamic stimulation. *Circulat. Res.*, 32, Suppl I: 17—27.

Alpha and Beta Blockers: Effects on Renin Release

ROBERT H. McDONALD, Jr., CLINTON N. CORDER and F.H.H. LEENEN

Departments of Medicine and Pharmacology, University of Pittsburgh School of Medicine, Pittsburgh, Pa. 15261 (U.S.A.)

The mechanisms controlling the release of renin appear to be intimately bound to a variety of parts of the adrenergic nervous system. Indeed, there is ample evidence to suggest that the interrelationship extends from hypothalamic centers to the juxtaglomerular cell itself. Furthermore, that each point of regulation and modulation between the initiating areas and the end organ may by receptor inhibition or stimulation modify the interrelationship. The presence of alpha and beta receptors at a variety of sites in the chain further complicates the analysis of alpha and beta receptors, their role in renin release and the efficacy of receptor blockade.

While Claude Bernard is credited with the discovery that the sympathetic nervous system exercised control over blood vessel tone, studies of the role of the sympathetic nervous system in maintenance of normal or elevated pressures are of more recent vintage. The realization that pheochromocytomas, by their secretion of epinephrine and norepinephrine generally presented with severe hypertensive episodes, served as an added spur to such investigations.

Collections of urine from normals and patients with essential hypertension have, at best, been equivocal. Thus while a number of authors have deduced a positive correlation between urinary excretion of catecholamines or their metabolites, other studies have either shown no correlation or, on occasion, a negative relationship. In such studies when plasma renin activity has also been evaluated, no consistent relationship has emerged. Possible explanations for such conflicting data are that: (1) there is a spectrum of types of norepinephrine excretors just as there is a spectrum of plasma renin activity responses, (2) the majority of studies of urinary norepinephrine excretion are done utilizing 24 hr collections and thus reflect an integrated value rather than a measure of responsivity.

While some studies have suggested a negative relationship between plasma renin activity and blood pressure levels, most such studies have been based on the stimulated response. While as noted, the catecholamine collections are an integration of supine and stimulated values. The data seem to be further complicated by the fact that there is an age dependent decline in both basal and response determined plasma renin activity. A similar decline has been reported for catecholamine excretion. Since blood pressure is known to rise with age, simple positive correlations are clearly not possible.

In individual studies, however, some correlations emerge. Esler et al. (1973) present data on 41 hypertensives and 20 normal subjects which indicate that while supine plasma renin activity (PRA) and basal epinephrine excretion are similar in the two groups, basal norepinephrine excretion is elevated. With tilting there is a positive change in both norepinephrine excretion and plasma renin activity in hypertensives but the change in normals, although directionally similar, was not significant. With other stresses, such as mental "stress" and hypoglycemia, there were increases in epinephrine but not in norepinephrine or plasma renin activity. In contrast, Jose et al. (1970) found no correlation between upright PRA and norepinephrine excretion.

While the studies referred to above suggest that stimuli which provoke epinephrine release are not associated with changes in plasma renin activity, contrary evidence has been educed from studies of patients with pheochromocytoma (Vetter et al., 1976). In such patients, if the tumor is secreting excesses of epinephrine as well as norepinephrine, plasma renin activity is enhanced. However, while a simple explanation would be that epinephrine has greater beta activity than norepinephrine, the elevated PRA returns to, or near, normal with phenoxybenzamine treatment.

More recently a number of methods have been developed by which reproducible measurements of plasma catecholamines can be obtained. Through such measurements recent data have suggested that patients with essential hypertension have elevations in, and that there is a direct correlation between, diastolic blood pressure and plasma norepinephrine levels. Since other studies have shown an inverse correlation between plasma renin activity and diastolic blood pressure, it is clear that a one to one relationship can not be said to exist. At the present time there do not appear to be studies in which both plasma renin activity and plasma catecholamines have been measured at rest and in response to a variety of stresses.

Any analysis of the effects of catecholamines on renin release is clouded by the variations in doses used as well as a variety of experimental preparations. At the most basic level epinephrine, norepinephrine, isoproterenol, cyclic AMP and glucagon cause efflux of renin in isolated renal tubule preparations (Michelakis et al., 1969), and in renal cortical slices (Nolly et al., 1974). While theophylline addition does not cause renin release, it enhances the effect of norepinephrine. Increases in release by all of these maneuvers, except glucagon, are blocked by propranolol. Thus, the cellular receptor appears to be a classic beta adrenergic receptor which activates cyclic AMP for the ultimate effect.

In the isolated perfused kidney, renin release is evoked by norepinephrine, epinephrine, isoproterenol, glucagon, and is blocked by L-propranolol but not D-propranolol or phenoxybenzamine (Vandongen et al., 1973). In the intact anesthetized dog with a non-filtering kidney, epinephrine administration causes significant increase in renin secretion which was blocked by simultaneous infusion of papaverine (Johnson et al., 1971). However, the effects of norepinephrine and renal nerve stimulation were not affected by papaverine. It should be noted that this is the only experimental study found in which norepinephrine effects were separated from epinephrine effects. In the intact animal and in man, a variety of other factors seems to modify the response. One of the major causes for differing results is the variation in experimental approach and in the dose used as well as attempts to compare anesthetized dogs and rats with normal and hypertensive humans. Both responses were blocked by DL -propranolol. In the anesthetized dog, Chokshi et al. (1972) found a slight but significant decline in PRA during dopamine infusion, 3 μg/kg/min, and an increase with isoproterenol infusion. The isoproterenol response was blocked by DL -propranolol. When dopamine was given in a dose sufficient to cause a 30% rise in systolic blood pressure, 9.5 μg/kg/min, there resulted mean rise of PRA of 53% in normals (Wilcox et al., 1974). An equipressor dose of norepinephrine (75 μg/min/kg) caused a fall in PRA. Previous work by Hollenberg et al. (1973) has demonstrated that maximal renal vasodilatation with dopamine in man is achieved at about 3 μg/kg/min and that above 7 μg/kg/min the effect is pressor and vasoconstrictor. In a separate study using head up tilt, Hollenberg et al. (1969) demonstrated that although mean blood pressure did not change, decreases in renal blood flow, particularly of the cortical component, result in an increase of the secretion of renin.

Ayers et al. (1969), using dogs who had developed hypertension secondary to right nephrectomy and partial occlusion of the left renal artery, demonstrated that two possible outcomes existed. In all dogs there was an initial rise in PRA following constriction, but survival could be equated with a return of resting PRA to preoperative levels. In such animals as well as trained unanesthetized dogs, both dopamine at 12 μg/kg/min, and isoproterenol at 0.25 μg/kg/min, resulted in significant rises in PRA. This finding is in distinct contrast to the effects of reserpine, trimethapan ganglionic blockage, or hydralazine, which although resulting in a greater fall in blood pressure, had a smaller effect on renin release. Reid et al. (1972) have performed experiments suggesting that systemically administered isoproterenol is more effective than intrarenal when changes in renal flow are held constant.

The response to dopamine and to isoproterenol were greater in hypertensive than in normotensive animals and men (Ayers et al., 1969; Hollenberg et al., 1969). In what is probably the most controversial report, Winer et al. (1969) presented data indicating that phentolamine was effective in blocking increases in renin release induced by diazoxide and ethacrynic acid. However, no estimates of the effect of these agents on intrarenal blood flow distribution were made, and since such are known to occur with these agents, the results should be viewed with caution.

Plasma renin release has been shown to be attenuated following ganglionic blockade (Božović et al., 1967a; Ayers et al., 1969) and following spinal transection (Božović et al., 1967b). Such findings might well argue for a direct sympathetic innervation rather than effect of circulating neurohumors.

In a variety of studies of the central nervous system control of peripheral renin release, the results have been in part dependent upon the area stimulated. Medullary stimulation in pentobarbital anesthetized dogs results in a rise in peripheral renin activity which is blocked by renal denervation and partially blocked by propranolol alone and completely blocked by a combination of propranolol and phenoxybenzamine (Passo et al., 1971). Mesencephalic stimulation in the dog in an area previously shown to effect renal blood flow as well as systemic blood pressure and pulse rate causes a marked increase in renin release as long as the renal nerves are intact (Ueda et al., 1967). Electrical stimulation of the dorsolateral pons in pentobarbital anesthetized cats results in a 28% decrease in renal blood flow despite a sharp systemic pressure rise (Richardson et al., 1974). Renin release rises sharply. Such release is blocked by propranolol although the decrease in renal blood flow is more marked. In contrast, in unanesthetized dogs, hypothalamic stimulation reduces renin release at a time when renal blood flow appears unchanged (Zehr et al., 1973). Ventriculocisternal perfusion of hyponatremic solutions has also been shown to cause large increases in renin release (Mouw et al., 1970).

In work from our laboratory (Leenen et al., 1975), we have been able to demonstrate in normal men that doses of methoxamine which caused reflex decreases of heart rate of 10 beats/min and the other cardiovascular manifestations of alpha adrenergic stimulation caused the same magnitude of increases in peripheral renin activity as did a dose of isoproterenol which caused a mean heart rate rise of 27 beats/min and the expected cardiovascular manifestations of beta adrenergic stimulation. We concluded that there was not one extrarenal factor which controlled renin release. In the second phase of the study we found that while the cardiovascular responses were modified in the expected manner by beta blockade with propranolol (i.e. methoxamine effect was enhanced and isoproterenol blocked), all changes in plasma renin activity were blocked.

More recently we have repeated similar studies in mild hypertensives. Certain differences emerged. When compared to the normals who were of the same age, significantly smaller doses of isoproterenol were required to evoke similar heart rate changes in the hypertensives. Equal sized doses of methoxamine were required to achieve the same heart rate changes. Changes in PRA were also of the same magnitude in normal and hypertensives. However, when the isoproterenol was administered to the hypertensives, increases in both diastolic and mean blood pressure were seen rather than the expected declines. The comparison of results is summarized in Table I.

Several possible explanations exist for the data suggesting that renin release is evoked by alpha and beta adrenergic stimuli. (1) There are several types of receptors on the J-G cell. This would make that cell similar to intestinal smooth muscle. (2) There are several receptors within the kidney. (3) Systemic adrenergic stimulation results reflexly in renin release and the infusion studies are manifestations of such an effect. (4) While the isoproterenol effect is a direct one, the alpha stimulating effect of methoxamine causes a reflex response. What is very clear is that this is not as pure a response as the chronotropic or inotropic stimulation of the myocardium.

These data led us to believe that no one unitary factor affected renin release but that the end-organ (the J-G cell) was beta receptor responsive. Further, that studies in normals were not necessarily transferable to hypertensives and that the latter are less able to systemically dilate but show similar renin release. To us this suggests that vasodilatation is not critical for renin release under these conditions.

There is evidence that alpha agonists can induce renin release and a strong indication that alpha antagonists can modify renin release. In the studies of renal slices (Nolly et al., 1974), phenoxybenzamine enhanced the norepinephrine effect. The enhancement may have been due to reduction of tissue

TABLE I

EFFECTS OF METHOXAMINE AND ISOPROTERENOL IN NORMAL AND HYPERTENSIVE SUBJECTS

	Control value		Change from control at 15 min		Change from control at 30 min		Change from control at 60 min	
	Normal	Hypertensive	Norm.	Hyper.	Norm.	Hyper.	Norm.	Hyper.
Heart rate (beats/min)								
Control infusion	69 ± 2.8	65.7 ± 3.8	-1.1	+3.3	+1.4	+4.5	-1.4	+3.7
Methoxamine	71 ± 3.4	66.7 ± 3.0	-10.4	-15.3	-13.9	-21.2	-9.9	-13.5
Isoproterenol	74 ± 5.6	66.2 ± 1.6	+19.2	+21.1	+27.4	+26.0	+1.5	+0.5
Plasma renin activity (ng of angiotensin I/ml/3 hr)								
Control infusion	3.76 ± 0.73	3.16 ± 0.84	-0.06	-0.70	-0.00	-0.64	+0.99	+0.74
Methoxamine	2.13 ± 0.66	2.74 ± 0.66	+4.65	+5.27	+2.71	+4.85	+0.84	-0.40
Isoproterenol	3.42 ± 1.23	4.76 ± 1.49	+4.44	+3.20	+7.80	+3.76	+1.44	-0.50
Presystolic ejection period (μsec)								
Control infusion	84.6 ± 7.0	91.7 ± 9.6	-9.7	+1.4	-11.4	-1.6	-9.2	-3.4
Methoxamine	84.4 ± 4.6	83.0 ± 10.0	+1.6	+4.9	+4.4	+11.3	+1.2	-10.8
Isoproterenol	88.6 ± 6.8	84.2 ± 6.1	-48.6	-36.7	-44.6	-29.1	+5.4	+3.4
Mean blood pressure (mm Hg)								
Control infusion	95 ± 2.6	105 ± 8.1	+4.2	-1.2	+2.4	-1.8	+3.4	-2.2
Methoxamine	99 ± 2.2	111 ± 7.4*	+4.8	+7.0	+11.4	+10.0	+2.2	+1.68
Isoproterenol	95 ± 3.7	95 ± 5.8	-5.4	+1.1*	-5.4	+8.3*	+0.2	+10.4*
Diastolic blood pressure (mm Hg)								
Control infusion	76 ± 3.4	98 ± 9.3	+1.5	+0.8	+0.2	+1.6	+3.4	+0.2
Methoxamine	84 ± 4.6	83 ± 9.9	+5.6	+6.7	+11.0	+10.3	+3.6	+2.3
Isoproterenol	78 ± 3.9	71 ± 6.4	-18.0	-2.06*	-18.0	+13.8*	+1.6	+22.7*

*Significantly different from normal ($P < 0.05$); 5 subjects in each group.

414

binding of norepinephrine (uptake 2) (Rand et al., 1975) and thus a relative increase in the amount available to stimulate the juxtaglomerular cell. In the studies by Vandongen et al. (1973), one-half of the isolated perfused kidney preparations studied also showed increases in norepinephrine induced renin release following phenoxybenzamine blockade. That phenoxybenzamine may enhance the effect of catecholamines on renin release is also suggested in the work of Assaykeen et al. (1974).

Mechanisms such as blockade of tissue uptake of catecholamine can be used as an explanation for enhancement of renin release by phenoxybenzamine but the explanation for the reported efficacy of alpha blockers in modifying renin release remains obscure.

Current evidence strongly suggests that the juxtaglomerular cell is principally responsive to beta adrenergic stimuli. There are no studies showing in vitro response to pure alpha stimulation and all agents used to stimulate release with the exception of glucagon have been blocked by L- but not D-propranolol when so tested. Studies with progressively more intact preparations are increasingly more difficult to interpret. Shifts in intrarenal blood flow which are difficult to measure have been shown to occur with catecholamines, denervation, renal artery stenosis, adrenergic blocking drugs and diuretics. Such changes will affect both perfusion of the juxtaglomerular cell as well as sodium filtration and distal tubular delivery of sodium. While studies have shown that there is a very narrow therapeutic range of vasodilatation for dopamine, further study may reveal similar effects with epinephrine and other catecholamines. Much of the data is clouded by an attempt to compare results from different species under different conditions of anesthesia as well as comparison of systemic versus intrarenal infusion of drugs and finally comparison of normals and hypertensives.

SUMMARY

A growing body of evidence has demonstrated the intimate relationship between the adrenergic nervous system and renin release. Changes in activity of either appear to be reflected in activity changes of the other. Present evidence suggests that such a relationship exists within certain areas of the central nervous system, within the kidney, and at peripheral adrenergic vascular termination. A variety of modes of interaction have been proposed but none have been confirmed. Adrenergic receptor blocking agents have been used in an attempt to clarify mechanisms of action. Because of nuances in experimental design, results appear equivocal. Stimulation of renin release can be evoked by both alpha and beta adrenergic agonists but beta blockade appears to be far more consistent in modification of renin release. Early studies in man have suggested relationships by means of parallel changes in blood levels of renin activity and urinary excretion of norepinephrine. Further dissection of the interrelationship is dependent upon elucidation of each of the feedback loops involved and specification of receptor types.

REFERENCES

Assaykeen, T.A., Tanigawa, H. and Allison, D.J. (1974) Effect of adrenoceptor-blocking agents on the renin response to isoproterenol in dogs. *Europ. J. Pharmacol.*, 26: 285—297.

Ayers, C.R., Harris, R.H. and Lefer, L.G. (1969) Control of renin release in experimental hypertension. *Circulat. Res.*, 24 and 25, Suppl. I: I-103—I-112.

Božović, L. and Castenfors, J. (1967a) Effect of ganglionic blocking on plasma renin activity in exercising and pain-stressed rats. *Acta physiol. scand.*, 70: 290—292.

Božović, L. and Castenfors, J. (1976b) Plasma renin activity after bleeding in rats with transected or destroyed medulla spinalis. *Acta physiol. scand.*, 71: 253—254.

Chokshi, D.S., Yeh, B.K. and Samet, P. (1972) Effects of dopamine and isoproterenol on renin secretion in the dog. *Proc. Soc. exp. Biol. (N.Y.)*, 140: 54—57.

Esler, M.D. and Nestel, P.J. (1973) Renin and sympathetic nervous system responsiveness to adrenergic stimuli in essential hypertension. *Amer. J. Cardiol.*, 32: 643.

Hollenberg, N.K., Epstein, M., Basch, R.I., Merrill, J.P. and Hickler, R.B. (1969) Renin secretion in the patient with hypertension. *Circulat. Res.*, 24 and 25, Supp. I: I-113—I-122.

Hollenberg, N.K., Adams, D.F., Mendell, P., Abrams, H.L. and Merrill, J.P. (1973) Renal vascular responses to dopamine: haemodynamic and angiographic observations in normal man. *Clin. Sci. molec. Med.*, 45: 733—742.

Johnson, J.A., Davis, J.O. and Witty, R.T. (1971) Effects of catecholamines and renal nerve stimulation on renin release in the nonfiltering kidney. *Circulat. Res.*, 29: 646—653.

Jose, A., Crout, J.R. and Kaplan, N.M. (1970) Suppressed plasma renin activity in essential hypertension. *Ann. int. Med.*, 72: 9—16.

Leenen, F.H.H., Redmond, D.P. and McDonald, R.H., Jr. (1975) Alpha and beta adrenergic-induced renin release in man. *Clin. pharmacol. (Kbh.)*, 18: 31—38.

Michelakis, A.M., Caudle, J. and Liddle, G.W. (1969) In vitro stimulation of renin production by epinephrine, norepinephrine, and cyclic AMP. *Proc. Soc. exp. Biol. (N.Y.)*, 130: 748—753.

Nolly, H.L., Reid, I.A. and Ganong, W.F. (1974) Effect of theophylline and adrenergic blocking drugs on the renin response to norepinephrine in vitro. *Circulat. Res.*, 35: 575—579.

Mouw, D.R. and Vander, A.J. (1970) Evidence for brain Na receptors controlling renal Na excretion and plasma renin activity. *Amer. J. Physiol.*, 219: 822—832.

Passo, S.S., Assaykeen, T.A., Goldfien, A. and Ganong, W.F. (1971) Effect of α- and β-adrenergic blocking agents on the increase in renin secretion produced by stimulation of the medulla oblongata in dogs. *Neuroendocrinology*, 7: 97—104.

Rand, M.J., McCulloch, M.W. and Story, D.F. (1975) Pre-junctional modulation of noradrenergic transmission by noradrenaline, dopamine and acetylcholine. In *Central Action of Drugs in Blood Pressure Regulation*, D.S. Davies and J.L. Reid (Eds.), Pitman, London. pp. 94—132.

Reid, I.A., Schrier, R.W. and Earley, L.E. (1972) An effect of extrarenal beta adrenergic stimulation on the release of renin. *J. clin. Invest.*, 51: 1861—1869.

Richardson, D., Stella, A., Leonetti, G., Bartorelli, A. and Zanchetti, A. (1974) Mechanisms of renal release of renin by electrical stimulation of the brainstem in the cat. *Circulat. Res.*, 34: 425—434.

Ueda, H., Yasuda, H., Takabatake, Y., Iizuka, M., Iizuka, T., Ihori, M., Yamamoto, M. and Yoshiyuki, S. (1967) Increased renin release evoked by mesencephalic stimulation in the dog. *Jap. Heart J.*, 8: 498—506.

Vandongen, R., Peart, W.S. and Boyd, G.W. (1973) Adrenergic stimulation of renin secretion in the isolated perfused rat kidney. *Circulat. Res.*, 32: 290—296.

Vetter, H., Vetter, W., Warnholz, C., Bayer, J.M., Kaser, H., Vielhaber, K. and Kruck, F. (1976) Renin and aldosterone secretion in pheochromocytoma. *Amer. J. Med.*, 60: 866.

Wilcox, C.S., Aminoff, M.J., Kurtz, A.B. and Slater, J.D.H. (1974) Comparison of the renin

416

response to dopamine and noradrenaline in normal subjects and patients with autonomic insufficiency. *Clin. Sci. molec. Med.*, 46: 481—488.

Winer, N., Chokshi, D.S., Yoon, M.S. and Freedman, A.D. (1969) Adrenergic receptor mediation of renin secretion. *J. clin. Endocr.*, 29: 1168—1175.

Zehr, J.E. and Feigl, E.O. (1973) Suppression of renin activity by hypothalamic stimulation. *Circulat. Res.*, 32 and 33, Suppl. I: I-17—I-27.

Differential Influence of Neonatal Sympathectomy on the Development of DOCA-Salt and Spontaneous Hypertension in the Rat

ABRAHAM P. PROVOOST, BÉLA BOHUS and WYBREN DE JONG

Rudolf Magnus Institute for Pharmacology, Medical Faculty, University of Utrecht, Utrecht (The Netherlands)

An important way how the brain exerts control over the circulation is by increasing and decreasing the functional activity of the sympathetic nervous system. A disregulation of this sympathetic control could result in an abnormally high or low blood pressure. Direct evidence for the involvement of an overactive sympathetic nervous system is lacking in both human essential hypertension and experimental hypertension in animals (De Quattro and Miura, 1973). Indirect evidence obtained by studying the mechanism of action of a great many of antihypertensive drugs, however, indicates that the sympathetic nervous system is involved in hypertension (Frohlich, 1974). Profound orthostatic hypotension, on the other hand, is a common finding when the efferent part of the baroreceptor reflex arc is interrupted in patients with an autonomic nervous dysfunction as in the Shy-Drager syndrome (Ibrahim et al., 1975). The same phenomenon is observed during treatment with ganglion blocking agents and may occur also with adrenergic neuron blocking agents such as guanethidine.

In order to assess the degree to which experimental hypertension is dependent on the integrity of the sympathetic nervous system, various forms of sympathectomy have been applied (for references see Provoost, 1976; Provoost and De Jong, 1976). These studies did not lead to a uniform conclusion on the role of the sympathetic nervous system in experimental hypertension, most probably due to the variability of the degree of sympathectomy.

Therefore, experiments were carried out to study the development of hypertension in neonatally sympathectomized (SX) rats in which complete sympathetic denervation of the vascular system had been assured by both biochemical and functional tests (Provoost et al., 1973, 1974; Provoost, 1976). Neonatal sympathectomy was produced by the administration of 6-hydroxy-dopamine HCl (Labkemi AB, Göteborg) to newborn male rats. On the day of birth (day 1) and on day 2, 100 μg/g was injected subcutaneously (s.c.). Two further doses of 250 μg/g were administered s.c. on days 8 and 15. Littermates receiving vehicle (0.9% NaCl) were used as controls. Most of the experiments were carried out when the animals were 3 months old.

Noradrenaline levels were very low in peripheral tissues of SX rats with exception of the adrenals. The high degree of sympathectomy was further indicated by the greatly reduced pressor response to intravenously (i.v.)

418

administered tyramine, especially after concomitant adrenalectomy. This was observed despite a 5-fold increase in sensitivity to i.v. administered noradrenaline, which also accompanies sympathetic denervation (Provoost et al., 1973).

Electrical stimulation of different parts of the central nervous system (CNS) was performed to ascertain whether central stimulation of sympathetic activity could still raise the blood pressure in SX rats. Pressor responses were obtained by stimulation at three different sites in the CNS: (a) the spinal cord sympathetic outflow (Provoost et al., 1974); (b) the medulla oblongata at obex level (De Jong et al., 1975a); and (c) the posterior hypothalamus (Provoost et al., 1974). Markedly reduced pressor responses were evoked by stimulation at these sites in SX rats as compared to the responses in control animals (Fig. 1). Adrenalectomy in SX rats caused a further reduction of the blood pressure increase after electrical stimulation of the spinal cord sympathetic outflow or the posterior hypothalamus to very low values (Provoost et al., 1974). Stimulation of the reticular formation in the medulla oblongata of SX rats did not result in an elevation of blood pressure, even without removing the adrenals (Fig. 2D). These findings probably indicate that stimulation of the hypothalamus or the spinal cord but not of the medulla oblongata causes release of catecholamines from the adrenal medulla.

Fig. 2 depicts examples of blood pressure recordings during electrical stimulation of the medulla oblongata in control animals and SX rats. A rise in blood pressure normally occurring in control rats by stimulating the reticular formation was absent in SX rats, while the blood pressure lowering effect by stimulating the area of the nucleus tractus solitarii was of similar magnitude in both controls and SX rats. It should be noted that, in intact rats, stimulation of

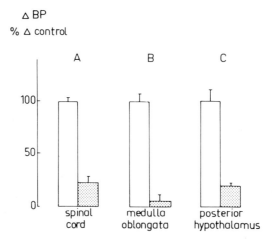

Fig. 1. Rise in systolic blood pressure (ΔBP) following electrical stimulation of (A) the spinal cord sympathetic outflow (stimulation parameters: 100 V, 10 Hz, 15 sec), (B) the reticular formation of the medulla oblongata at obex level (6 V, 50 Hz, 5 sec) and (C) the posterior hypothalamus (10 V, 50 Hz, 5 sec) in controls (open bars) and neonatally sympathectomized rats (stippled bars). Bars indicate mean increase in systolic blood pressure in % of the increase in controls ± S.E.M. for 5 anesthetized rats. The control values were 124 ± 5 mm Hg for spinal cord, 43 ± 3 mm Hg for medulla oblongata and 78 ± 9 mm Hg for hypothalamus stimulation.

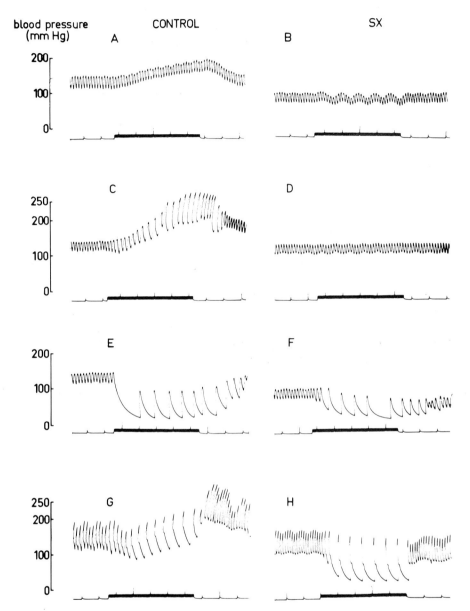

Fig. 2. Examples of blood pressure recordings of the effect of electrical stimulation of the medulla oblongata just caudally of the obex level in an anesthetized control animal (left panel) and in a neonatally sympathectomized rat (SX; right panel). Electrode locations were 0.5 mm lateral of the midline at a depth of 1.8 mm (A,B), 0.9 mm (C,D) and 0.6 mm (E,F; the area of the nucleus tractus solitarii) and 1.5 mm lateral of the midline in the area of the nucleus ambiguus (G,H). Note the absence of any increase in blood pressure after electrical stimulation in the SX rat. Neither a direct rise, nor a secondary rise in blood pressure, as occurred after the mainly bradycardic response to stimulation in the area of the nucleus ambiguus in controls, was observed in the SX rat. A current intensity of 150—200 μA (5—6 V) with a frequency of 50 Hz was employed during a 5 sec period.

the area of the nucleus ambiguus caused a secondary rise in blood pressure after the stimulation was ceased. This may be due to a reflex activation of the sympathetic nervous system following the initial bradycardic and hypotensive response. Although a similar initial response was observed in SX rats, a secondary blood pressure rise did not occur.

The data summarized above show that pressor responses in SX rats were practically absent after central electrical stimulation of sympathetic activity. Furthermore, in SX rats blood pressure did not increase at all after the application of increased intracranial pressure (Cushing response) (De Jong et al., 1974). These functional tests indicated that neonatally SX rats may serve as a useful model for detecting forms of experimental hypertension mainly dependent on an increased sympathetic drive. Hypertension may also be caused by several other factors, such as elevated activity of the renin-angiotensin system, sodium retention and an increase in plasma and extracellular volume, increased secretion of adrenocortical steriods and increased release of adreno-medullary catecholamines. The role of the sympathetic nervous system in the development of these forms of hypertension is not yet fully understood. Therefore, it was of interest to study whether various forms of experimental hypertension could develop in SX rats.

Spontaneous hypertensive rats (SHR) with Wistar—Kyoto rats as normo-tensive controls (Okamoto and Aoki, 1963; De Jong et al., 1975b) were used to study a genetic form of hypertension. Furthermore, hypertension was induced in normotensive Wistar TNO rats by s.c. implantation of 40 mg deoxycorti-costeroneacetate (DOCA) and replacing tap water with 0.9% NaCl as the drinking fluid.

Blood pressure was assessed directly, since indirect blood pressure measure-ments on the tail were impossible in effective sympathectomized rats due to an absence of detectable pulsations (Provoost et al., 1974). Mean blood pressure of normotensive SX rats was significantly lower than that of controls under pentobarbital, urethane or ether anesthesia. However, when measured directly without anesthesia, via a permanent indwelling cannula in an iliac artery, mean blood pressure of normotensive SX rats was not significantly different from that of control animals (Fig. 3). Anesthesia seems to attenuate compensatory mechanisms which assure a near normal basal blood pressure in SX rats. Observations on anesthetized SX rats may accordingly lead to false conclusions. Therefore, in all further experiments the use of anesthesia in determining basal blood pressure levels was avoided.

In SHR an intact sympathetic nervous system appears essential for the development of hypertension, since no development of hypertension was observed in SX SHR. At the age of 3 months, when high blood pressure has already developed in control SHR, mean blood pressure of SX SHR was only slightly higher than that of normotensive Wistar—Kyoto rats (Fig. 3A). Even up to the age of one year, mean blood pressure of SX SHR did not increase further. Heart rate did not differ significantly from control SHR. It has been reported that hypertension in SHR is caused by an elevation of the peripheral resistance (Frohlich et al., 1975; Iriuchijima et al., 1975). This and our experimental data indicate that an important contribution to the hypertension in SHR stems from an increased activity of the sympathetic nervous system to

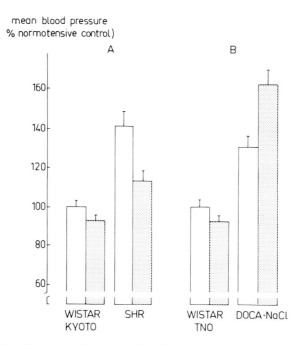

mean blood pressure
% normotensive control)

Fig. 3. A: mean blood pressure in 3-month-old unanesthetized control (open bars) and neonatally sympathectomized (SX; stippled bars) normotensive Wistar—Kyoto rats and 3-month-old control and SX spontaneous hypertensive rats (SHR). B: mean blood pressure in unanesthetized control and SX normotensive Wistar TNO rats and in control and SX rats 3 weeks after implantation of 40 mg DOCA with 0.9% NaCl as drinking fluid. Bars represent mean blood pressure in % of the normotensive control rats for 6—12 animals.

the vascular system, which is probably of central origin. (Provoost and De Jong, 1976). The importance of the medulla oblongata for the high blood pressure in SHR has already been suggested by Japanese workers (Okamoto et al., 1967, Okamoto, 1969). Recently, Judy et al. (1976) reported an increased sympathetic nerve activity in SHR. They suggested that central sympathetic centers, uninhibitable by the baroreceptor system, become active during the development of hypertension in SHR.

An enhanced development of DOCA-salt hypertension in SX rats was observed in contrast to the absence of development of hypertension in SHR after sympathectomy. DOCA-salt hypertension not only developed much more rapidly, but was in fact potentiated in the absence of an intact sympathetic nervous system. Mean blood pressure in SX rats rose faster and to a higher level after implantation of DOCA with 0.9% NaCl as the drinking fluid as compared to control rats. After one week, when blood pressure in control rats showed only a moderate increase of 20 mm Hg, mean blood pressure in SX rats had already reached an extremely high level of 195 mm Hg. This high blood pressure level was also seen in SX rats 3 weeks after DOCA implantation, while at that time hypertension stabilized at 155—160 mm Hg in control DOCA-salt hypertensive rats (Fig. 3B).

This rather unique observation of a potentiated hypertensive mechanism in

SX rats suggests that an intact sympathetic nervous system may somehow protect against extreme chronic increase in blood pressure. An inappropriate functioning of the baroreceptor reflex in SX rats following a rise in blood pressure may be a possible explanation of the observed phenomenon. Sympathectomy could also influence the regulation of blood volume. In the dog, thoracic sympathectomy reduced the sensitivity of atrial receptors to increases in blood volume, while it also accelerated the development of hypertension after wrapping one kidney with contralateral nephrectomy, which was accompanied by an increase in blood volume (Ferrario and McCubbin, 1976). Acute sympathectomy by 6-hydroxydopamine in dogs has been reported to increase plasma volume (De Champlain et al., 1975). In SX rats the effect of a rise in blood volume, which normally occurs after administration of DOCA and salt, could be exaggerated because of an already existing elevated plasma volume. The DOCA-salt induced hypertension in SX rats was accompanied by a marked tachycardia, which may suggest an increased venous return caused by an elevated circulating volume.

Other types of experimental hypertension also developed in SX rats. Hypertension after administration of 9-α-fluorohydrocortisone was slightly potentiated in SX rats (Provoost and De Jong, 1976). Renal hypertension, caused by unilateral renal artery constriction with an intact contralateral kidney, did also develop in SX rats (De Jong et al., 1974; Provoost, 1976). In some SX rats with renal hypertension a very high mean blood pressure level (ca. 200 mm Hg) associated with a tachycardia was observed. This combination was comparable, in both blood pressure and heart rate, with the values observed with DOCA-salt hypertension in SX rats.

Taken together, our data indicate that an intact sympathetic nervous system appears to be essential in the development of hypertension in SHR. Other models of experimental hypertension, steroid and renal hypertension, could develop after neonatal sympathectomy. In fact, a marked potentiation of DOCA-salt hypertension was seen in the absence of an intact sympathetic nervous system.

SUMMARY

The development of various kinds of experimental hypertension was studied in sympathectomized (SX) rats. Sympathectomy, produced by injection of neonatal rats with 6-hydroxydopamine, was biochemically and functionally ensured. No substantial increases in blood pressure could be obtained by stimulating the sympathetic nervous system indirectly via electrical stimulation of the spinal cord sympathetic outflow, the medulla oblongata or the posterior hypothalamus in SX rats.

Mean blood pressure in conscious SX rats was not significantly different from controls. Since blood pressure in anesthetized SX rats was significantly lower than that of controls, blood pressure measurements were made in conscious rats when the development of hypertension was studied.

Hypertension did not develop in SX spontaneous hypertensive rats (SHR), suggesting that hypertension in SHR is caused by a centrally evoked hyperactivity of the sympathetic nervous system. In contrast, DOCA-salt hypertension was potentiated in SX rats. This may indicate that in intact rats the sympathetic nervous system may under some conditions protect against the evolution of hypertension caused by factors other than an increase in sympathetic activity.

ACKNOWLEDGEMENT

This work was supported by the Dutch Medical Research Foundation FUNGO (No. 13-45-10).

REFERENCES

De Champlain, J., Gauthier, P., Porlier, G., Van Ameringen, M.R. and Nadeau, R.A. (1975) Compensatory mechanisms following peripheral sympathectomy. In *Chemical Tools in Catecholamine Research. I. 6-Hydroxydopamine as a Denervation Tool in Catecholamine Research*, G. Jonsson, T. Malmfors and Ch. Sachs (Eds.), North-Holland, Amsterdam, pp. 231—238.
De Jong, W., Provoost, A.P. and Zandberg, P. (1974) Effects of adrenalectomy and of neonatal sympathectomy in normotensive, renal hypertensive and spontaneously hypertensive rats. *Arch. int. Physiol. Biochem.*, 82: 324—326.
De Jong, W., Zandberg, P. and Bohus, B. (1975a) Central inhibitory noradrenergic cardiovascular control. In *Hormones, Homeostasis and the Brain, Progr. in Brain Res. Vol. 42*, W.H. Gispen, Tj.B Van Wimersma Greidanus, B. Bohus and D. De Wied (Eds.), Elsevier, Amsterdam, pp. 285—298.
De Jong, W., Nijkamp, F.P. and Bohus, B. (1975b) Role of noradrenaline and serotonin in the central control of blood pressure in normotensive and spontaneously hypertensive rats. *Arch. int. Pharmacodyn.*, 213: 272—284.
De Quattro, V. and Miura, Y. (1973) Neurogenic factors in human hypertension: mechanism or myth. *Amer. J. Med.*, 55: 362—378.
Ferrario, C.M. and McCubbin, J.W. (1976) Reduction in sensitivity of atrial receptors following sympathectomy. In *The Nervous System in Arterial Hypertension*, S. Julius and M.D. Esler (Eds.), Thomas, Springfield, Ill., pp. 236—247.
Frohlich, E.D. (1974) Inhibition of adrenergic function in the treatment of hypertension. *Arch. intern. Med.*, 33: 1033—1048.
Frolich, E.D., Pfeffer, M.A. and Pfeffer, J.M. (1975) Hemodynamics of SHR hypertension: evidence against autoregulatory theory. In *Recent Advances in Hypertension, Vol. 2*, P. Milliez and M. Safar (Eds.), Boehringer, Ingelheim, pp. 173—179.
Ibrahim, M.M., Tarazi, R.C. and Dustan, H.P. (1975) Orthostatic hypotension: mechanisms and management. *Amer. Heart J.*, 90: 513—520.
Iriuchijima, J., Numao, Y. and Suga, H. (1975) Effect of increasing age on hemodynamics of spontaneously hypertensive rats. *Jap. Heart J.*, 16: 257—264.
Judy, W.V., Watanabe, A.M., Henry, D.P., Besch, H.R., Murphy, W.R. and Hockel, G.M. (1976) Sympathetic nerve activity. Role in regulation of blood pressure in the spontaneously hypertensive rat. *Circulat. Res.*, 38, Suppl. II: II-21—II-29.
Okamoto, K. (1969) Spontaneous hypertension in rats. *Int. Rev. exp. Pathol.*, 7: 227—270.
Okamoto, K. and Aoki, K. (1963) Development of a strain of spontaneously hypertensive rats. *Jap. Circulat. J.*, 27: 282—293.
Okamoto, K., Nosaka, S., Yamori, Y. and Matsumoto, M. (1967) Participation of neural factors in the pathogenesis of hypertension in the spontaneously hypertensive rat. *Jap. Heart J.*, 8: 168—180.
Provoost A.P. (1976) *Hypertensie en het sympatisch zenuwstelsel. Een onderzoek naar de invloed van neonatale sympathectomie op het ontstaan van experimentele hypertensie bij de rat*. Ph.D. thesis, University of Utrecht.

Provoost, A.P. and De Jong, W. (1977) Influence of neonatal chemical sympathectomy on the development of hypertension in spontaneously hypertensive rats and in rats with renal or corticosteroid hypertension. *Clin. exp. Pharmacol. Physiol.*, 3, Suppl.: in press.

Provoost, A.P., De Kemp, J.A. and De Jong, W. (1973) Effect of neonatal 6-hydroxydopamine treatment on the blood pressure response to noradrenaline and tyramine in rats. *Europ. J. Pharmacol.*, 23: 297—301.

Provoost, A.P., Bohus, B. and De Jong, W. (1974) Neonatal chemical sympathectomy: functional control of denervation of the vascular system and tissue noradrenaline level in the rat after 6-hydroxydopamine. *Naunyn-Schmiedeberg's Arch. exp. Path. Pharmak.*, 284: 353—363.

A Pharmacological Analysis of Cushing's Response in Rats

N.Th. P. ROOZEKRANS and P.A. VAN ZWIETEN

Department of Pharmacy, Division of Pharmacotherapy, University of Amsterdam,
Amsterdam (The Netherlands)

INTRODUCTION

Cushing (1901) demonstrated that acute elevation of intracranial pressure (ICP) to levels above the initial mean arterial pressure (MAP) provokes an increase in blood pressure. This effect, now known as the Cushing response, is accompanied by tachycardia. The pressor response during the Cushing reflex is a result of a strong sympathetic discharge (Freeman and Jeffers, 1940; Hoff and Mitchell, 1972). It was the purpose of our investigations to subject the Cushing response to a pharmacological analysis.

METHODS

Male Wistar rats (180—200 g) were anaesthetized with pentobarbital sodium (50—75 mg/kg, i.p.). The ICP was raised by perfusing saline rapidly into the left lateral ventricle under constant elevated pressure. For this purpose a cannula was introduced into the ventricle according to the method described by Noble et al. (1967). The cannula was connected to a saline-containing system, hence pressure could be established at every elevated level desired. Blood pressure was taken from a carotid artery and recorded by means of a Statham transducer and a Hellige HE 17 device. Drugs were injected into a cannulated jugular vein. The rats were subjected to artificial respiration and body temperature was kept constant. ICP was elevated abruptly. The elevation was maintained until the response had ceased. The response was evoked only once in each rat. An ICP/blood pressure curve was established in order to choose a suitable ICP for the rest of our experiments.

We studied the influence of bilateral vagotomy, with and without atropine pretreatment (1 mg/kg i.v.) on the Cushing response. Moreover, the effect of the following drugs, administered prior to the increase in ICP, was established: the β-blocking agents L(—)propranolol (3 and 10 mg/kg i.v.) and practolol (3 mg/kg i.v.), the antihypertensive drugs clonidine (25 μg/kg i.v.) and hydralazine (3 mg/kg i.v.), the α-sympathicolytic agents phentolamine (10, 30 and 60 mg/kg i.v.) and piperoxane (10 and 30 mg/kg i.v.), while we also studied the effect of a combination of L(—)propranolol (3 mg/kg) and phentolamine (10 mg/kg).

Pretreatment with reserpine (5 mg/kg i.p., 24 hr before the experiment) and with 6-hydroxydopamine (6-OHDA ; dosage schedule see Thoenen and Tranzer, 1968) and guanethidine (dosage schedule see Douglas et al., 1975) was studied in relationship to the Cushing response with and without the combination of bilateral adrenalectomy. In all control experiments we injected the same volume of saline instead of the drug.

RESULTS AND DISCUSSION

From the ICP/blood pressure curve we chose an ICP of 160 mm Hg for all our further experiments, because this pressure always yielded maximal pressor responses which were reproducible and prolonged (>5 min). Like other investigators (Cushing, 1901; Sagawa et al., 1961; Hoff and Reis, 1969) we also found that there was an ICP threshold below which the Cushing response could not be provoked. This threshold was in the approximate range of the diastolic blood pressure.

Bilateral vagotomy, with or without atropine pretreatment, had no effect on the blood pressure response after acute elevation of the ICP to 160 mm Hg. The detailed results have been listed in Table I.

The β-blocking agents L(−)propranolol and practolol (both infused intravenously during 20 min) did not significantly influence the blood pressure response, although the increase in systolic pressure was less and the duration of the response was much shorter than without pretreatment with the β-adrenolytic agents. The antihypertensive drugs clonidine and hydralazine produced a strong initial hypotension, but after elevation of the ICP to 160 mm Hg we saw an increase of the blood pressure to the same levels as in the untreated controls. The α-sympathicolytic agents phentolamine and piperoxane also reduced the initial blood pressure, but inhibited the Cushing reflex in a dose-dependent matter as well.

The combination of phentolamine and L(−)propranolol did not influence the blood pressure response in a manner significantly different from that induced by pretreatment with the same dose of phentolamine alone. Pretreatment with reserpine did not change the blood pressure response after elevation of the ICP to 160 mm Hg. However, the combination of reserpine pretreatment and bilateral adrenalectomy inhibited the Cushing response almost completely, while bilateral adrenalectomy without any pretreatment did not give rise to values different from the controls. Similar observations were made after 6-OHDA pretreatment and after repeated administration of guanethidine.

These drugs which induce pharmacological sympathectomy did not influence the Cushing response significantly, but in combination with bilateral adrenalectomy, there occurred a clear cut inhibition of the pressor response. All these results would suggest that in order to provoke the Cushing response, not only the intact peripheral sympathetic nervous system but also the adrenal medulla is highly relevant.

Freeman and Jeffers (1940) demonstrated with surgical techniques that a rise in blood pressure from cerebral compression can be obtained in dogs with

TABLE I

MEAN ARTERIAL PRESSURE (MAP) RESPONSE TO ACUTELY
ELEVATION OF INTRACRANIAL PRESSURE TO 160 mm Hg
IN RATS (= CUSHING RESPONSE)

See text for details.

(Pre)Treatment	n	Initial MAP ± S.E.M.	Max. response MAP ± S.E.M.
Controls	11	118 ± 5.6	186 ± 3.3
Vagotomy (bilateral)	12	121 ± 4.8	187 ± 2.7
+ 1 mg/kg atropine	5	101 ± 1.9	179 ± 2.6
L(−)propranolol 3 mg/kg	6	110 ± 10.8	170 ± 7.2
” 10 mg/kg	5	97 ± 6.6	166 ± 2.2
Practolol 3 mg/kg	7	106 ± 8.8	179 ± 2.9
Hydralazine 3 mg/kg	6	40 ± 2.2	169 ± 2.1
Clonidine 25 μg/kg	6	57 ± 4.6	181 ± 6.4
Phentolamine 10 mg/kg	8	63 ± 3.0	140 ± 6.5
” 30 mg/kg	6	48 ± 3.0	92 ± 11.2
” 60 mg/kg	5	45 ± 1.5	54 ± 2.7
Piperoxane 10 mg/kg	4	80 ± 7.1	173 ± 3.7
” 30 mg/kg	6	57 ± 5.5	90 ± 9.7
Phentolamine 10 mg/kg + L(−)propranolol 3 mg/kg	5	47 ± 4.8	120 ± 8.5
Reserpine 5 mg/kg	5	86 ± 4.7	172 ± 5.2
+ adrenalectomy	5	38 ± 2.9	47 ± 5.1
6-OHDA	5	91 ± 6.5	174 ± 2.0
+ adrenalectomy	5	73 ± 3.5	105 ± 9.6
Guanethidine	5	107 ± 4.8	170 ± 5.2
+ adrenalectomy	4	52 ± 6.5	68 ± 6.7
Adrenalectomy (bilateral)	5	84 ± 7.2	184 ± 4.0

sympathetic cardiac denervation, only if the medullary-adrenal secretion is present.

The blood pressure response to ICP depends upon the integrity of one component of the sympathetic system, because neither bilateral adrenalectomy nor chemical sympathectomy could prevent the Cushing response completely. De Champlain and Van Ameringen (1972) suggested that the removal of the component of the sympathetic system can be compensated for by a hyperactivity of the remaining component. Brown (1956) concluded that vasoconstriction was the dominant factor in the Cushing response and our experiments with the α- and β-blocking agents would underline his conclusion.

SUMMARY

The blood pressure response after acute elevation of the intercranial pressure was studied in anaesthetized rats. After establishing an ICP/blood pressure curve we studied the influence on this response of bilateral vagotomy, with and without atropine pretreatment and that of L(−)propranolol, practolol, phentolamine, piperoxane, clonidine and hydralazine. The influence of reserpine, 6-OHDA and guanethidine, with or without bilateral adrenalectomy, has been studied as well. The results suggest that in order to be able to inhibit a pressor response due to a rise in ICP both the peripheral sympathetic system and the adrenal medulla should be dysfunctional.

REFERENCES

Brown, F.K. (1956) Cardiovascular effects of acutely raised intracranial pressure. *Amer. J. Physiol.*, 185: 510—514.

Cushing, H. (1901) Concerning a definite regulation of the vasomotor centre which controls blood pressure during cerebral compression. *Bull. Johns Hopkins Hosp.*, 12: 290—292.

De Champlain, J. and Van Ameringen, M.R. (1972) Regulation of blood pressure by sympathetic nerve fibers and adrenal medulla in normotensive and hypertensive rats. *Circulat. Res.*, 31: 617—627.

Douglas, J.R., Johnson, E.M., Marshall, G., Heist, J., Hartman, J.K. and Needleman, P. (1975) Development and maintenance of renal hypertension in normal and guanethidine sympathectomized rats. *Circulat. Res.*, 36—37, Suppl. I: 171—178.

Freeman, N. and Jeffers, W. (1940) Effect of progressive sympathectomy on hypertension produced by increased intracranial pressure. *Amer. J. Physiol.*, 128: 662—671.

Hoff, J.T. and Mitchell, R. (1972) The effect of hypoxia on the Cushing response. In *Intracranial Pressure*, M. Brock and H. Dietz (Eds.), Springer, Heidelberg, pp. 205—209.

Hoff, J.T. and Reis, D.J. (1970) Localisation of regions mediating the Cushing response in the central nervous system of the cat. *Arch. Neurol. (Chic.)*, 22: 228—240.

Noble, E.P., Wurtman, R. and Axelrod, J. (1967) A simple and rapid method for injecting H^3-noradrenaline into the lateral ventricle of the rat brain. *Life Sci.*, 6: 281—291.

Sagawa, K., Ross, J.M. and Guyton, A.C. (1961) Quantitation of cerebral ischemic pressor response in dogs. *Amer. J. Physiol.*, 200: 1164—1168.

Thoenen, H. and Tranzer, J. (1968) Chemical sympathectomy by selective destruction of adrenergic nerve endings with 6-hydroxy-dopamine. *Naunyn-Schmiedeberg's Arch. exp. Path. Pharmak.*, 261: 271—288.

SUBJECT INDEX